The Dentist's Drug and Prescription Guide

The Dentist's Drug and Prescription Guide

Second Edition

Mea A. Weinberg, DMD, MSD, RPh
Diplomate of the American Board of Periodontology;
Clinical Professor
Ashman Department of Periodontology and Implant Dentistry
New York University College of Dentistry
New York, NY, USA

Stuart J. Froum, DDS
Diplomate of the American Board of Periodontology;
Diplomate of the International Congress of Oral Implantologists;
Adjunct Clinical Professor and Director of Clinical Research
Ashman Department of Periodontology and Implant Dentistry
New York University College of Dentistry
New York, NY, USA;
Private Practice, New York, NY, USA

Stuart L. Segelnick, DDS, MS
Diplomate of the American Board of Periodontology;
Diplomate of the International Congress of Oral Implantologists;
Adjunct Associate Professor of Oral Medicine
University of Pennsylvania School of Dental Medicine;
Adjunct Clinical Professor
Ashman Department of Periodontology and Implant Dentistry
New York University College of Dentistry
New York, NY, USA;
Private practice, Brooklyn, NY, USA

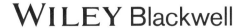

Registered Office
John Wiley & Sons, Inc., 111 River Street, Hoboken, NJ 07030, USA

Editorial Office
111 River Street, Hoboken, NJ 07030, USA
For details of our global editorial offices, customer services, and more information about Wiley products visit us at www.wiley.com.

Wiley also publishes its books in a variety of electronic formats and by print-on-demand. Some content that appears in standard print versions of this book may not be available in other formats.

Library of Congress Cataloging-in-Publication Data

Names: Weinberg, Mea A., author. | Froum, Stuart J., author. | Segelnick,
    Stuart L., author.
Title: The dentist's drug and prescription guide / Mea A. Weinberg, Stuart J. Froum,
    Stuart L. Segelnick.
Description: Second edition. | Hoboken, NJ : Wiley-Blackwell, 2020. |
    Includes bibliographical references and index.
Identifiers: LCCN 2019048454 (print) | LCCN 2019048455 (ebook) | ISBN
    9781119539346 (paperback) | ISBN 9781119539353 (adobe pdf) | ISBN
    9781119539360 (epub)
Subjects: LCSH: Dental pharmacology–Handbooks, manuals, etc. |
    Drugs–Prescribing–Handbooks, manuals, etc. | Drugs–Dosage–Handbooks,
    manuals, etc.
Classification: LCC RK701 .W44 2020 (print) | LCC RK701 (ebook) | DDC
    617.6/061–dc23
LC record available at https://lccn.loc.gov/2019048454
LC ebook record available at https://lccn.loc.gov/2019048455

Cover Design: Wiley
Cover Images: Empty medical prescription © Makistock/Shutterstock,
Packaging of tablets © VonaUA/Shutterstock,
Prescription drug bottle © Tomas Nevesely/Shutterstock

Set in 9.5/12.5pt STIXTwoText by SPi Global, Pondicherry, India
Printed and bound in Singapore by Markono Print Media Pte Ltd

10 9 8 7 6 5 4 3 2 1

Contents

List of Contributors

The author would like to thank the following people for their contributions to chapters and assistance while writing this book.

Cheryl Barber, MPH, MSOD
Senior Research Scientist
HIV/AIDS Research Program
New York University
New York, NY, USA

Edgard El Chaar, DDS, PC
Clinical Associate Professor
Department of Periodontology and Implant
  Dentistry
Director, Advanced Education Program
Former Director and Founder of
  Advanced Education Program
  in Periodontics
Lutheran Medical Center
New York University College of Dentistry
New York, NY, USA;
Private Practice, New York, NY, USA

James B. Fine, DMD
Senior Academic Dean, Postgraduate,
  Graduate & CE Programs
Professor of Dental Medicine (Periodontics)
College of Dental Medicine
Columbia University Irving
  Medical Center
New York, NY, USA

Johnathan M. Gordon, PharmD, DDS
Private practice
Naples, FL, USA

Aaron Greenstein, MD
Resident Doctor
Harvard Medical School
Brookline, MA, USA

Johnathan Love, MD
Resident Doctor
Harvard Medical School
Brookline, MA, USA

Dena M. Sapanaro, MS, DDS
Clinical Assistant Professor
Department of Pediatric Dentistry
Dental Anesthesiology
New York University College of Dentistry
New York, NY, USA

Marc A. Singer, MD
Internal medicine, Cardiology;
Private practice;
On staff, Long Island Jewish Medical Center
New Hyde Park;
North Shore University Hospital
Manhasset, NY, USA

Preface

The Dentist's Drug and Prescription Guide, 2nd edition, is a much-needed update to the first edition. Change has occurred in both the dental and pharmacology field and we have striven to imbue this edition with the same scientific basis for the sensible and appropriate use of drugs in the dental patient.

Keeping this book in easy reach will enable you to answer the most common and uncommon questions the dental professional has. Whether you are a dentist, dental specialist, dental hygienist, dental assistant, or dental lab technician, this drug guide will make a valuable addition to your knowledge base.

Today, the dental provider interacts with an increasing population of medically treated and possibly medically compromised patients. According to the US Department of Health and Human Services Centers for Disease Control and Prevention National Center for Health Statistics, "During 2015–2016, almost one-half of the U.S. population used one or more prescription drugs in the past 30 days (45.8%)." Dentists will surely be faced with daily decisions on treating people on medications. The importance of understanding potential drug interaction with our health care is essential for dental practice.

The proliferation of computer software programs providing drug interaction advice is helpful but we do not recommend thoughtlessly basing your treatment decisions on these algorithms. In this new edition, we have built for you a solid foundation allowing you to interact with the most up-to-date techniques and technologies in the dental and pharmacological world.

We have thoroughly updated most sections, including the most recent peer-reviewed publications. We have added completely new sections on the new classification of periodontal disease including antimicrobial treatment, the opioid crisis in dentistry, and HIV/AIDS research and medications.

Features of the book still include the following.

- Readability: short, easy question and answer format linking pharmacy theory to clinical dental practice.
- Need-to-know information: the content of this book was written in regard to the many questions practitioners have about prescribing drugs to patients.
- Drug tables: there are many tables in the book which not only summarize the main pharmacological features of the different disciplines but also allow the reader to review the key drugs and theories at a quick glance.

We sincerely hope you enjoy *The Dentist's Drug and Prescription Guide,* 2nd edition, and that it becomes a highly useful addition in your professional practice.

1

Introduction to Pharmacology

1.1 Definition of Terms

Absorption	the movement of a drug from its site of administration into the systemic circulation.
Adverse drug event (ADE)	injury resulting from the use of a drug. It is an unfavorable and unintentional response resulting from an administered medication. Includes medication errors such as miscalculation of dosage or misreading a prescription by the pharmacist, doctor, and/or patient.
Adverse drug reaction (ADR) (also known as side effect)	harm to the body due to a medication that was properly prescribed (e.g., drug taken at normal doses and via the correct route of administration), or an allergic reaction to a drug. There is a causal relationship between the drug and an ADR.
Affinity	the ability of a drug to bind to the receptor to cause a therapeutic response.
Antibiotic prophylaxis	antibiotic given to prevent an infection.
Bioavailability	the amount of a drug (expressed as a percentage) that reaches the systemic circulation. For example, any drug administered intravenously has 100% bioavailability
Biologics	agents that are naturally produced in an animal or human body.
Clearance	quantitative measure of the rate of drug elimination from the body divided by the concentration.
Creatinine	a waste product in skeletal muscle produced by the breakdown of creatinine phosphate.
Creatinine clearance (CrCl)	a test that compares the level of creatinine in the urine with that of creatinine in the blood and determines normal functioning of the kidneys.
Cytochrome P450 (CYP) enzymes	found primarily in the liver and are responsible for the metabolism of many drugs. Many drug interactions occur because some drugs are inhibitors or inducers of the substrate (drug being metabolized) resulting in high or low blood levels of one or the other drug.

The Dentist's Drug and Prescription Guide, Second Edition. Mea A. Weinberg, Stuart J. Froum and Stuart L. Segelnick.
© 2020 John Wiley & Sons, Inc. Published 2020 by John Wiley & Sons, Inc.

Distribution	movement of a drug through the body to the various target tissues/organs (site of action) after entering the bloodstream.
Dosage	the amount of drug required to produce the desired effect.
Dose	the amount of drug taken at any one time.
Drug	any substance which changes a physiological function or modifies a disease process.
Drug action	the response of living matter to administered chemicals. Levels of drug action include cellular or molecular. Cellular site of drug action is defined as all foreign parts that enter the body will react with at least one portion of the cell. The initial reaction occurs here. At the molecular level, the molecules of the drug will react with the molecules of the body.
Efficacy	the ability of a drug to stimulate the receptor and produce the maximum response achievable by the drug. Two drugs can have the same efficacy but different potencies where one drug is more potent (lower dose required to produce desired effect) than the first drug but both will have the same effect.
Elimination half-life ($t_{1/2}$)	the time required to reduce the amount of drug in the body or concentration of drug in blood by 50%. However, once the first 50% is gone, it will take the body more time to clear 50% of the remaining medication. Usually, it takes about five half-lives to clear 99% of the medication. To determine the time it takes for a drug to be 99% eliminated from the body, multiply the half-life of the drug by five.
First-pass effect (or first-pass metabolism)	before an orally administered drug enters the systemic circulation, it goes to the liver to be metabolized or biotransformed. Some oral drugs can undergo extensive first-pass effect so that they are ineffective by the time of entering the bloodstream while other drugs undergo little first-pass effect and maintain their original efficacy. Drugs that undergo extensive first-pass effect cannot be given orally because they become pharmacologically ineffective by the time they enter the general circulation. Lidocaine is an example of a drug that cannot be given orally because it undergoes extensive first-pass effect.
First-order kinetics	the rate of drug elimination decreases with time. That is, the rate of drug elimination falls as the concentration falls. Most drugs are removed from the body by first-order kinetics.
Loading dose (LD)	an initial higher dose of a drug that may be given at the beginning of a course of treatment (to more quickly reach adequate plasma levels) before dropping down to a lower maintenance dose (MD) afterwards. A LD is given on the first day of drug treatment.
Maintenance dose (MD)	a lower drug dose that keeps the plasma drug concentration continuously within the therapeutic range. The MD is given starting after the LD on day 1 of drug therapy and is usually half the dose of the LD.
Metabolism (biotransformation)	the primary mechanism of drug elimination from the body. Biotransformation will usually end the pharmacological action of the drug.

Pharmacodynamics	describes how the drug works, its mechanism of action. How a drug interacts with receptors and what happens once the drug binds to the receptor.
Pharmacogenetics	the convergence of pharmacology and genetics that deals with genetic factors that influence an organism's response to a drug.
Pharmacognosy	study of drugs derived from herbal and other natural sources.
Pharmacokinetics	study of the action of a drug once it is in the patient. It describes the absorption, distribution, metabolism, and elimination of the drug from the body
Pharmacology	the science dealing with drugs and their interaction with the body's components.
Pharmacotherapeutics	the medical use of drugs in the prevention, diagnosis, and treatment of diseases.
Polypharmacy	when many different medications including over-the-counter (OTC) and prescription drugs are taken by the patient.
Potency	strength of the drug relative to therapeutic effect.
Prodrug	a drug that becomes active only after it is ingested and metabolized in the liver. Codeine is converted from an inactive form to the pharmacologically active form morphine by first-pass metabolism.
Protein binding	attachment of a drug to proteins in the plasma. Drugs that are protein bound are inactive and become active in the free unbound form.
Steady state	the point at which the rate of drug input into the body is equal to the rate of elimination. As such, the amount or concentration in the body reaches a plateau.
Therapeutic index (TI)	a measure of the relative safety of a drug. For example, lithium has a narrow TI so if the plasma levels are slightly above the therapeutic range, toxicity can occur quickly. Patients must be on chronic lithium maintenance treatment to avoid toxicity. On the other hand, penicillin has a wide TI so that slightly more than the usual dose will not cause toxicity.
Therapeutic range	the dosage range of a drug that achieves the desired pharmacological response.
Therapeutics	branch of medicine that deals with the treatment of disease.
Toxicology	study of poisons and poisonings.
Zero-order kinetics	the drug is removed at a constant rate regardless of the drug concentration; it is linear with time. The elimination from the body of a large concentration of alcohol is an example of a drug that follows zero-order kinetics. (Gossel 1998a,b; Weinberg 2013).

1.2 Pharmacokinetics

Q. What is the definition of pharmacokinetics and why is it important to know?

A. Pharmacokinetics describes the actions of the drug as it moves through the body and how the body influences drug concentrations. It is easiest to remember pharmacokinetics by the acronym: ADME (A = absorption into the systemic circulation; D = distribution to the target tissues and organs; M = metabolism or biotransformation; E = elimination from the body). It is important to know the basics of pharmacokinetics in order to understand the basic principles of prescribing medications (Doogue and Polasek 2013). Pharmacokinetics (e.g., absorption of the drug into the blood) may be altered when certain antibiotics prescribed in dentistry are taken with food. Instructions must be verbally expressed to the patient and documented in the patient's chart on how to take medications that are prescribed by dentists (e.g., antibiotics, antimicrobial agents, analgesics, antifungal agents, antiviral agents, fluorides).

Q. What factors affect the rate of drug absorption?

A. In the gastrointestinal tract, many factors can influence the rate of drug absorption into the systemic circulation such as acidity of the stomach and food in the stomach. Some medications used in dentistry should be taken with food to reduce gastrointestinal irritation, some medications should be taken on an empty stomach because the food could delay the absorption of the drug, and some can be taken with or without food because food does not interfere with absorption. Usually, the absorption of the total amount of drug is not reduced but rather it will just take longer to be absorbed. Usually, antibiotics have the most restrictions regarding taking with meals. Nonsteroidal antiinflammatory drugs such as ibuprofen must be taken with food to avoid gastric irritation. Specific drugs will be discussed within the relevant chapters.

Q. What does "take on an empty stomach" mean?

A. "Take on an empty stomach" means to take the drug within one hour before eating or two hours after eating. Take on an empty stomach is not interpreted as not eating.

Q. What is the pharmacokinetics of an orally administered drug?

A. The pharmacokinetics of a drug administered orally such as penicillin VK is as follows (Gossel 1998a,b; Weinberg 2013).

1) An orally administered drug is swallowed and goes down the esophagus. It is important to take a tablet/capsule with a full glass of water to facilitate its passage through the esophagus into the stomach.

2) In the stomach, the tablet/capsule must be released or liberated from its formulation. Once a tablet is "broken up" and a capsule is "opened," and the active ingredients are released, there is dissolution of the drug from the liberated drug particles. Some acidic drugs are enteric coated to protect the stomach lining. Dosage forms such as syrups or solutions are liquids, which are immediately available for absorption and transport. A liquid gel capsule (Aleve®, Advil®) is formulated to dissolve quickly, allowing the liquid inside the capsule to be absorbed fast.

3) Drug goes into the upper part of the small intestine (duodenum) where most absorption into the systemic circulation occurs. This is because the small intestine has a large surface area due to microvilli, through which drugs may diffuse.

4) From the small intestine, the drug molecules are absorbed into the bloodstream. Many factors can affect the rate and extent of drug absorption, including foods and minerals. For example, tetracycline should not be given at the same time as dairy products or minerals (e.g., iron, calcium, magnesium) because insoluble complexes form in the intestinal tract, which slows down absorption. This can be avoided by taking the tetracycline 1–2 hours before or after the dairy/mineral product. Some antibiotics (e.g., tetracycline) must be taken

on an empty stomach (one hour before or two hours after meals), which increases the rate of absorption. Most antibiotics can be taken without regard to meals (with or without food) but if stomach upset occurs, these antibiotics can be taken with food (Huang et al. 2009).

5) Absorption occurs when a drug is in a nonionized or charged form and if it is more lipid soluble. Most drugs are combined with a salt to enhance absorption (e.g., lidocaine HCl, tetracycline HCl, doxycycline hyclate, amoxicillin trihydrate).

6) Before an orally administered drug reaches the systemic circulation, it goes to the liver via the portal vein whereby it is immediately exposed to metabolism by liver enzymes (Huang et al. 2009). This first exposure is referred to as the *first-pass effect*. Some drugs such as lidocaine and morphine that undergo extensive first-pass embolism will become inactive so they cannot be given orally. Diazepam (Valium®) has close to 100% bioavailability (low first-pass metabolism) so it has similar oral and intravenous doses. Alternate routes of drug administration that bypass the first-pass effect include sublingual, rectal, and parenteral (intravenous, intramuscular, subcutaneous) (Fagerholm 2007; Pond and Tozer 1984; Robertson 2017).

7) Once it reaches systemic circulation, the drug is distributed in the blood to the various organs. Many drugs are bound to circulating proteins such as albumin (acidic drugs) and glycoproteins (basic drugs). Highly protein-bound drugs are not active and only the free drug that is not bound to proteins is active.

8) Once the drug has exerted its actions, it must then be eliminated from the body. The first part of drug elimination involves *metabolism* or *biotransformation*, which occurs mostly in the liver. It may take a drug several passes through the liver before it is entirely metabolized. Biotransformation converts lipid-soluble drug molecules to metabolites or endproducts that are more water soluble and therefore easier to eliminate from the body. Most of the conversion of drugs occurs in the liver by metabolizing enzymes called microsomal enzymes. These enzymes, which are also called *cytochrome P450 (CYP)* enzymes, are the primary enzymes responsible for the oxidation of many drugs. There are many different isoenzymes for different drugs (e.g., CYP3A4 is involved with many dental drugs). Many drug–drug and drug–food interactions occur via the microsomal enzymes. Some *prodrugs* have no pharmacological activity unless they are first metabolized to the active form in the body (e.g., codeine is metabolized by the liver enzyme CYP2D6 to the active morphine) (Weinberg 2013).

9) *Drug elimination*: now the more water-soluble metabolite must be eliminated from the body. The main route of drug elimination is excretion via the kidneys so diseases of the kidney can significantly prolong the duration of drug action. Therefore, dosage adjustments may be needed from the patient's physician. Some elimination occurs through the lungs, breast milk, sweat, tears, feces, and bile. Some drugs (e.g., tetracycline) undergo biliary excretion whereby the drug is eliminated in the bile and enters the small intestine and eventually leaves the body in the feces. Most bile is then circulated back to the liver by *enterohepatic recirculation* and eventually metabolized by the liver and excreted via the kidneys. This route of reabsorption is helpful in prolonging the activity (increasing the half-life) of some antibiotics (Weinberg 2013).

Q. What is the definition of drug absorption?

A. Drug *absorption* is the movement of a drug from the site of administration to the systemic circulation.

Q. What does it mean when a drug has 100% bioavailability?

A. *Bioavailability* describes the portion of an administered drug that reaches the systemic circulation. It is the rate and extent of absorption and how fast and how much of the drug is absorbed. It indicates that the drug is 100% absorbed into the blood. Only intravenously administered drugs have 100% bioavailability because 100% of the drug enters directly into the blood. A drug administered orally that undergoes extensive first-pass metabolism (or first-pass effect) by traveling first to the liver, where it is metabolized, and can become almost inactive by the time it reaches the systemic circulation, is a drug with low bioavailability.

Q. What is the first step involved in drug absorption?

A. The first step before a drug can be absorbed in the small intestine is disintegration of the dosage formulation into a formulation that can easily be absorbed. The stomach might be expected to be the first site of absorption but in reality, very little absorption occurs in the stomach because the surface area is very small. A tablet must break up to expose the active ingredient, which takes some time. A capsule must open up, which takes less time than a tablet. A solution is already in a liquid, easily absorbed form and takes the least time for disintegration and absorption. The order of bioavailability is oral solution > oral suspension > capsule > tablet (Lloyd et al. 1978).

Q. Is there any systemic absorption of a topical anesthetic applied on the surface of the gingiva?

A. Yes. The purpose of topical agents is to maximize the concentration of the drug at the target site while minimizing potential systemic adverse effects. Although drug absorption is not desired, there could be some systemic absorption, especially if the agent is applied on abraded gingiva or skin. Because of its lipophilic nature, the stratum corneum of the skin may act as a reservoir for many drugs. Consequently, the local effects of the drug may persist long enough to allow once-daily application. For example, once-daily application of corticosteroid preparations is as effective as multiple applications in most circumstances. Direct access to the skin may predispose the patient to frequent topical applications, increasing the risk of systemic adverse effects.

Q. How does a drug get absorbed into the systemic circulation?

A. A drug must pass through many cell membranes to get into the blood. A drug must have some water solubility to go through aqueous fluids and some lipid solubility to get through the cell membrane, which is composed of two layers of phospholipids.

Q. What is the purpose of epinephrine added to local anesthetics?

A. Epinephrine is a vasoconstrictor that acts to constrict blood vessels to decrease blood flow in the submucosal area via activating alpha-1 receptors (Becker and Reed 2012). This allows the anesthetic solution to stay at the site of action longer, which slows absorption of the anesthetic solution.

Q. What is drug distribution and what factors affect distribution?

A. Drug *distribution* is the movement of an agent through the blood or lymph to various sites of action in the body. An important factor affecting drug distribution is *protein binding*. Many drugs in the blood are bound to circulating proteins such as albumin for acidic drugs (e.g., penicillin, barbiturates, aspirin, vitamin C) and acid glycoproteins and lipoproteins for basic drugs (e.g., narcotic analgesics, erythromycin). When drugs are bound to plasma proteins, they are inactive while circulating in the blood. This binding to proteins is temporary, reversible, and can convert to free drug. Only drugs that are not bound to plasma proteins are "freely active" and bind to specific receptors on the target tissue/organ. Another factor that affects drug distribution is blood flow to the target organs.

Q. What is the minimum effective concentration (MEC) of a drug?

A. The *minimum effective concentration (MEC)* is the amount of drug required to produce a thera-peutic effect. This is important to know because a drug should not be given above the MEC as this will produce toxic concentrations. The ideal concentration of a drug should be between the MEC and the toxic concentration. This is referred to as the *therapeutic range*. For example, after periodontal surgery, it is recommended that the patient take ibuprofen (Motrin®, Nuprin®). If the patient decides to take only one 200 mg tablet during the day, they will still experience pain because the therapeutic range was not reached. The patient should take two or three tablets which will increase the plasma level of ibuprofen into the therapeutic range. If the patient takes five or more tablets at one time, then adverse effects may occur because the plasma level of ibuprofen is outside the therapeutic range and the maximum dose has been exceeded. Beyond the maximum dose, the analgesic effect does not increase.

Q. What does the term "dose" mean?

A. The *dose* of a drug is the amount of drug taken at any one time. Dose is expressed as the weight of drug (e.g., 500 mg), the number of dosage forms (e.g., one capsule), or the volume of liquid (e.g. two drops).

Q. What is the elimination half-life of a drug?

A. The *elimination half-life ($t_{1/2}$)* of a drug is essentially the duration of action of a drug. Also, it is used to determine the dosing of a drug. The elimination half-life of a drug is the amount of time required for a drug to decrease its original concentration by 50%. The second half-life is when it removes another 50%, leaving 25% in the blood. The third half-life is when it removes another 50%, leaving 12.5% in the blood. Drugs have different predetermined half-lives. As repeated doses of a drug are administered, the plasma concentration builds up and reaches "steady state." Steady state occurs when the amount of drug in the plasma builds up to a level considered therapeutically effective. In order to achieve steady state, the amount of drug administered must balance the amount being cleared from the body. It usually takes about between four and five half-lives to reach clinical steady state and about six half-lives before 98% of the drug is eliminated from the body (Ito 2011). For example, if a drug has a $t_{1/2}$ of 2 hours, it will take about 8–10 hours to reach clinical steady state (Ito 2011).

Drugs with a short $t_{1/2}$ are eliminated faster than drugs with a long $t_{1/2}$. For example, tetracy-cline HCl has a $t_{1/2}$ of 6–12 hours and doxycycline hyclate has a $t_{1/2}$ of 14–24 hours. Thus, tetra-cycline dosing is one capsule every four hours while doxycycline is dosed 100 mg every 12 hours on day 1, then 100 mg every day. On average, doxycycline's half-life is around 19 hours. By multiplying 19 hours by six hours (average $t_{1/2}$ to be 98% eliminated from the body) ($19 \times 6 = 114$ hours), it takes 114 hours, or about five days, before 98% of the doxycycline has been removed from the body. Penicillin VK has a $t_{1/2}$ of 30 minutes and amoxicillin's $t_{1/2}$ is 1–1.3 hours. Thus, penicillin is given every six hours and amoxicillin is dosed every eight hours (Thomson 2004a,b).

Ibuprofen has a short $t_{1/2}$ and is cleared from the body more rapidly than a drug with a longer $t_{1/2}$. Ibuprofen requires a more frequent, regular dosing regimen of 200–400 mg (OTC strength) q4–6h or prescription ibuprofen 600–800 q6–8h in order to build up and maintain a high enough concentration in the plasma to be therapeutically effective.

Q. What is the volume of distribution (V_D)?

A. *Apparent volume of distribution (V_D)* refers to the amount of drug in the various tissues of the body. Volume of distribution is a calculated value referring to the volume of fluid (e.g., plasma, interstitial fluid [fluid between the cells], and lymph) in which a drug is able to distribute to the organs. The volume of distribution can be used to calculate the LD, MD, and clearance of a drug (Aki et al. 2010; Thomson 2004a, b; Wesolowski et al. 2016).

Q. What is drug biotransformation?

A. *Drug biotransformation* (or metabolism, as it is sometimes called) terminates the action of a drug. It is a process by which a substance changes from one chemical form to another via a reaction in the body. Usually, biotransformation occurs in the liver but can also occur in the plasma and kidney.

Q. What is the importance of drug clearance?

A. *Clearance* refers to the volume of fluid (e.g., plasma) that would be completely cleared of drug if the entire drug being excreted were removed from that volume of fluid. Essentially, clearance is the removal of a drug from the plasma. It is a calculated value and measured in liters/hour. Clearance indicates the ability of the liver and kidney to eliminate a drug from the body (Doogue and Polasek 2013). Clearance may be reduced in the elderly. Both clearance and V_D are important values in determining the half-life of a drug (Gossel 1998a,b).

Q. What must happen to a drug in the body in order for a drug effect to occur?

A. The rate of absorption must be greater than the rate of elimination for the drug to have an effect on the body. Usually, the rate of elimination is slower than the rate of absorption so that the rate of elimination is the controlling factor in the presence of the drug in the body (Fujimoto 1979).

1.3 Pharmacodynamics

Q. What is the definition of pharmacodynamics and what is its significance in dentistry?

A. *Pharmacodynamics* deals with the mechanism of action of drugs or how the drug works in the body to produce a pharmacological response and the relationship between drug concentration and response. It is important to know the mechanism of action of drugs because it will help with understanding the reason for prescribing the drug.

Q. What is the definition of drug affinity?

A. *Affinity* is the ability of a drug to bind to the receptor to elicit a therapeutic response. If one drug has a greater affinity than another drug, it means that drug binds more readily to the receptor. If a drug has a high affinity, this means that a smaller dose can produce a therapeutic effect compared to a drug with a lower affinity for the same receptor.

Q. Do drugs bind strongly to a receptor?

A. Most drugs bind weakly to their receptors via hydrogen, hydrophobic and ionic bonds. Because these are relatively weak bonds, the drug can bind and unbind the receptor. Some drugs do bind strongly to the receptor via covalent bonds.

Q. Can drugs bind to other receptors besides their specific receptors?

A. Yes. For example, atypical antipsychotic drugs bind to dopamine receptors for their antipsychotic response but also bind to alpha receptors which cause adverse effects such as weight loss while binding to muscarinic receptors causes xerostomia.

Q. How do most drugs cause a therapeutic response?

A. Most drugs have an affinity for a specific receptor. Most receptors are proteins. Once the drug binds to the receptor, a therapeutic response occurs. Receptors have a steric or three-dimensional structure so when the substrate or drug binds to that receptor, the receptor undergoes steric realignment which allows the drug to bind more precisely to the receptor with better efficacy.

Q. Do all drugs interact with receptors to cause a therapeutic response?

A. No. Epinephrine binds to alpha and beta receptors on the organs but also produces some of its effects by activating an enzyme called adenyl cyclase. Also, anesthetic gases do not bind to receptors in the central nervous system. Antacids do not work by interacting with receptors.

Q. What are drug agonists and antagonists?

A. Drugs produce their effects by altering the function of cells and tissues in the body or organisms such as bacteria. Most drugs have an affinity for a target receptor, which is usually a protein on the cell surface. Once a drug binds to a receptor, it can act as either as an *agonist* (produces a stimulatory response) or an *antagonist* (sits on the receptor site and prevents an agonist from binding to the receptor; an antagonist does not produce a therapeutic response).

For example, epinephrine in low doses as used in dentistry is an agonist that binds to and activates beta-2 receptors, resulting in vasodilation of systemic arterioles (Becker and Reed 2012). This vasodilation tends to reduce peripheral resistance and therefore diastolic blood pressure. At the same time, the beta-1 receptors in the heart are activated to increase cardiac output and systolic blood pressure. These two influences cancel each other out regarding mean blood pressure (Becker and Reed 2012).

An example of an antagonist is flumazenil (Romazicon®), which is a benzodiazepine receptor antagonist used as rescue medication in the event of benzodiazepine overdose. It will bind the benzodiazepine receptor (BZR) and prevent the benzodiazepine from attaching. Naloxone (Narcan®) is a narcotic receptor antagonist.

Q. What is the difference between drug potency and efficacy?

A. *Potency* is the relationship between the dose of a drug and the therapeutic effect; it is the strength of drug required to produce the desired response. *Efficacy* refers to the ability of a drug to exert an effect. For example, 500 mg of acetaminophen and 200 mg of ibuprofen both produce the same analgesia and have the same efficacy, but ibuprofen is more potent because it requires a lower dosage.

Q. What is the TI of a drug?

A. The *therapeutic index* (TI) is the dose range within which the drug is effective without causing adverse events/effects (Tamargo et al. 2015). The TI or ratio equates the blood level at which a drug causes a therapeutic effect compared to the dose that causes death. To determine drug safety, the drug's TI is calculated by dividing LD_{50} by ED_{50}. The ED_{50} is the median effective dose, which is the dose required to produce a specific therapeutic response in 50% of patients. The median lethal dose (LD_{50}) refers to the dose of drug that will be lethal in 50% of a group of animals, not humans. Some drugs (e.g., lithium, digoxin) have a narrow TI so that routine blood tests are necessary to assure the plasma drug level is within the therapeutic range.

Q. What is an ADR and why is it important to know?

A. An *adverse drug reaction* (ADR) is defined by the World Health Organization (WHO) as any response to a drug that is noxious, unintended, and *occurs when a drug is properly prescribed at doses normally* used in humans for the prophylaxis, diagnosis, or therapy of disease. Medical errors are not included in this definition. Bisphosphonate-induced osteonecrosis of the jaws is an ADR. Other examples of ADRs include drug interactions, allergic reactions and irritating adverse effects of a drug such as gastrointestinal problems (nausea, diarrhea). A drug interaction occurs when the effects of one drug are altered by the effects of another drug, resulting in an increase or decrease in the blood levels of the drug. An allergic reaction due to a drug is an abnormal and unwanted response that ranges from a mild rash to life-threatening anaphylaxis. An allergic reaction does not often happen the first time you take a medication but is much more likely to occur the next time you take that medication (Shamna et al. 2014). ADRs have a great effect on quality of life and continue to be challenging in prevention and treatment because of the increased use of alternative medications and an increase in the elderly population (Coleman and Pontefract 2016; Rieder and Ferro 2015).

Q. How does an ADR differ from an adverse effect or allergy?

A. An adverse effect is a type of ADR mediated by an immune response and is not the intended therapeutic outcome. It has been suggested to avoid using the term "side effect" and use the term "adverse effect" or "adverse drug reaction" instead (Riedl and Casillas 2003; VA Center for Medication Safety and VHA Pharmacy Benefits Management Strategic Healthcare Group and the Medical Advisory Panel 2006).

Q. What is an ADE and is it the same as an ADR?

A. An *adverse drug event* (ADE) is an unfavorable and unintended response to a drug that includes medical errors (e.g., miscalculations, misinterpretation of handwritten prescriptions). The dentist has the responsibility to report any ADE that occurs through the FDA's Adverse Event Reporting System (MedWatch; www.fda.gov/Safety/MedWatch/default.htm) (Mayer et al. 2010). The terms ADE and ADR are often used interchangeably but should not be (Leheny 2017). Adverse drug events are not desired and usually require medical intervention. On the other hand, the majority of ADRs are undesirable but are usually predictable. The majority of cases resolve on their own (Leheny 2017).

Q. What is the definition of tolerance?

A. *Tolerance* is the development of resistance to the effects of a drug. Therefore, in order to achieve the desired response, more of the drug must be taken. Overdose is very common. Narcotics and alcohol are common examples of drugs that produce tolerance.

References

Aki, T., Heikkinen, A.T., Korjamo, T. et al. (2010). Modelling of drug disposition kinetics in in vitro intestinal absorption cell models. *Basic and Clinical Pharmacology and Toxicology* 106 (3): 180–188.

Becker, D.E. and Reed, K.L. (2012). Local anesthetics: review of pharmacological considerations. *Anesthesia Progress* 59 (2): 90–102.

Coleman, J.J. and Pontefract, S.K. (2016). Adverse drug reactions. *Clinical Medicine* 16 (5): 481–485.

Doogue, M.P. and Polasek, T.M. (2013). The ABCD of clinical pharmacokinetics. *Therapeutic Advances in Drug Safety* 4 (1): 5–7.

Fagerholm, U. (2007). Prediction of human pharmacokinetics – gastrointestinal absorption. *Journal of Pharmacy and Pharmacology* 59: 905–916.

Fujimoto, J.M. (1979). Pharmacokinetics and drug metabolism. In: Practical Drug Therapy, 1e (ed. R.I.H. Wang), 11–16. Philadelphia: J.B. Lippincott Company.

Gossel, T.A. (1998a). Pharmacology back to basics. *US Pharmacist* 23: 70–78.

Gossel, T.A. (1998b). Exploring pharmacology. *US Pharmacist* 23: 96–104.

Huang, W., Lee, S.L., and Yu, L.X. (2009). Mechanistic approaches to predicting oral drug absorption. *AAPS Journal* 11: 217–224.

Ito, S. (2011). Pharmacokinetics 101. *Paediatrics and Child Health* 16 (9): 535–536.

Leheny, S. (2017). 'Adverse Event,' Not the Same as 'Side Effect.' www.pharmacytimes.com/contributor/shelby-leheny-pharmd-candidate-2017/2017/02/adverse-event-not-the-same-as-side-effect.

Lloyd, B.L., Greenblatt, D.J., Allen, M.D. et al. (1978). Pharmacokinetics and bioavailability of digoxin capsules, solutions and tablets after single and multiple dose. *American Journal of Cardiology* 2: 129–136.

Mayer, M.H., Dowsett, S.A., Brahmavar, K. et al. (2010). Reporting adverse drug events. *US Pharmacist* 35: HS-15–HS-19.

Pond, S.M. and Tozer, T.N. (1984). First-pass elimination. Basic concepts and clinical consequences. *Clinical Pharmacokinetics* 9: 1–25.

Rieder, M. and Ferro, A. (2015). Adverse drug reactions. *British Journal of Clinical Pharmacology* 80 (4): 613–614.

Riedl, M.A. and Casillas, A.M. (2003). Adverse drug reactions: types and treatment options. *American Family Physician* 68: 1781–1790.

Robertson, D. (2017). First pass metabolism. *Nurse Prescribing* 15 (6): 303–305.

Shamna, M., Dilip, C., Ajmal, M. et al. (2014). A prospective study on adverse drug reactions of antibiotics in a tertiary care hospital. *Saudi Pharmaceutical Journal* 22 (4): 303–308.

Tamargo, J., Le Heuzey, J.Y., and Mabo, P. (2015). Narrow therapeutic index drugs: a clinical pharmacological consideration to flecainide. *European Journal of Clinical Pharmacology* 71 (5): 549–567.

Thomson, A. (2004a). Back to basics: pharmacokinetics. *Pharmaceutical Journal* 272: 796–771.

Thomson, A. (2004b). Variability in drug dosage requirements. *Pharmaceutical Journal* 272: 806–808.

VA Center for Medication Safety and VHA Pharmacy Benefits Management Strategic Healthcare Group and the Medical Advisory Panel (2006). Adverse drug events, adverse drug reactions and medication errors. Frequently asked questions. www.pbm.va.gov/PBM/vacenterformedicationsafety/tools/AdverseDrugReaction.pdf.

Weinberg, M.A. (2013). Fundamentals of drug action. In: Oral Pharmacology, 2e (eds. M.A. Weinberg, C. Westphal and J.B. Fine), 18–40. New Jersey: Pearson Education Inc.

Wesolowski, C.A., Wesolowski, M.J., Babyn, P.S., and Wanasundara, S.N. (2016). Time varying apparent volume of distribution and drug half-lives following intravenous bolus injections. *PLoS One* 11 (7): e0158798. https://doi.org/10.1371/journal.pone.0158798.

2

The Prescription and Drug Names

2.1   Parts of a Prescription

Q. What are the different parts of a written prescription?
A. • Heading:
  – Prescriber's name, address, phone number, license number, Drug Enforcement Administration (DEA) number and NPI (national provider identifier) (the DEA number can also be located at the bottom of the prescription by the prescriber's signature)
  – Patient's information (name, address, age, weight)
  – Date of the order (must be written or it is not legal).
  • Body:
  – Rx symbol
  – Medication prescribed (drug name, strength, and formulation) and quantity to be dispensed
  – Instructions to the pharmacist. For example: Dispense 10 capsules.
  • Closing:
  – Signature (Sig): directions to the patient
  – Signature of prescriber
  – Whether or not substitution is permissible
  – Number of refills
  – Label (informs the pharmacist how to label the medication).

Q. What does "Rx" mean?
A. Rx is a symbol referring to "prescription." Rx stands for the Latin word "recipe" or "take thou" or "take thus" or "to take." Essentially, it is a command to take a specific compound.

Q. What does "Sig" mean?
A. Sig is an abbreviation for the Latin *signatura*, meaning "write," "make" or "label." These should always be written in English; however, prescribers sometimes use Latin abbreviations, e.g., "1 cap tid pc," which the pharmacist translates into English as "take one capsule three times daily after meals."

The Dentist's Drug and Prescription Guide, Second Edition. Mea A. Weinberg, Stuart J. Froum and Stuart L. Segelnick.
© 2020 John Wiley & Sons, Inc. Published 2020 by John Wiley & Sons, Inc.

Q. Does the age of the patient need to be written on the prescription?

A. Yes. Generally, it is helpful to write in the age (in years) of the patient. For pediatric prescriptions, it is recommended to write in the age of the child if the patient is less than 12 years of age and the age in years and months if less than 5 years of age. Including the weight of the child is also helpful. For Schedule II drugs, it is mandatory to include the age of the patient on the prescription. The reason for writing the age of the patient is that in some cases dose adjustments may be needed.

Q. What is the NPI?

A. NPI stands for national provider identifier. It is an identification number given to healthcare providers by the CMS (Centers for Medicare and Medicaid Services). Healthcare providers must apply for an NPI number through an application process on the CMS website. Health practitioners need to have this number in order to receive reimbursement from insurance companies and to prescribe medicines.

Q. What does the label box at the bottom of the prescription mean?

A. Any information about the medication to be dispensed is provided on the label that is affixed to the drug container.

2.2 Generic Substitution

Q. When does a brand name drug become generic?

A. A brand name drug can become generic when the patent for that drug expires. Once the brand name drug goes off-patent, several drug companies can begin to manufacture a generic equivalent drug. In the United States, one company is given 180 days of exclusivity to manufacture a generic version of a drug. After 180 days, other manufacturers of generic medications can then start to make their own generic form of the drug. For example, the patent on Celebrex® expired in 2013. Until 2013, Celebrex was not available in a generic form (www.fda.gov/Drugs/DevelopmentApprovalProcess/ucm079031.htm).

Q. At the bottom of the prescription there is a section that says "dispense as written" or "substitution permissible." What is the difference between a generic drug and a brand name drug?

A. A generic drug is manufactured and distributed usually without a patent. However, the generic drug may still have a patent on the entire formulation but not on the active ingredient. A drug that has a trade (brand) name is protected by a patent whereby it can only be manufactured and sold by the company holding the patent. Once the patent expires (between seven and 12 years) on a brand name drug, the generic form becomes available (Welage et al. 2001).

Q. What is generic equivalency?

A. Generic equivalency was developed to save consumers and insurance companies high costs. Generic drugs are much cheaper because of competition between drug manufacturers once the patent has expired. Also, it costs less to manufacture generic drugs. Many brand name drugs have less expensive generic substitutes that according to the FDA are therapeutically and biochemically equivalent to the brand name drug. The FDA requires the bioequivalence of the generic drug (active ingredient) to be between 80% and 125% of that of the brand name drug.

Generics are considered by the FDA to be identical in dose, strength, safety, efficacy, and intended use (Balthasar 1999; Greene et al. 2001; Meridith 2003).

Q. Is a generic drug always equivalent to a brand name drug?

A. According to the law, drug companies are required to prove bioavailability. Many drugs that are available generically are equally efficacious with the equivalent brand name (Birkett 2003).

Q. What is generic substitution and how do I know if a generic drug substitute is available?

A. Generic substitution is the process by which a brand name drug is dispensed by a different form of the same active substance (Posner and Griffin 2011). There is a book called the "Orange Book: Approved Drug Products with Therapeutic Equivalence Evaluations" that all pharmacies have, and since February 2005, there has been a daily Electronic Orange Book (EOB) product information for new generic drug approvals. The downloaded Annual Edition and Cumulative Supplements are also available in a paper version (Approved Drug Products with Therapeutic Equivalence Evaluations, ADP 2008) from the US Government Printing Office: http://bookstore.gpo.gov; toll free telephone number 866-512-1800.

Q. How do I write for a generic substitute on a prescription?

A. Prescriptions have instructions on whether the prescriber will allow the pharmacist to substitute a generic version of the drug. This instruction is communicated in several different ways which differ among states. Usually, the prescription contains two signature lines. One line has "substitution permitted" or "substitution permissible" printed at the bottom of the prescription and the other line has "dispense as written" or "do not substitute." The prescriber signs either line. Some states have a "daw" (dispense as written) box printed at the bottom of the prescription. This means that the prescription will be filled generically unless the prescriber writes "daw" in the box, in which case the prescription will be filled the way it is written by the prescriber. For example, if you write a prescription for the trade name of a drug such as Vibramycin® (the patient only wants to take a brand name drug) and sign the line "do not substitute" or write "daw" in the box, the prescription will be dispensed with the brand name drug rather than the generic substitute (doxycycline) (Meridith 2003).

Q. When should a generic drug rather than a brand name drug be prescribed?

A. Any time. It is the decision of the patient. Most drugs today are dispensed as generic. Generic substitution is intended for the pharmacist to use a form of the drug which may be less expensive to the patient. It is usually the cheaper drug yet still has the same FDA guidelines in manufacturing and should be equal in efficacy to the brand name drug. However, if the prescriber writes a prescription for the brand name drug and signs "do not substitute," the patient cannot request the generic (Food and Drug Administration [FDA] – Center for Drug Evaluation and Research [CDER]. Statistical approaches to Establishing Bioequivalence 2001).

Q. Who decides to choose a generic substitute?

A. The patient makes the decision as long as the prescription is signed by the prescriber to allow for substitution. If the prescriber does not sign the appropriate place to allow for generic substitution, the pharmacist must dispense the generic.

2.3 Controlled Drugs

*Note: Always confirm any drug laws with your state regulations because *the most restrictive clause will prevail, whether state or federal.*

Q. What are controlled substances?

A. Controlled substances come under the jurisdiction of the Controlled Substances Act of 1970. The federal agency is the DEA and the State agency is the Division of Narcotics and Dangerous Drugs of the DHHR. The Controlled Substances Act 1970 was developed to educate and monitor the prescribing and dispensing of potentially addictive substances into five Schedules according to their potential for abuse or physical or psychological dependence.

Q. What is the schedule for marijuana?

A. Even though marijuana is legal in some states and many groups want it rescheduled, the government says it is still a dangerous drug and should not be rescheduled. However, Epidiolex® (a drug derived from cannabidiol which is contained in the marijuana plant and indicated for Lennox–Gastaut syndrome) has been rescheduled to a Schedule V controlled substance.

Q. What is the definition of physical dependence?

A. Physical dependence is a physiological state characterized by the development of an abstinence syndrome on abrupt withdrawal of the medication. Physical dependence does not imply abuse or addiction.

Q. Sometimes controlled substances are written as Schedule III or "C-III." Is there a difference?

A. No. The *C* refers to controlled substance. Drugs which are subject to control under the Controlled Substances Act are assigned to one of five schedules, referred to as controlled substance schedules: Schedule I controlled substance, Schedule II controlled substance, Schedule III controlled substance, Schedule IV controlled substance and Schedule V controlled substance, depending on the abuse potential. These schedules are commonly shown as C-I, C-II, C-III, C-IV, and C-V.

Q. What are the different controlled (scheduled) drugs?

A. Refer to Table 2.1.

Q. Is a DEA number required to prescribe an opioid?

A. Yes. A dentist is required by law to register with the DEA in Washington, to dispense, store or prescribe controlled drugs. A DEA number will be issued to the prescriber in the state where they are practicing dentistry. If the state requires that the dentist have a State Controlled Substance Number, in addition to the DEA number, then the DEA will require that this number be issued before the DEA number can be issued. Twenty-six states that require a Controlled Substance Number and a DEA number are New Jersey, Alabama, South Carolina, Nevada, Iowa, District of Columbia, Utah, Oklahoma, Massachusetts, Michigan, Illinois, Connecticut, South Dakota, Louisiana, Guam, Wyoming, Puerto Rico, Rhode Island, Missouri, Indiana, Delaware, Texas, New Mexico, Maryland, Hawaii, and Idaho. There must be a space on the prescription to write in the DEA number.

Table 2.1 Controlled drugs

Schedule	Abuse potential	Examples
C-I	Highest	Not accepted for medical purposes: heroin, lysergic acid diethylamide (LSD), methaqualone, peyote, 3,4,methylenedioxymethamphetamine ("Ecstasy"), marijuana
C-II	High	Oxycodone/acetaminophen (Percocet®, Tylox®), hydrocodone/acetaminophen (Vicodin®, Lorcet®), meperidine (Demerol®), codeine, cocaine, morphine, oxycodone (OxyContin®), methadone (Dolophine®)
C-III	Less potential than C-II	Acetaminophen w/codeine, phenobarbital
C-IV	Less potential than C-III	Zolpidem (Ambien®), diazepam (Valium®), alprazolam (Xanax®)[a]
C-V	Limited abuse	Cough syrups with codeine, antidiarrheals such as diphenoxylate/atropine (Lomotil®)

[a] In certain states like New York, Schedule IV benzodiazepines (e.g., Valium, Xanax) are treated as Schedule II.

Q. Are prescription writing rules for controlled substances state or federal regulated?

A. Both. Regulations can be under state or federal law. The prescriber must review individual laws in their state. For example, under federal law, a prescription for Schedule II substances must be filled within 30 days of writing. *A state could establish rules tighter than the federal rules and the most restrictive clause will prevail, whether state or federal.*

Q. According to state and federal law, are there limits to the quantity of controlled drugs that can be prescribed?

A. While states may have more restrictive rules, the federal law does not limit the amount prescribed. *The most restrictive clause will prevail, whether state or federal.*

Q. Can Schedule I substances be prescribed by a private practitioner?

A. No. Schedule I substances have the highest abuse potential and no medical uses, thus no indications to be prescribed, and are not legally available to the public. This is a federal law and does not vary from state to state.

Q. Can Schedule II substances be prescribed by a private practitioner?

A. Yes. Schedule II drugs have a high abuse potential and include narcotics and amphetamines. There cannot be any refills and prescriptions are invalid after a certain number of days which is state regulated. For example, in New Jersey any controlled substance prescription can be filled in a pharmacy within 30 days of writing the prescription. After the limit, a new prescription is required. A Schedule II drug can be phoned into the pharmacy only in emergency situations and must be followed up by a written prescription within 72 hours. Only a three-day supply can be dispensed.

Q. What are the regulations for Schedule III drugs?

A. Schedule III drugs have a lower abuse potential than Schedule II drugs. Prescriptions for Schedule III substances expire six months after the date written. Refills are allowed but only five refills within six months. A practitioner may issue a new prescription for the Schedule III substance within a six-month period if necessary.

Q. What is the refill regulation for Schedule IV and V drugs?

A. Five refills in six months.

Q. Can the prescriber presign prescriptions for controlled substances?

A. No. Federal law prohibits prescribers from presigning prescriptions. All prescriptions for controlled substances must be dated and manually signed on the day the prescription was written.

Q. What are prescription drug monitoring programs (PDMPs)?

A. Diversion of controlled substances that have a high potential for abuse or profit when sold illegally is a serious problem. Different methods of diversion include illegal selling of controlled substance by physicians, dentists, and pharmacists; prescription theft; and inappropriate prescribing by physicians and dentists to themselves, family members or others. Drug monitoring programs were developed to control diversion. The program is run via an electronic database that tracks controlled substance prescriptions in a state. These monitoring programs are intended to improve opioid prescribing and protect patients at risk. Some states that have a drug monitoring system include California, Hawaii, Idaho, Illinois, Indiana, Massachusetts, Michigan, New York, Oklahoma, Rhode Island, Texas, New York, and New Jersey. Information on controlled drugs, primarily Schedule II substances, prescribing, dispensing, and purchasing is sent via electronic means to the state and analyzed. New York State also has extended its program to include benzodiazepines that are federally scheduled as C-IV controlled substances. Therefore, in New York State, all benzodiazepines, such as alprazolam (Xanax®) or diazepam (Valium®) require a new prescription every month and no refills.

2.4   Principles of Prescription Writing

Q. What is a legend drug?

A. A legend drug is a drug that can only be dispensed by a pharmacist with a prescription. Labels on these medications carry the legend: "Caution! Federal law prohibits dispensing without a prescription."

Q. What is the chemical name of a drug?

A. The chemical name describes the chemical make-up of a drug. For example, the chemical name for acetaminophen is *N*-acetyl-*p*-aminophenol.

Q. What is the proprietary name of a drug?

A. Other terms for proprietary name are brand or trade name and refer to the drug name assigned by the specific manufacturer which is protected by copyright. For example, one of the brand names for ibuprofen is Motrin® (McNeil).

Q. How long is a prescription valid until it is filled?

A. Every state has different rules which apply to prescriptions. A nonnarcotic prescription is valid for 365 days (one year) from the date on the prescription. Check with the local state boards for state-specific laws.

Q. How is the quantity of the drug being dispensed written?

A. The symbol # is acceptable to indicate *number* and informs the pharmacist to dispense tablets, capsules or liquid ounces. Sometimes the prescriber will write Disp: before the #, meaning "dispense." For example: Disp: # 12.

Q. What does "Sig" refer to?

A. Sig refers to the Latin word *signatura*, meaning "write," "make" or "label." This is the direction to the patient on how to take the medication.

Q. Should the dosage form of the drug be indicated on the prescription?

A. Yes. Tablets, capsules, suspension, or solution must be indicated on the prescription. For example, amoxicillin 500 mg Disp: # 28 capsules.

Q. Should the drug strength be written on the prescription?

A. Yes. The correct strength of the drug prescribed must be clearly written on the prescription. For example, amoxicillin 500 mg.

Q. Should the route of administration be specified on the prescription?

A. Yes. The dentist must indicate the correct route of administration of the drug prescribed even if it is orally.

Q. Should the duration of the drug prescribed be specified on the prescription?

A. Yes. The number of days or weeks must be written on the prescription. For example, penicillin V, 500 mg tid for seven days.

Q. Does the number of refills need to be written on the prescription?

A. Yes. If no refills are required, then "NR" or "zero" should be checked or written on the prescription. The number of refills should be spelled out. Do not just write "0." Some prescriptions have a checkoff box for "None."

Q. How many refills are allowed for nonscheduled and scheduled drugs?

A. The prescriber can write for no refills, indicated by NR (no refills). Prescription drugs may be refilled for only one year after the date of the prescription. A prescription for a controlled substance listed in Schedule III–V can only be refilled for six months or five refills, whichever comes first, after the date on such a prescription. After five refills or six months, whichever occurs first, a new prescription is required. For Schedule II drugs, there are no refills allowed.

Q. What is the law for dispensing a controlled substance for office use?

A. A blanket prescription cannot be written to provide a medical/dental office with medications for administration. If the office requires C-II medications, a DEA 222 form must be used to transfer the C-II stock. For all other medications, an invoice must be utilized.

Q. What does "label" on the prescription mean?

A. When the prescriber wants the patient to know the name of the drug, the box on the prescription form marked "label" should be checked.

Q. Can I phone in a prescription for a medication?

A. Yes. A nonnarcotic medication (e.g., antibiotics, nonsteroidal antiinflammatory drugs [NSAIDs]) can be phoned into the pharmacist and does not require a follow-up written prescription to be sent to the pharmacist.

When phoning in a controlled substance (e.g., Vicodin® C-II, Tylenol® with codeine C-III, Percocet C-II), the rules are different. Schedule II drugs cannot be phoned into the pharmacy except in an emergency and must be followed up with a written prescription usually within 72 hours (states may require that the prescription be sent to the pharmacist in a shorter time frame and the more restrictive clause prevails) and only for a three-day supply. Schedule III drugs can be dispensed by an oral (verbal) or written prescription and does not need a follow-up written prescription (the pharmacist writes all information which is equivalent to a written prescription). Renewal of Schedule III–V drugs can be called in to the pharmacy.

Q. Is there a limit on the quantity prescribed for a Schedule II, III, or V narcotic?

A. Although some states and many insurance companies limit the quantity of controlled substances dispensed to a 30-day supply or 120 doses, whichever is less, there are no specific federal limits to quantities of drugs dispensed by a prescription. Review the law in individual states. Remember the most restrictive clause will prevail, whether state or federal.

Q. Can a Schedule II narcotic (e.g., Percocet) be phoned into the pharmacy?

A. Yes, but only for emergency situations. Federal law requires the prescriber to follow up with a written prescription sent to the pharmacy within 72 hours, but different states have different time limits. No refills are allowed.

Q. What is the purpose of e-prescribing?

A. In 2010, the DEA legalized e-prescribing of controlled substances to reduce drug fraud and abuse. All nonnarcotic prescriptions can be e-prescribed. New York has the I-STOP law (Internet System for Tracking Over Prescribing) which requires *all* prescriptions to be sent to pharmacies through e-prescribing. In addition, as of 2016, all prescribers have to monitor patient use of controlled substance prescriptions via the PDMP.

According to the DEA, as of 1 June 2010, it is permissible to have e-prescribing for controlled substances in all 50 states; however, not all states are using it. E-prescribing software must meet the DEA requirements and have the required certifications before e-prescribing is allowed. In addition, some state laws and regulations will require changes before controlled substance e-prescribing will be fully legal. E-prescribing helps to reduce medication errors associated with prescribing (https://decisionresourcesgroup.com/drg-blog/health-reform/states-require-e-prescribing-combat-fraud-abuse).

Q. Can a Schedule II prescription be faxed to the pharmacy?

A. According to the DEA, in order to expedite the filling of a prescription, a prescriber may transmit a Schedule II prescription to the pharmacy by fax, but the original prescription must be presented to the pharmacist before the drug can be dispensed. The faxed copy is just an alert to the pharmacist that the patient is on the way with an original prescription. Otherwise, a fax for a Schedule II drug is not accepted.

Q. In which situations can a faxed C-II prescription serve as an original prescription?

A. A faxed C-II prescription can serve as an original for patients in a long-term care facility (LTCF), community-based care, enrolled in hospice, or receiving home infusion/IV pain management therapy. The fax *must* be signed by the prescriber.

Q. Can a Schedule III–V prescription be faxed to the pharmacist?

A. It depends. According to federal law, Schedule III–V substances can be faxed but certain states do not allow faxing of prescriptions for any controlled substance. The most restrictive clause will prevail. So, if federal law allows faxing but state law does not, the state law will succeed. According to the DEA, Schedule III–V prescriptions can be communicated orally, in writing, or by fax to the pharmacist and may be refilled (not more than five times within six months) as written on the prescription or by call-in.

Q. Are preprinted prescriptions for controlled substances allowed?

A. No.

Q. What are the more common Latin abbreviations used in prescription writing?

A. See Table 2.2.

Table 2.2 Common Latin abbreviations used in dental prescription writing

Abbreviation	Meaning
q	every hour
qhs	every night
qd	every day
q8h	every 8 hours
bid	twice a day
cap	capsule
tid	three times a day
qid	four times a day
stat	immediately
ac	at meal times
h	hour
hs	at bedtime
NR	no refills
pc	after meals
po	orally (by mouth)
prn	as needed
tab	tablet

Q. What are the different measurement systems used in pharmacy and for writing prescriptions?

A. The *metric system* which bases calculations on the base of 10. There is a metric unit of weight (gram [g]) and a metric unit of volume (liter [L]). The *apothecary system*, which is becoming obsolete, uses old measures of weights and volumes such as grains (gr). This system is also confusing because the abbreviation "gr" can be mistaken for gram, which is abbreviated "g." The *avoirdupois system* or household system of weights is used for ordinary commodities such as ounce, teaspoonful, and tablespoonful.

Q. What is a milligram (mg)?

A. A milligram (mg) is a unit (metric system) of mass equal to one thousandth of a gram. Thus, 1 gram (g) equals 1000 milligrams (mg). It is advised to write "g" instead of "gm" as an abbreviation for gram because "gm" can easily be misinterpreted as "mg."

Q. What is a grain?

A. A grain (gr) is a unit of (apothecary) measurement of mass and $1 g = 64.79 mg = 0.06479 g$. It is often confused with grams, which is abbreviated "g."

Q. What does the term "parts per million" mean when expressing permissible exposure to fluorides?

A. Parts per million when referring to permissible exposure to fluorides means the number of grams (g) per million mL of solution. For example, one part per million (ppm) is interpreted as one gram per million mL of solution.

Q. What does a 1 : 100 solution mean?

A. In calculating the amount of a drug that must be administered, especially if it is in solution, there is specific information that is required to do the calculations. The concentration of the drug in solution is expressed as gm/mL, or as a percent or as a ratio such as 1 : 100, 1 : 1000 and so on. A percent solution means what percentage of a drug is in 100 mL of solution.

- For example: 1 : 100 means that there is 1 g of drug in 100 mL of solution (1 g/100 mL) = 0.01 g/mL = 10 mg/mL = 1%
- 1 : 100 000 = 1 mg/100 mL = 0.01 mg/mL = 0.001%
- 5% solution means that there is 5000 mg/100 mL or 50 mg/mL. A simple way to figure this out is just to move the decimal one place to the right of the percent.
- 3% hydrogen peroxide means 3 g of hydrogen peroxide in 100 mL of solution or 3000 mg/100 mL or 30 mg/mL.

Q. What is a **Black Box Warning** regarding certain drugs?

A. A **Black Box Warning** (sometimes called a boxed warning) is a warning found on the package insert of a drug. It is given this name because there is a black border around the text of the warning. According to the FDA, a boxed warning is given to drugs that have a significant risk of serious or life-threatening adverse reactions. Note that every Black Box Warning has the date that the warning was announced by the FDA. Not all drugs have a boxed warning. Examples of some drugs related to dentistry with boxed warnings include the following.

- *March 2011*: fluoroquinolone antibiotics including levofloxacin (Levaquin®) can exacerbate muscle weakness in persons with myasthenia gravis.
- *January 2011*: the FDA asked drug manufacturers to voluntarily limit the strength of acetaminophen in prescription drug products, which are predominantly combinations of acetaminophen and opioids. This action will limit the amount of acetaminophen in these products to 325 mg per tablet, capsule, or other dosage unit, making these products safer for patients.

In addition, a *Boxed Warning* highlighting the potential for severe liver injury and a *Warning* highlighting the potential for allergic reactions (e.g., swelling of the face, mouth, and throat, difficulty breathing, itching, or rash) are being added to the label of all prescription drug products that contain acetaminophen. These actions will help to reduce the risk of severe liver injury and allergic reactions associated with acetaminophen.

Note: over-the-counter (OTC) products containing acetaminophen (e.g. Tylenol) are not affected by this action. Information about the potential for liver injury is already required on the label for OTC products containing acetaminophen. The FDA is continuing to evaluate ways to reduce the risk of acetaminophen-related liver injury from OTC products.

- *April 2009*: onabotulinumtoxinA (marketed as Botox®/Botox Cosmetic®) and rimabotulinumtoxinB (marketed as Myobloc®) have the possibility of experiencing potentially life-threatening distant spread of toxin effect from the injection site after local injection to produce symptoms consistent with botulism. Symptoms such as unexpected loss of strength or muscle weakness, hoarseness or trouble talking (dysphonia), trouble saying words clearly (dysarthria), loss of bladder control, trouble breathing, trouble swallowing, double vision, blurred vision, and drooping eyelids may occur. The other botulinum toxin product in this class, abobotulinumtoxinA (marketed as Dysport®), was approved on April 29, 2009 and included the Boxed Warning.
- *July 2008*: fluoroquinolone antibiotics (ciprofloxacin [Cipro®], levofloxacin [Levaquin®]) have an increased risk of tendonitis and tendon rupture that could cause permanent injury. This risk is further increased in patients over 60 years of age, in patients taking corticosteroid drugs, and in those with kidney, heart or lung transplants.
- *November 2005*: *Clostridium difficile*-associated diarrhea (CDAD) has been reported with use of nearly all antibacterial agents, including clindamycin HCL, and may range in severity from mild diarrhea to fatal colitis. Treatment with antibacterial agents alters the normal flora of the colon, leading to overgrowth of *C. difficile*. *C. difficile* produces toxins A and B, which contribute to the development of CDAD. Hypertoxin-producing strains of *C. difficile* cause increased morbidity and mortality, as these infections can be refractory to antimicrobial therapy and may require colectomy. CDAD must be considered in all patients who present with diarrhea following antibiotic use. Careful medical history is necessary since CDAD has been reported to occur over two months after the administration of antibacterial agents. If CDAD is suspected or confirmed, ongoing antibiotic use not directed against *C. difficile* may need to be discontinued. Appropriate fluid and electrolyte management, protein supplementation, antibiotics or surgical intervention may be required.
- *April 2005*: the FDA concluded that the benefits of Celebrex® outweigh the potential risks in properly selected and informed patients. Accordingly, the FDA allowed Celebrex to remain on the market and asked the manufacturer Pfizer to take the actions listed below. According to the FDA requirements, the Celebrex label must:
  - include a Boxed Warning containing the class NSAID warnings and contraindication (see below) about cardiovascular (CV) and gastrointestinal (GI) risk, plus specific information

on the controlled clinical trial data that demonstrate an increased risk of adverse CV events for celecoxib (Messerli and Sichrovsky 2005)

- encourage prescribers to discuss with patients the potential benefits and risks of Celebrex and other treatment options before a decision is made to use Celebrex
- encourage practitioners to use the *lowest effective dose* for the shortest duration consistent with individual patient treatment goals.

- *April 2005*: the FDA asked manufacturers of all OTC products containing ibuprofen (Motrin, Advil®, Ibu-Tab 200®, Medipren®, Cap-Profen®, Tab-Profen®, Profen®, Ibuprohm®), naproxen (Aleve®), and ketoprofen (Orudis®, Actron®) to revise their labeling to include more specific information about the potential CV and GI risks and instructions about which patients should seek the advice of a physician before using these drugs.
- *July 2001*: warning about the abuse potential of OxyContin, a Schedule II controlled substance.

Q. How do I write for a prescription for doxycycline?

A. See Figure 2.1.

Interpretation of prescription: the salt form of doxycycline is hyclate or monohydrate. Doxycycline monohydrate is used in the treatment of acne. Doxycycline hyclate is used for other bacterial infections. So it is necessary to identify the correct salt form. Also, in order to write a prescription, it must be known whether to write for capsules or tablets. Doxycycline is supplied as 50, 75, and 100 mg capsules or tablets. In this prescription, the prescriber prescribed capsules. Latin abbreviations were used but they were written legibly. It is probably safest not to use Latin abbreviations but rather write the prescription in English. The number of days the patient should take the medication for was indicated (× 10 days; the × refers to "for"). Also, it is important for the safety of the patient to write on the prescription "for dental infections" because the patient may be taking many different medications and may have a lot of pill containers in the medicine cabinet. Identifying this prescription bottle for use for a dental infection will make it easier for the patient to pick up that container. Directions for use (Sig:): Take one capsule orally every 12 hours on day 1, then one capsule every day for 10 days for dental infections.

2.5 How to Avoid Prescription Errors

Q. How can I prevent medication errors when writing a prescription?

A. If your handwriting is poor, consider faxing or e-prescribing. Also, many drug names are very similar. To avoid misinterpretation, names should be written clearly and the use of abbreviations should be avoided. Also, before sending, review the prescription and make sure the drug, strength, and directions are correct.

Q. What else can I do to avoid prescribing errors?

A. Always interview your patient thoroughly about allergies. For example, a patient with asthma who is allergic to aspirin may experience an acute bronchospasm after taking an NSAID such as ibuprofen (Advil, Nuprin®) or naproxen sodium (Aleve). In adults, this reaction is called Samter's triad and it is a condition consisting of asthma, nonallergic aspirin sensitivity, and nasal polyps. Recently, a fourth symptom has been added, hyperplastic sinusitis,

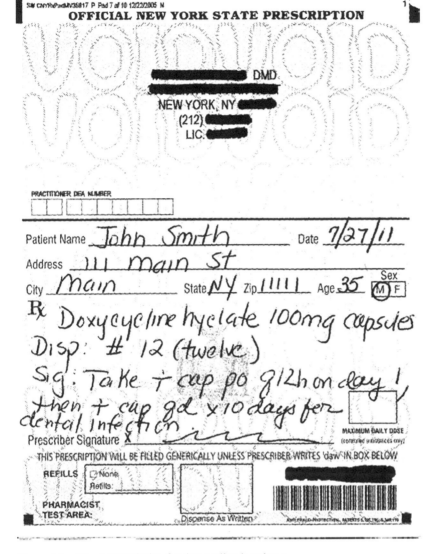

Figure 2.1 How a prescription for doxycycline is written.

and instead of Samter's triad, it can also be called aspirin-exacerbated respiratory disease. This occurs because NSAIDs block the production of prostaglandins and leukotrienes, which are chemical substances involved in the inflammatory response resulting in severe allergy-like symptoms. It is best to avoid aspirin and NSAIDs in asthmatics.

Another example: clindamycin is prescribed to a patient who is allergic to penicillin. A review of the patient's history confirms she has a history of ulcerative colitis. Clindamycin is contraindicated in an individual with a history of ulcerative colitis. An alternative would be azithromycin (Zithromax®). Refer to Chapter 4.

Q. Can there be errors when writing decimal points and zeros on a prescription?

A. Yes. To avoid prescription misinterpretations, avoid unnecessary decimal points. For example, when writing for 5 mL of a suspension or solution, it should be written as 5 mL not 5.0 mL because the 5.0 could be understood as 50. Also, always place a zero before quantities. For example, write 0.25 mg and not .25 mg because this could be misinterpreted as 25 mg.

Q. Should I review the prescription with the patient?

A. Definitely. The dentist should go over the medication and how to take it, including the number, frequency, and with meals or on an empty stomach. Also, make sure the patient is not allergic to the medication. Don't just review the medical history in the chart. You must ask the patient if he/she is allergic. If the patient confirms allergy, ask what happened when that drug was taken. Ask if there was a rash or difficulty breathing or just gastrointestinal upset (diarrhea). Document in the chart that you reviewed how to take the medication with the patient, whether history of allergies was denied, and if the patient had or did not have any questions and that they understood everything.

Q. Is it OK to use the Latin abbreviations on how to take the medicine?

A. Yes, but it is not advised because misinterpretation of abbreviations is a common source of error. Overdoses have occurred when "qd" used for every day was interpreted as "qid," four times a day. It is recommended not to abbreviate and to write out all instructions in English and avoid Latin abbreviations.

Q. Is it acceptable to write abbreviations of drugs?

A. No. The full name should be written legibly. For instance, do not write PCN for penicillin V.

Q. Is it acceptable to write "take as directed"?

A. No. The instruction "take as directed" or "take as needed" is not satisfactory and should be avoided. Patients may fail to understand or forget the instructions given in the prescriber's office. Similarly, most insurance companies will only reimburse the patient or pharmacist for a specific number of doses or duration of treatment. The same thing holds true with writing "as needed." The directions to the patient should include a reminder of the intended purpose of the medication by including such phrases as "for relief of dental pain" or "for dental infection" (Warner and Mitchell 2008).

Q. What about recommending over-the-counter drugs?

A. Even though OTC drugs are not prescription or legend drugs, if the dentist recommends an OTC in the dental office the same responsibilities for proper prescribing apply. For example, after a surgical procedure the patient asks which OTC analgesic is good to take. Do not recommend any OTC drug without reviewing the medical history. If the patient has controlled hypertension and is taking a beta-blocker, NSAIDs (e.g., ibuprofen, naproxen sodium) in doses adequate to reduce inflammation and pain can increase blood pressure in both normotensive and hypertensive individuals. In addition, NSAID use may reduce the effect of all antihypertensive drugs except calcium channel blockers (nifedipine [Procardia®], amlodipine [Norvac®]). The manufacturer recommends that NSAIDs be used for a maximum of five days in patients taking any antihypertensive drugs except for calcium channel blockers (White 2007).

Q. Is there any special labeling of OTC drugs?

A. Yes. In the Federal Register of March 1999, the FDA published the OTC Drug Facts Label regulation. This regulation required most OTC drug products to comply with the new format and content requirements by May 2002. This "new" drug labeling of OTC was intended to inform the consumer about the medication in an easy-to-read label. OTC medicines also differ from prescription drugs in their labeling. The OTC Drug Facts label contains all the information a consumer needs in order to select an appropriate OTC medicine, to use the medicine safely and effectively, and to decide when to consult a physician, if needed. Some changes to the labeling include the word "uses" which replaces "indications," and terms such as "precautions" and "contraindications" have been replaced with more easily understood words. The label is written in large font and formatted with bullet points, so it is easier to read.

References

Balthasar, J. (1999). Bioequivalence and bioequivalency testing. *American Journal of Pharmaceutical Education* 63: 194–198.

Birkett, D. (2003). Generics – equal or not? *Australian Prescriber* 26: 85–87.

Food and Drug Administration (2008). Approved Drug Products with Therapeutic Equivalence Evaluations. www.fda.gov/drugs/resources-information-approved-drugs/approved-drug-products-therapeutic-equivalence-evaluations-orange-book.

Food and Drug Administration – Center for Drug Evaluation and Research (CDER) (2001). Statistical Approaches to Establishing Bioequivalence. www.fda.gov/downloads/Drugs/GuidanceComplianceRegulatoryInformation/Guidances/ucm070244.pdf.

Greene, W.L., Concato, J., and Feinstein, A.R. (2001). Claims of equivalence in medical research: are they supported by the evidence. *Annals of Internal Medicine* 132: 715–722.

Meridith, P. (2003). Bioequivalence and other unresolved issues in generic drug substitution. *Clinical Therapeutics* 25: 2875–2890.

Messerli, F.H. and Sichrovsky, T. (2005). Does the pro-hypertensive effect of cyclooxygenase-2 inhibitors account for the increased risk in cardiovascular disease? *American Journal of Cardiology* 96: 872.

Posner, J. and Griffin, J.P. (2011). Generic substitution. *British Journal of Clinical Pharmacology* 72 (5): 731–732.

Warner, T.D. and Mitchell, J.A. (2008). COX-2 selectively alone does not define the cardiovascular risks associated with non-steroidal anti-inflammatory drugs. *Lancet* 371: 270–273.

Welage, L.S., Kirking, D.M., Ascione, F.J. et al. (2001). Understanding the scientific issues embedded in the generic drug approval process. *Journal of the American Pharmaceutical Association* 41: 856–867.

White, W.B. (2007). Cardiovascular effects of the cyclooxygenase inhibitors. *Hypertension* 49: 408–418.

Additional Resources

www.deadiversion.usdoj.gov/pubs/manuals/pract/section5.htm

www.fda.gov/Drugs/DrugSafety/ucm239821.htm

www.blackboxrx.com

FDA Guidance for Industry. Dissolution Testing for Immediate Release Solid Oral Dosage Forms. US Department of Health and Human Services. www.fda.gov/regulatory-information/search-fda-guidance-documents/dissolution-testing-immediate-release-solid-oral-dosage-forms

3

Basic Prescribing and Drug Dosing for the Dental Patient

3.1   Basic Principles of Drug Dosing

Q. What is the difference between dose and dosage form?

A. The dose of a drug is a specified quantity of a drug – the size or frequency at which the drug doses are administered. The dosage form of a drug is the drug formulation such as a tablet, capsule, syrup, liquid suspension, solution, ointment, or cream that generally contains the active drug substance in association with one or more inactive ingredients. The FDA has stated that a dosage form is the way of identifying the drug by its physical form, which is linked both to physical appearance of the drug product and to the way it is administered (www.fdalawblog. net/fda_law_blog_hyman_phelps/2009/05/fda-petition-response-reaffirms-fda-orange-book-dosage-form-nomenclature-policy.html).

  If a patient is instructed to take one 500 mg capsule po (orally) qid (four times a day), the total dose is calculated from the dose multiplied by the number of times a day the dose is administered; one tablet (500 mg) qid is 2000 mg or 2 g.

Q. Why are some tablets "candy coated"?

A. These "candy-coated" tablets are what is known as enteric coated. Some drugs are either irritating to the stomach lining or are inactivated, to different degrees, by acid in the stomach. To prevent the drug from being inactivated or destroyed in the stomach and allow it to travel to the intestine where it will ultimately be absorbed, enteric-coated buffered tablets protect the drugs from gastric juices. Examples include erythromycin base, ibuprofen, and aspirin.

Q. Is it important to know the patient's baseline hepatic and renal function when deciding on the proper dosage?

A. Yes. Most drugs require adequate hepatic function for metabolism and adequate renal function for elimination. It is important to review the medical history and specifically ask the patient if they have any liver or kidney problems.

Q. What is the principle of selection of a therapeutic regimen?

A. Since the outcome of drug therapy is the product of a multifaceted interaction between drug and patient, the selection of an appropriate drug and dosing regimen is dependent on a thorough evaluation of the patient's medical and dental status and the actions and effects of the drugs to be used in treatment.

The Dentist's Drug and Prescription Guide, Second Edition. Mea A. Weinberg, Stuart J. Froum and Stuart L. Segelnick.
© 2020 John Wiley & Sons, Inc. Published 2020 by John Wiley & Sons, Inc.

Q. What are the variabilities in drug dosage requirements?

A. There are many variabilities relating to alterations in drug dosing. The age of the patient, their renal and liver function, and pregnancy status can change the way the body reacts to medications.

Q. What are loading doses and maintenance doses of drugs?

A. Most drugs are not administered as a single dose. Rather, repeated doses resulting in an accumulation of the drug in the blood are needed to reach a plateau whereby the level of drug in the plasma is maintained constantly within the therapeutic range and there are no fluctuations in the concentration-time profile. A *steady state* is achieved when the amount of drug absorbed into the body equals the amount of the drug leaving the body. To keep a proper steady state, the drug dosing must be consistent and the drug must be taken at the same time every day. Not achieving and maintaining steady state may make the drug therapy ineffective. It must be emphasized to the patient that the drug must be taken as prescribed. The drug should be taken at the same time every day and without any missed doses. In order to reach steady state, a *loading dose* is first administered on day 1, which is a higher amount of drug needed to quickly reach a therapeutic plasma drug concentration. Without a loading dose, it takes longer to reach steady state. After the loading dose is administered and before the plasma levels drop, a *maintenance dose* is given to maintain plasma drug levels within the therapeutic range. This maintenance dose is given in lower doses after the loading dose. For example, penicillin V is usually given as "1000 mg initially, followed by 500 mg every 6 hours." Doxycycline is given as "100 mg every 12 hours on day 1, then 100 mg every day afterward."

Q. How much loading dose is administered?

A. The loading dose is usually twice the regular dose.

Q. What drugs are given as an initial loading dose followed by a maintenance dose?

A. Antibiotics that are administered every 6–8 hours (including azithromycin, which is dosed once every 24 hours) usually require a loading dose in order to rapidly achieve a high tissue concentration for acute dental infections.

Q. How is a loading dose, followed by a maintenance dose, administered?

A. The loading dose is given on day 1, followed by the maintenance dose on day 1, day 2 etc....

Q. What is the proper duration of antibiotic treatment for dental infections?

A. Generally, the duration of antibiotic therapy has been variable and not evidence based. The current theory focuses on shortening the course of antibiotics, which might limit antibiotic resistance. Generally, most private practice and hospital-based dentists empirically prescribe antibiotics for 7–10 days. However, high-dose, short-term therapy has also been advocated in medical guidelines. Prescribing antibiotics for three days has been shown to reduce the incidence of antibiotic resistance (Paterson et al. 2016). It is also important to take the antibiotic for the full course prescribed, even if the patient is clinically responding, in order to minimize the chance of the resistant bacteria not being targeted, thus preventing a relapse. However, there are no specific guidelines or recommendations regarding the duration of dental antibiotic therapy.

Q. What is the importance of knowing the peak concentration of a drug?

A. Peak concentration is the maximum plasma concentration of a drug which is seen during dosing intervals. At the time (usually hours) of peak concentration, the drug has the highest concentration in the plasma. Knowing the peak concentration of a drug is important because this is the time required if antibiotic prophylaxis is to be achieved. Antibiotic prophylaxis is defined as prevention of development of an infection at the surgical site (Munckoff 2005). For example, antibiotic prophylaxis is recommended by the American Heart Association (AHA) before a sinus graft is performed in anticipation of possible perforation of the Schneiderian membrane (creating signs and symptoms of sinusitis). Having the antibiotic already in the systemic circulation before the surgical procedure is performed is ideal for optimum therapeutic effects. Thus, before performing surgical procedures, the antibiotic needs to be administered only during the peak hours before the surgery and not days before.

Q. What are the peak blood levels of antibiotics used in dentistry?

A. See Table 3.1.

Table 3.1 Peak blood levels of antibiotics

Drug	Time to peak
Amoxicillin	1–2 hours
Azithromycin (Zithromax®)	2.5–4 hours
Clindamycin	45–60 minutes
Doxycycline	1–2 hours
Penicillin VK	30–60 minutes
Tetracycline	2–4 hours

Q. What are the peak levels of common analgesics used in dentistry?

A. See Table 3.2

Table 3.2 Peak levels of common analgesics

Drug	Time to peak
Acetaminophen	0.5–2 hours
Codeine	1–1.5 hours
Diflunisal (Dolobid®)	2–3 hours
Ibuprofen	1–2 hours
Meperidine (Demerol®)	1 hour
Naproxen sodium (Aleve, Anaprox®)	1 hour
Oxycodone	30–60 minutes

Q. What is the difference in prescribing capsules or tablets (e.g., doxycycline 100 mg comes in tablets and capsules)?

A. If a patient has difficulty swallowing capsules, prescribe tablets. To be absorbed, capsules need to undergo dissolution or to be opened (usually takes about four minutes) and tablets need to undergo disintegration or to break up (takes slightly longer than a capsule) to release the active ingredient that will be absorbed. Both processes take time and absorption will occur in the duodenum (small intestine). A liquid gel capsule (Aleve®, Advil®) is formulated to dissolve quickly which allows the liquid inside the capsule to be absorbed fast. A gel capsule is a capsule-shaped tablet coated with gelatin for easy swallowing. Basically, it is a tablet and not a capsule. That means it will be absorbed like a tablet, but it may take longer to disintegrate because the gelatin must disintegrate first and then the tablet. Liquid drug (e.g., solution) is absorbed most rapidly, followed by liquid gel capsule, capsule, tablet, and then gel capsule.

Q. What happens if a patient misses a dose of an antibiotic?

A. It is important not to miss doses because drugs that require daily administration are only effective when they achieve steady state in the blood, which is required for a medication to reach therapeutic and effective levels. This means that steady state occurs when the amount of drug entering the blood equals the amount of drug being eliminated from the body. Ideally, doses should be equally spaced throughout the day and taken at the same times each day. This will help to maintain a constant level of antibiotic in the bloodstream. If the patient misses a dose of an antibiotic, it is best not to double the next dose because this could increase the incidence of adverse effects. If you miss a dose, take it as soon as remembered; do not take if it is almost time for the next dose. Instead, skip the missed dose and resume your usual dosing schedule. Do not "double up" the doses.

Q. What does first-pass effect have to do with drug dosing?

A. First-pass effect is defined as the biotransformation of a drug in the liver that occurs before the drug enters the systemic circulation. For example, sublingual nitroglycerin has a high first-pass metabolism because 90% of it is inactivated by the liver before it enters the blood. Morphine and lidocaine are other drugs with high first-pass effect when administered orally. Because this, they cannot be given orally because they would be totally inactivated before reaching the target site.

Q. How does age affect drug metabolism?

A. Age often affects drug metabolism and drug dosages may need to be adjusted in children and the elderly. Years ago, pediatric dosing was determined using pediatric formulas such as Clark's Rule, Young's Rule and Fried's Rule, which were based on the weight of the child in pounds or on their age in months. Today, these formulations are not used but rather the dose is based on body surface area or weight of the infant/child. In order to calculate the proper dosage, the manufacturer's safe dose (in mg/kg) of the prescribed drug must be known. This dose is predetermined by the manufacturer.

Children and the elderly require lower drug doses due to differences in their response to drugs.

3.2 Pediatric Patients

*Note: The prescriber should use their own judgment in prescribing for pediatric patients. The prescriptions in this section are not absolute numbers, only suggestions.

Q. Are there standardized dosage recommendations for children?

A. Yes. The dosage is dependent on the age and weight of the child. It should be noted that there is a wide range of correct dosages for a drug. Usually, drug information for pediatric dosage (mg/kg) is supplied by the drug manufacturer. For example, the dose recommendations for children on amoxicillin range from 20 to 45 mg/kg body weight per day depending on weight and height of the patient and the severity (mild or severe infection) of the medical condition. (www.emiphysicians.com/calculator1.html).

Q. Should a solid dose form or liquid suspension or solution be given to a pediatric patient?

A. It depends on the age and weight of the child but always ask the parent if the child can swallow a pill. Sometimes when calculating dosage, it may be more accurate to give a liquid dosage form.

Q. What is the difference between mL and cc?

A. mL (milliliters) is sometimes referred to as cc or cubic centimeters. Sometimes, a medical dropper will have markers in cc; cc is the same as mL.

Q. How does the parent accurately measure out teaspoonfuls or mL?

A. Medicine droppers and spoons are available in the pharmacy. The dropper and spoon have measurements in medical teaspoonful (tsp) and mL. The patient should be cautioned not to use a household teaspoon because it can vary in size.

Q. What should be prescribed if the calculation for a pediatric dose is, for example, 275 mg for penillicin V?

A. Since there is no dosage strength available for 275 mg, it is recommended to always use the lower dose and then increase the number of days of therapy (prescribe the antibiotic for 10 days rather than seven days) *or* to use the suspension instead.

Q. What directions should be given to the parent about oral suspensions?

A. Oral suspensions should be shaken very well and stored in the refrigerator. Any unused medicine should be discarded after 14 days.

Q. Given the following case, what dosage of penicillin V should be prescribed to this child?

A. *10-year-old male patient who weighs 32 kg (70 lbs) has an endodontic abscess that is not draining. An antibiotic should be prescribed. Penicillin V is the drug of choice. The antibiotic can be prescribed as an oral suspension or as a tablet.*

3.2.1 Penicillin V Oral Suspension

Steps to follow when prescribing for a pediatric patient: www.drugguide.com/ddo/ub/view/Davis-Drug-Guide/109514/0/Pediatric_Dosage_Calculations

- What is the dose for the age of the child? This information can be obtained from a drug reference source. This is a set dosage for a child of that age and weight.
  - Dose required: <12 year: 15–30 mg/kg/d q6–8 h; max. 3 g/day × 7–10 days (this is an established dosage obtained from a drug reference source).
- If it is decided to give an oral suspension, the amount of active ingredient in the suspension must be known. This information is also obtained from a drug reference book.
  - How supplied: oral suspension 125 mg/5 mL; 250 mg/5 mL (100 mL bottle).

Table 3.3 Calculation for correct dose to give to a pediatric patient

Step 1 Convert pounds to kg:	70 lb × 1 kg/2.2 lb = 31.8 kg
Step 2 Calculate the dose in mg:	31.8 kg × 15 mg/kg/day = 477 mg/day
Step 3 Divide the dose by the frequency:	477 mg/day ÷ 3 (tid) = 159 mg/dose q8h
Step 4 Convert the mg dose to mL:	159 mg/dose ÷ 125 mg/5 mL = 6.36 mL qid
Step 5 Convert mL to teaspoonfuls[a]	6.36 mL ÷ 5 mL = 1.27 teaspoonful (round to 1¼ teaspoonful)

[a] Each teaspoonful is 5 mL.
Calculation for 159 mg/dose ÷ 125 mg/5 mL is the following: 159 x 5 ÷ 125 = 6.36.

Table 3.4 How the prescription is written

Rx Penicillin V oral suspension 250 mg/5 mL
Disp: 1 bottle (100 mL)
Sig: Take 1¼ teaspoonful orally three times a day for 7 days for dental infectio

Advise the parent to use a medicine dropper/spoon rather than an ordinary teaspoon because of variations in measurements. After penicillin V solution is mixed, it is best to store it in a refrigerator between 2 °C and 7 °C (36–46 °F); do not freeze. Throw away any unused medicine after 14 days.

- Now, the correct dose to give to the pediatric patient must be calculated (Table 3.3).
- How is the prescription written (Table 3.4)?

3.2.2 How is the Dose Calculated if the Child can Swallow Tablets (Table 3.5)?

3.2.2.1 Penicillin V Tablets

- Dose required: <12 year: 15–30 mg/kg/d q6–8 h; max. 3 g/day × 7–10 days (this is an established dosage. There is a dose range, so it depends on the weight of the patient and severity of the infection).
- How supplied: 250, 500 mg tabs.

3.2.3 If Amoxicillin Is To Be Prescribed

3.2.3.1 Amoxicillin Oral Suspension

Calculate the dose of amoxicillin suspension in mL for a 10-year-old child weighing 32 kg (70 lbs) (Table 3.6).

- Dose required: 25–45 mg/kg/day divided bid or 20–40 mg/kg/day q8h (this is given by the manufacturer).

Table 3.5 How to calculate dose if the child can swallow tablets

Step 1 Convert pounds to kg:	70 lb × 1 kg/2.2 lb = 31.8 kg
Step 2 Calculate the dose in mg:	31.8 kg × 15 mg/kg/day = 477 mg/day
Step 3 Divide the dose by the frequency:	477 mg/day ÷ 3 (tid) = 159 mg/dose q8h

The total dose is 159 mg every 8 hours. Since the tablets only come in 250 and 500 mg, it is probably best to prescribe the oral suspension to be more precise.

Table 3.6 Calculating the dose of amoxicillin suspension in mL for a 10-year-old child weighing 70 lb

Step 1 Convert pounds to kg:	70 lb × 1 kg/2.2 lb = 31.8 kg
Step 2 Calculate the dose in mg:	31.8 kg × 40 mg/kg/day = 1272 mg/day
Step 3 Divide the dose by the frequency:	1272 mg/day ÷ 3 (tid) = 424 mg/dose bid
Step 4 Convert the mg dose to mL:	424 mg/dose ÷ 125 mg/5 mL = 3.39 mL bid
Step 5 Convert mL into teaspoonfuls[a]	3.39 mL ÷ 5 mL = 0.68 teaspoonful

Rx: amoxicillin oral suspension 125 mg/5 mL

Disp: 100 mL bottle

Sig: Take 3.4 cc orally three times a day for 7 days for dental infection

Note: mL (milliliters) is sometimes referred to as cc or cubic centimeters. Usually, a medical dropper will have markers in cc which is the same as mL. There is probably less misinterpretation when mL is used rather than cc.

[a] Each teaspoonful is 5 mL.

- How supplied: suspension comes in concentrations of 125 mg/5 mL, 250 mg/5 mL, 250 mg/mL, 400 mg/mL (100 mL bottle).

Advise the parent to get a medicine dropper/spoon rather than using an ordinary teaspoon because of variations in measurements of a teaspoonful. After amoxicillin solution is mixed, it is best to store it in a refrigerator between 2 °C and 8 °C (36–46 °F); do not freeze. Throw away any unused medicine after 14 days.

3.2.3.2 Amoxicillin Chewable Tablets (Table 3.7)
- Dose required: 25–45 mg/kg/day divided bid or 20–40 mg/kg/d q8h (this is given by the manufacturer).
- How supplied: chewable tabs 125, 400 mg.

3.2.3.3 Amoxicillin Capsules (Table 3.8)
- Dose required: 25–45 mg/kg/day divided bid (given by the manufacturer).
- How supplied: capsules 250, 500 mg.

Table 3.7 Calculating the dose of amoxicillin chewable tablets in mg for a 10-year-old child weighing 70 lb

Step 1 Convert pounds to kg:	70 lb × 1 kg/2.2 lb = 31.8 kg
Step 2 Calculate the dose in mg:	31.8 kg × 30 mg/kg/day = 954 mg/day
Step 3 Divide the dose by the frequency:	954 mg/day ÷ 3 (tid) = 378 mg/dose bid

Since chewable tablets only come in strengths of 125 and 400 mg, it is recommended to always use the lower dose and then increase the number of days of therapy *or* to use the suspension instead, which may be more precise.

Table 3.8 Calculating the dose of amoxicillin capsules in mg for a 10-year-old child weighing 70 lb

Step 1 Convert pounds to kg:	70 lb × 1 kg/2.2 lb = 31.8 kg
Step 2 Calculate the dose in mg:	31.8 kg × mg/kg/day = 1272 mg/day
Step 3 Divide the dose by the frequency:	1272 mg/day ÷ 2 (bid) = 636 mg/dose bid

The dose is 636 mg bid; either 500 mg capsules can be prescribed and increase the number of days of therapy or it may be best to use the oral suspension.

Q. If the child in Case 1 (above) were allergic to penicillin, what other antibiotics could be prescribed?

A. Clarithromycin (Biaxin®) (Table 3.9)

- Dose required: 15 mg/kg/day divided q12h (Table 3.10).
- How supplied: oral suspension comes in concentrations of 125 mg/5 mL, 250 mg/5 mL (100 mL bottle) (Table 3.11).

Table 3.9 Calculating the dose of clarithromycin (Biaxin) in mL for a 10-year-old child weighing 70 lb

Step 1 Convert pounds to kg:	70 lb × 1 kg/2.2 lb = 31.8 kg
Step 2 Calculate the dose in mg:	31.8 kg × 15 mg/kg/day = 477 mg/day
Step 3 Divide the dose by the frequency:	477 mg/day ÷ 2 (bid) = 238.5 mg/dose bid
Step 4 Convert the mg dose to mL:	238.5 mg/dose ÷ 250 mg/5 mL = 4.77 mL q12h
Step 5 Convert mL into teaspoonfuls[a]	4.77 mL ÷ 5 mL = 0.954 teaspoonful bid

[a] Each teaspoonful is 5 mL.

Table 3.10 Pediatric dosage schedule

Weight (kg)	Weight (lb)	Dosage (q12h) (tablets)	125 mg/5 mL[a] (suspension)	250 mg/5 mL (suspension)
9	20	67.5 mg q12h	2.7 mL q12h	1.35 mL q12h
18	40	136 mg q12h	5.4 mL q12h	2.7 mL q12h
25	55	187.5 mg q12h	7.5 mL q12h	3.75 mL q12h
34	75	255 mg q12h	10 mL q12h	5 mL q12h

Source: Adapted from www.rxlist.com/biaxin-drug.htm
[a] A teaspoonful is 5 mL.
This is an easy-to-follow table for prescribing clarithromycin to pediatric patients; the usual recommended dosage is 15 mg/kg/day divided q12h for 10 days.

Table 3.11 How the clarithromycin (Biaxin) prescription should be written

Rx: clarithromycin oral suspension 250 mg/5 mL
Disp: 1 bottle (100 mL)
Sig: Take 1 teaspoonful orally twice a day for 7 days for dental infection

3.2.4 Azithromycin

3.2.4.1 Oral Suspension (Table 3.12)

- Dose required: 10 mg/kg/day q24h × 3 days.
- How supplied: oral suspension comes in concentrations of 100 mg/5 mL, 200 mg/5 mL, 1 g powder packet.

Q. When should the 100 mg/5 mL suspension be prescribed?

A. The 100 mg/5 mL strength is prescribed for younger children weighing less than 44 lb (20 kg).

Table 3.12   Calculating the dose of azithromycin oral suspension in mL for a 10-year-old child weighing 70 lb and how the prescription should be written

Step 1 Convert pounds to kg:	70 lb × 1 kg/2.2 lb = 31.8 kg
Step 2 Calculate the dose in mg:	31.8 kg × 10 mg/kg/day = 318 mg/day
Step 3 Divide the dose by the frequency:	318 mg/day once a day = 318 mg/dose
Step 4 Convert the mg dose to mL:	318 mg/dose ÷ 200 mg/5 mL = 7.9 mL q24h

Rx: azithromycin oral suspension 200 mg/5 mL

Disp: 1 bottle (100 mL)

Sig: Take 7.9 mL orally once a day for 3 days for dental infection

Table 3.13   Calculating the dose of azithromycin tablets in mg for a 10-year-old child weighing 70 lb

Step 1 Convert pounds to kg:	70 lb × 1 kg/2.2 lb = 31.8 kg
Step 2 Calculate the dose in mg:	31.8 kg × 10 mg/kg/day = 318 mg/day
Step 3 Divide the dose by the frequency:	318 mg/day once a day = 318 mg/dose once a day

The strengths of tablets are 250, 500, or 600 mg. Since the dose is 318 mg once a day, it is probably more precise to prescribe the oral suspension.

Table 3.14   Calculating the dose of clindamycin oral solution in mL for a 10-year-old child weighing 70 lb and how the prescription should be written

Step 1 Convert pounds to kg:	70 lb × 1 kg/2.2 lb = 31.8 kg
Step 2 Calculate the dose in mg:	31.8 kg × 10 mg/kg/day = 318 mg/day
Step 3 Divide the dose by the frequency:	318 mg/day ÷ 3 (tid) = 106 mg/dose q8h
Step 4 Convert the mg dose to mL:	106 mg/dose ÷ 75 mg/5 mL = 7 mL tid
Step 5 Convert mL into teaspoonfuls[a]	7 mL ÷ 5 mL = 1.4 teaspoonful

Rx: Clindamycin oral solution 75 mg/5 mL

Disp: 1 bottle

Sig: Take 1.4 teaspoonful orally three times a day for 7 days for dental infection

[a] Each teaspoonful is 5 mL.

3.2.4.2   Azithromycin Tablets (Table 3.13)
- Dose required: 10 mg/kg/day q24h × 3 days.
- How supplied: 250 mg, 500 mg, 600 mg tablets.

3.2.5   Clindamycin

3.2.5.1   Clindamycin Oral Solution (Table 3.14)
- Dosage required: 10–30 mg/kg/day q6–8 h.
- How supplied: oral solution 75 mg/5 mL (100 mL bottle).

3.2.5.2   Clindamycin Capsules (Table 3.15)
- Dosage required: 10–30 mg/kg/day q6–8 h.
- How supplied: 75, 150, 300 mg capsules.

Table 3.15 Calculating the dose of clindamycin capsules in mg for a 10-year-old child weighing 70 lb

Step 1 Convert pounds to kg:	$70\,lb \times 1\,kg/2.2\,lb = 31.8\,kg$
Step 2 Calculate the dose in mg:	$31.8\,kg \times 10\,mg/kg/day = 318\,mg/day$
Step 3 Divide the dose by the frequency:	$318\,mg/day \div 4\,(qid) = 80\,mg/dose\,q6h$

The dose is 80 mg; either 75 mg capsules can be prescribed and increase the number of days of therapy, or it may be best to use the oral suspension.

3.3 Pregnant and Nursing Patients

Q. Why may dosage adjustment be required in the pregnant patient?

A. Pregnancy and the first weeks of life represent two physiological situations in which there are continuous and significant changes in the levels of plasma proteins, and it may therefore be necessary to adjust the doses of medication during these times (Moore 1998).

Q. Why is it important to be aware of the effect of drugs in the nursing mother?

A. Nearly all drugs pass into human milk by passive diffusion. Almost all medication appears in very small amounts, usually less than 1% of the maternal dose. The higher the dosage, the more the drug transfers into milk. Different features of drugs including molecular weight, fat solubility, and half-life will affect how much of the drug is transferred into the milk. The pH of milk is 7, which is slightly lower than plasma (pH 7.4) so that drugs that are weak bases (e.g., erythromycins, tetracyclines) will achieve high concentrations in breast milk and should be avoided.

Q. What are the "new" FDA pregnancy categories?

A. Approximately 30 years ago, the FDA required that all prescription drugs absorbed systemically or known to be potentially harmful to the fetus be given a pregnancy category of A, B, C, D or X. Table 3.16 lists all categories (Lynch et al. 1991). In 2014, the FDA replaced the letter categories with new labeling that is more explanatory to patients and clinicians and enables more effective patient counseling. This classification was revised in 2015. The new Pregnancy and Lactation Labeling Final Rule (PLLR) started on June 30, 2015 and can be found on the package insert of the medication. The PLLR consists of narrative sections and subsections which include the following (www.drugs.com/pregnancy-categories.html).

Table 3.16 FDA pregnancy categories

Drug category	Description
A	Controlled studies in women fail to show a risk to the fetus
B	Animal or human studies have not shown a significant risk to the fetus. No controlled studies in pregnant women. Drugs have been found to have adverse effects in animals but no well-controlled studies of humans
C	Drugs for which there are no adequate studies, either animal or humans, or drugs shown to have adverse fetal effects in animals but for which no human data are available
D	Fetal risk in humans is evident
X	Studies in animals or humans have shown definitive fetal risk. These drugs are contraindicated in women who are or may become pregnant

Pregnancy (includes labor and delivery)

- Pregnancy Exposure Registry
- Risk Summary
- Clinical Considerations
- Data

Lactation (includes nursing mothers)

- Risk Summary
- Clinical Considerations
- Data

Females and males of reproductive potential

- Pregnancy Testing
- Contraception
- Infertility

Q. What drugs used in dentistry are safe during pregnancy and breast feeding?

A. The "new" pregnancy label is not without debate (Walker 2018). *Since we cannot print all the statements of the drugs dentists use, the original letter categories will be used.* See Table 3.17 (Turner et al. 2006).

Table 3.17 List of dental drugs commonly used during pregnancy and nursing

Drug	FDA category	Can use during pregnancy?	Can use during nursing?
Antibiotics			
Amoxicillin	B	Yes	Yes
Penicillin VK	B	Yes	Yes
Erythromycin base or ethylsuccinate	B	Yes (except for estolate form)	Yes
Clarithromycin	C	No	No data available. Manufacturer cautions against its use in nursing mothers
Azithromycin	B	Yes; no human studies; give when benefits outweigh risk	Not enough information. Manufacturer advises caution
Ciprofloxacin	C	No	Discontinue breast feeding or do not use ciprofloxacin
Clindamycin	B	Yes; when benefit outweighs risk	Excreted in mother's milk. Discontinue nursing or choose another antibiotic
Metronidazole	B	Yes but not in first trimester	Discontinue breast feeding for 12–24 hours. Best to prescribe another antibiotic
Tetracyclines	D	No	No

(Continued)

Table 3.17 (Continued)

Drug	FDA category	Can use during pregnancy?	Can use during nursing?
Analgesics			
Acetaminophen	B	Yes	Yes
Aspirin	C/D (risk for use during third trimester)	No. Aspirin use in pregnancy has been associated with alterations in both maternal and fetal hemostasis	No
Ibuprofen (and all NSAIDs including Naprosyn® and naproxen)	B/D (D in third trimester; do not recommend during third trimester)	After first trimester for 24–72 hours only. Best to avoid in third trimester due to effects on fetal cardiovascular system (closure of ductus arteriosus)	No data available. Effects on nursing baby are not known
Codeine (e.g., acetaminophen with codeine)	C/D (in third trimester)	Only give if benefit outweighs risks. Codeine is the only narcotic analgesic which has shown a statistically significant association with teratogenicity (involving respiratory tract malformations; depression)	Codeine is metabolized to morphine, which can result in morphine overdose in the baby, especially if mothers are ultra-rapid metabolizers of codeine. Signs of morphine overdose in a nursing baby include limpness, increased sleepiness, and difficulty breathing
Hydrocodone (e.g., Vicodin®)	C/D (in third trimester)	Neonatal respiratory depression	Hydrocodone is metabolized to codeine isomer and a small percent to hydromorphone. Signs of morphine overdose in a nursing baby include limpness, increased sleepiness, and difficulty breathing
Antifungal agents			
Nystatin	B	Yes	Yes
Clotrimazole (topical)	B	Yes	Yes
Local anesthetics			
Lidocaine	B	Yes	Yes
Mepivacaine	C	No	Caution
Bupivacaine	C	No	Yes
Etidocaine	B	Yes	Yes
Prilocaine	B	Yes	Yes
Articaine	C	No	Caution
Marcaine	C	No	Caution
Anesthesia			
Nitrous oxide	Not classified	Not in first trimester; with caution in third trimester	Controversial; consult with patient's prenatal care provider
Antianxiety drugs			
Benzodiazepines (e.g., diazepam, alprazolam)	D	No	No
Triazolam and temazepam	X	No	No

Source: Adapted from New York State Department of Health (2006). Oral Health Care during Pregnancy and Early Childhood. Practice Guidelines. Moore (1998). www.drugs.com/pregnancy

Q. Why are there concerns about the use of antibiotics during pregnancy?

A. Some antibiotics have adverse effects on the developing fetus. Choosing the appropriate antibiotic requires consideration of the effects on both the mother and the fetus. The first trimester starts at conception and continues throughout the 11th week. During this period there is an increase in blood volume and hepatic and renal blood flow, which can alter the serum antibiotic concentrations. Thus, the safety of many antibiotics varies with the period of gestation and the maturity of the fetus. The embryo is most vulnerable to a teratogenic agent between days 18 and 60 (Moore 1998; Lynch et al. 1991; Lomaestro 2009).

Q. What antibiotics are the safest for pregnant patients?

A. First of all, it is best to avoid antibiotics during pregnancy. However, if an antibiotic must be prescribed, a narrow-spectrum drug is the safest (Kuperman and Koren 2016). Penicillin V (and amoxicillin) is thought to be safe to prescribe during pregnancy. If the patient is allergic to penicillin, erythromycin (except estolate form), metronidazole or clindamycin can be prescribed and these have been reported to have minimal risk. Tetracyclines including tetracycline HCl, doxycycline hyclate and minocycline HCl are category D and should never be used (Moore 1998). Also, clarithromycin is a category C, but azithromycin is a category B drug.

Q. Are dosage adjustments required when prescribing a "safe" antibiotic or analgesic for the pregnant patient?

A. No. It is not necessary to reduce the dose of an antibiotic prescribed to a pregnant patient.

Q. Is aspirin safe in pregnant patients?

A. Aspirin should be avoided especially late in pregnancy due to delivery complications and postpartum bleeding in the mother.

Q. Is ibuprofen safe in pregnant patients?

A. For much the same reason as aspirin, nonsteroidal antiinflammatory drugs (NSAIDs) may prolong pregnancy and should be avoided, especially in late pregnancy or after the first trimester, and can be used for 24–72 hours only.

Q. Which is the safest analgesic recommended for pregnant patients?

A. Acetaminophen alone is safe for the pregnant patient and nursing mother and is the analgesic drug of choice.

Q. Is epinephrine safe to administer in pregnant patients?

A. Yes. Epinephrine (also known as adrenaline) is a natural hormone and neurotransmitter produced by the adrenal medulla (part of the adrenal gland). It is generally considered to have no teratogenic effects when administered in dental anesthetics. It must be emphasized that since epinephrine stimulates cardiac function, when administering, careful technique (e.g., aspirate to avoid intravascular injection) and proper dosing are required (Fayans et al. 2010).

Q. Can acetaminophen and codeine combination be prescribed safely to a nursing patient?

A. On 17 August 2007, the FDA warned breastfeeding mothers who take codeine, either in combination with another analgesic or in any form of cough syrup, that babies are at increased risk for morphine overdose. Newborn babies are especially sensitive to the effects of the smallest dosages of narcotics. Codeine is metabolized to morphine and in women who are "ultra-rapid" metabolizers of codeine, adverse effects of morphine can be seen very quickly. Being an ultra-rapid metabolizer of codeine is due to a mutation in the gene coding for cytochrome P450 enzyme (CYP2D6) in the liver. It is relatively uncommon but does occur (www.fda.gov/drugs/postmarket-drug-safety-information-patients-and-providers/use-codeine-and-tramadol-products-breastfeeding-women-questions-and-answers).

3.4 Elderly Patients

Q. Are dosage adjustments necessary in the elderly patient?

A. Yes. Volume of drug distribution, drug clearance (renal function), protein binding, and metabolism are altered in the elderly, necessitating a reduction in drug dosage. If necessary, contact the patient's physician. Additionally, there is a difference in body composition (decreased muscle mass) and function. The elderly may also have increased sensitivity to drugs because the liver metabolizes and kidneys excrete the drug less efficiently.

Q. Is kidney function reduced in the elderly?

A. Yes. Renal function progressively declines as one ages even though there could be normal serum creatinine values. Since many drugs are excreted through the kidneys, a reduction in drug dosage is necessary.

Q. Is liver function reduced in the elderly?

A. Yes. There may be a significant reduction in hepatic function, and it is important to reduce the dose of drugs metabolized by the liver.

3.5 Patients with Renal Impairment

Q. What are the different types of chronic kidney disease?

A. Renal insufficiency, which is seen in the early phase, renal failure, which occurs when the kidneys cannot function in excretion, and end-stage renal disease (ESRD) with the nephrons losing function and uremia, which leads to malnutrition, altered drug metabolism, electrolyte imbalance, bleeding, anemia, and death.

Q. Does renal disease alter the response to drugs?

A. Yes. The use of drugs in patients with reduced kidney function (e.g., patients on dialysis) may produce toxicity because of impaired elimination from the body. Whether the dose must be reduced depends on if the drug is eliminated entirely by renal excretion or is partly metabolized. Because the kidney is the major regulator of the internal fluid environment, the physiological changes associated with renal disease have pronounced effects on the pharmacology of many drugs.

Either the dose does not have to be altered or the dosing interval is increased, or the dose is reduced while maintaining the same dosing interval (this is called dose reduction and is the preferred method because it maintains more constant plasma concentrations).

Q. What happens to the half-life of the drug in kidney disease?

A. As the plasma half-life of drugs excreted by the kidney is prolonged in renal failure, it may take many days for the reduced dosage to achieve a therapeutic plasma concentration. Therefore, the loading dose should usually be the same size as the initial dose for a patient with normal renal function, but the maintenance dose should be reduced. Consult with the patient's physician.

Q. What blood values must be known before prescribing for a patient with renal impairment?

A. Dose recommendations are based on the severity of renal impairment which is expressed in terms of glomerular filtration rate (GFR), measured by the creatinine clearance (CrCl). CrCl, which is measured as mL/min, indicates the function of the kidneys with regard to removing creatinine, a waste product, from the blood into the urine. Both blood and urine are required to determine CrCl. CrCl is not recommended for routine evaluation of kidney function. Normal CrCl is 80–120 mL/minute.

Glomerular filtration rate indicates how efficiently the kidneys are filtering wastes from the blood. GFR is used to determine the severity of kidney disease. Chronic kidney disease is defined as GFR <60 mL/min/1.73 m^2 or GFR ≥60 mL/min/1.73 m^2 together with kidney damage for more than three months. Serum creatinine levels are used to measure GFR (Brockmann 2010; Hassan et al. 2009).

Q. When should antibiotics be given to a patient undergoing dialysis?

A. Antibiotics should be administered after dialysis to allow for therapeutic concentrations to be maintained.

Q. What is the severity scale for renal disease?

A. Currently, according to the National Kidney Foundation, there is no uniform classification of the stages of chronic kidney disease (Table 3.18). A review of textbooks and journal articles clearly demonstrates ambiguity and overlap in the meaning of current terms.

Q. Can penicillin V be prescribed to patients with renal impairment?

A. Penicillin V is rapidly excreted through the kidneys in the urine. There is a delay in excretion in patients with impaired renal function. When GFR is <10 mL/min/1.73 m^2 then the dose of penicillin V should be reduced to 250 mg every six hours.

Q. Which antibiotics *do not* require a change in dosing adjustment in chronic kidney disease?

A. Azithromycin, clindamycin, doxycycline (www.remedirx.com/wp-content/uploads/2016/01/2016-01-M.R.-Antibiotic-Renal-Dosing.pdf)

Q. Why is it important to know about bleeding problems in renal disease patients?

A. There may be a prolonged bleeding time (altered platelet aggregation) due to uremia (syndrome associated with fluid, electrolyte, and hormone imbalances and metabolic abnormalities). The platelet and hematocrit levels should be known especially if bleeding during dental treatment is anticipated. Thus, a consultation with the patient's nephrologist is required before any type of dental surgery.

Q. If a patient with a kidney transplant requires antibiotic prophylaxis, which antibiotic is recommended?

A. For antibiotic prophylaxis, no dosing adjustments are required for azithromycin or clindamycin. Amoxicillin requires dosage adjustments. If the patient is taking cyclosporine after the kidney transplant, then clarithromycin and erythromycin should not be prescribed due to the risk of cyclosporine toxicity.

Q. Should fluoride topical products such as PreviDent® be prescribed to a patient with renal disease?

A. No. PreviDent contains 1.1% sodium fluoride, which is indicated for the prevention of tooth decay, reducing dentinal hypersensitivity and remineralization. Topical fluoride should never be swallowed; it is toxic. Topical fluorides should not be prescribed to a patient with kidney disease because fluoride is highly excreted by the kidneys so the risk of toxicity is greater in patients with impaired kidney function.

Q. What are the treatments for renal disease?

A. Treatments for renal disease include monitoring with diet control, hemodialysis or kidney transplant. Most patients undergo hemodialysis rather than peritoneal dialysis.

Q. How often does a patient usually have hemodialysis?

A. Every 2–3 days for 3–5 hours.

Q. How soon after a patient undergoes hemodialysis should they have dental procedures?

A. A consultation with the patient's nephrologist is necessary. Because of the increased risk of bleeding, it is best to see the patient on days when they are not undergoing dialysis. Heparin, an anticoagulant, is injected into the patient before dialysis to facilitate blood cycling through the dialyzer. If heparin has a half-life of four hours, then it takes about five half-lives to be completely eliminated from the body, about 20 hours. It is best to treat the patient one day after hemodialysis.

Q. Is antibiotic prophylaxis required for a patient having hemodialysis?

A. It is suggested to have a consultation with the nephrologist regarding this because there are many medical conditions that may require antibiotic prophylaxis. During hemodialysis, a surgically produced arteriovenous fistula is made, which may be susceptible to infection.

Q. How do I prescribe medications for a patient with kidney disease?

A. Inappropriate dosing in patients with chronic kidney disease can cause toxicity or ineffective therapy. Dosages of drugs cleared renally are based on renal function (calculated as GFR or CrCl). Dosing guidelines are divided into three broad GFR categories:

- $<10\,mL/min/1.73\,m^2$
- $10–50\,mL/min/1.73\,m^2$
- $50\,mL/min/1.73\,m^2$

It is advisable to contact the patient's physician and a pharmacist when prescribing medications. The type and severity of renal impairment must be determined. It is most important to obtain a copy of the patient's blood test to determine the GFR, which is the most reliable value for overall kidney function.

Q. Can local anesthetics be administered to patients with chronic kidney disease?

A. All amide local anesthetics including lidocaine and all other injectable anesthetics are metabolized by the liver. No adjustments are needed.

Q. Are most antibiotics safe to prescribe in renal disease?

A. See Table 3.18. Many antibiotics can induce renal dysfunction. Acute tubular necrosis (ATN) and interstitial nephritis are the most common types of acute renal failure associated with

Table 3.18 Severity scale for renal disease

Grade (severity)	Glomerular filtration rate (GFR)	Creatinine clearance (CrCl)
Mild	$20\text{–}50\,\text{mL/min/}1.73\,\text{m}^2$	$1.7\text{–}3.4\,\text{mg/dL}$
Moderate	$10\text{–}20\,\text{mL/min/}1.73\,\text{m}^2$	$3.4\text{–}7.9\,\text{mg/dL}$
Severe	$<10\,\text{mL/min/}1.73\,\text{m}^2$	$>7.9\,\text{mg/dL}$
Stage	**Severity**	**GFR**
Stage 1	Normal or increased GFR	$\geq 90\,\text{mL/min/}1.73\,\text{m}^2$
Stage 2	Mild	$60\text{–}89\,\text{mL/min/}1.73\,\text{m}^2$
Stage 3	Moderate	$30\text{–}59\,\text{mL/min/}1.73\,\text{m}^2$
Stage 4	Severe	$15\text{–}29\,\text{mL/min/}1.73\,\text{m}^2$
Stage 5	Kidney failure	$<15\,\text{mL/min/}1.73\,\text{m}^2$

Source: Adapted from National Kidney Foundation (https://renal.org/information-resources/the-uk-eckd-guide/ckd-stages).

antibiotic use. Acute interstitial nephritis may occur within minutes of drug exposure or may not develop for several months. Preexisting renal disease, dose, duration, and prior exposure to the offending antibiotic may increase the susceptibility of patients to acute interstitial nephritis. Some antibiotics that can cause this adverse effect include penicillin, amoxicillin, and fluoroquinolones. Tetracycline is contraindicated in patients with renal disease and may cause renal failure because it is 50–60% eliminated through the kidneys (Miller and McGarity 2009). Azithromycin, clindamycin, and doxycycline do not require a dosage or interval change and are safe to use. Doxycycline is only 20–30% eliminated through the kidneys, so no dosage adjustment is needed.

3.6 Patients with Hepatic Impairment

Q. Why is it important to consult a physician for a patient with chronic liver disease?

A. Liver disease can increase the risk of bleeding, especially in patients taking warfarin and low molecular weight heparins (LMWHs). It is important to get the results of the patient's liver function tests, which is an overview of how the liver is functioning. Albumin, bilirubin, and prothrombin time (PT) measure the function of the liver and the capacity to make enzymes. These enzymes include alkaline phosphatase (AP), aspartate aminotransferase (AST), and alanine aminotransferase (ALT), which indicate if there has been any damage to the liver cells but not the function of the liver. Elevated levels of enzymes indicate liver damage. A prolonged PT indicates a deficiency in one of the clotting factors.

A complete blood count (CBC) including platelets is important because in liver disease there is usually bleeding with a decrease in platelet count (thrombocytopenia). Additionally, many drugs are metabolized by the liver so if the patient has a compromised liver, some antibiotics and analgesics may need to have dosage adjustment or another drug must be prescribed.

Q. What is the mechanism of increased bleeding?

A. The liver produces clotting factors II, V, VII, IX, and X. Vitamin K is the cofactor required to synthesize these clotting factors. Severe liver disease leads to lower levels of vitamin K, resulting in less production of clotting factors. Bleeding will happen with an international normalized ratio (INR)>1.5. However, the prothrombin time (or INR) is considered to be abnormal when about 80% of liver function is lost, which is considered to be severe liver disease. Often, the patient will have gingival bleeding and bruises. Partial prothrombin time (PTT) is a test that determines how long it takes for the blood to clot and is measured in seconds.

Levels of albumin, a water-soluble, coagulable protein, may decrease, which will lead to a decrease in clotting ability.

Q. Does liver disease alter the response to drugs?

A. Yes. Liver disease, including hepatitis and cirrhosis, may alter the response to drugs. Drugs that are primarily cleared by the liver *may* require dosage adjustment in patients with hepatic impairment. However, before changes in drug metabolism occur, liver disease must progress to the level of "severe." Consultation with the patient's physician is necessary before drug prescribing.

Q. How can the dentist determine if dosage adjustment is necessary?

A. Unlike in renal disease, in which CrCl and GFR can be used as reliable indicators for adjustments in drug dosage, it is more difficult to determine indicators of liver function. The liver enzymes such as AST, ALT, gamma-glutamyl transferase (GGT) and AP only indicate if there is liver cell damage but does not relate to the ability of the liver to metabolize drugs. Either the dosage must be decreased or the dosing interval increased. Consult with the patient's physician for any dosage adjustments.

Q. Why do certain drugs require dosage adjustments in patients with liver insufficiency?

A. See Table 3.19. All drugs have to be eliminated from the body. Either the drug is metabolized into a water-soluble metabolite in the liver or it is eliminated unchanged (not metabolized). Most drugs are metabolized and excreted primarily by the kidneys in the urine. Other drugs that are not metabolized go through the liver unchanged and are excreted in the bile (fluid secreted by the liver and stored in the gallbladder). From there, the bile with the drug enters the gastrointestinal tract and then is either eliminated in feces or reabsorbed back to the liver by *enterohepatic recirculation* (or enterohepatic cycling) and eventually metabolized by the liver and excreted via the kidneys in the urine. Some drugs can also change into metabolites in the liver and are then excreted in the bile; these are eliminated in the feces and reabsorbed back into the blood. For example, tetracycline is not metabolized (unchanged) and undergoes enterohepatic recirculation being excreted in both the urine and bile and recovered in the feces. Doxycycline is also not metabolized in the liver but is partially deactivated in the intestines and primarily recovered in the feces.

If the liver is not functioning normally, the dosage of a drug that is eliminated primarily in the liver may need to be adjusted. But as mentioned earlier, there is no way to determine liver function.

Q. What drugs used in dentistry must have their dosages altered in patients with renal and liver impairment?

A. See Table 3.19.

Table 3.19 Drug dosages in renal and liver impairment

Drug	GFR >50 mL/min/1.73 m²	GFR 10–50 mL/min/1.73 m²	GFR <10 mL/min/1.73 m²	Liver impairment
Acetaminophen (Tylenol®)	No change (interval is q4–6h)	Every 6 hours	Every 8 hours	Limited, low-dose therapy is tolerated in hepatic cirrhosis. Maximum dose should be <2 g/day
Amoxicillin	No change (250–500 mg q8h interval)	Every 12 hours	Every 24 hours	Safe to use with usual dosage
Amoxicillin/clavulanate (Augmentin®)	No change (500 mg q12h or 250 mg q8h)	Every 12 hours	Every 24 hours	If history of amoxicillin/clavulanate-associated hepatic damage, then it is contraindicated
Aspirin	No change	No adjustment	Avoid	Avoid due to increased risk of bleeding
Azithromycin (Zithromax)	No change (500 mg once, then 250 mg qd × 4 days)	No adjustment	No adjustment	Avoid
Clarithromycin (Biaxin)	No change (250–500 mg q12h)	500 mg once, then 250 mg every 24 hours	Increase interval to every 24 hours or reduce dose by 50%	No adjustment
Clindamycin (Cleocin®)	No change (150–450 mg tid)	No adjustment	No adjustment	No adjustment with hepatitis; decrease dose by 50% in cirrhosis
Codeine (with acetaminophen)	No change (60 mg (no. 3) q4–6h)	Administer 50% of dose with same interval (15–30 mg)	Administer 75% of dose with same interval (7.5–15 mg)	Not recommended in severe liver disease because codeine will not be converted to morphine, resulting in inadequate analgesia
Diflunisal (Dolobid®)	No change (500–1000 mg followed by 250–500 mg q8–12h; maximum daily dose 1.5 g)	Best to avoid or decrease dose 50%	Best to avoid or decrease dose 50%	Avoid

(*Continued*)

Table 3.19 (Continued)

Drug	GFR >50 mL/min/1.73 m²	GFR 10–50 mL/min/1.73 m²	GFR <10 mL/min/1.73 m²	Liver impairment
Doxycycline	No change (100 mg q12h on day 1, then 100 mg qd)	No adjustment	No adjustment	Administered cautiously in patients with preexisting liver disease or biliary obstruction. Reduced dosages may be appropriate, since doxycycline undergoes enterohepatic recycling. Best to give alternative antibiotic
Erythromycin	No change (base: 250–500 mg q6h) (erythromycin ethylsuccinate 400 mg)	No adjustment	No adjustment	Avoid with the estolate – may cause hepatotoxicity
Hydrocodone and acetaminophen (Vicodin, Lorcet®, Lortab®)	One to two tabs q4–6h	Start conservatively and titrate dosage carefully to desired effect	Start conservatively and titrate dosage carefully to desired effect	Consider decreasing dose and use for 2–3 days, or avoid
Ibuprofen (Advil, Motrin®, Nuprin®)	No change (OTC: 200 mg q4–6h; max 1200 mg/24h)	Best to avoid, or reduce dose in significantly impaired renal function; caution advised	Best to avoid, or reduce dose in significantly impaired renal function; caution advised	Avoid in severe hepatic disease (hepatitis and cirrhosis)
Metronidazole (Flagyl®)	No change (500 mg q6–8h interval)	No adjustment	Every 12–24 hours	Reduce dose in severe liver disease because drug can accumulate. No dose adjustment needed with mild liver disease
Naproxen (Naprosyn) Naproxen sodium (Aleve)	Naprosyn: 250–500 mg bid Aleve: 220 mg q8h	Not recommended	Not recommended	Not recommended
Penicillin V	No change (250–500 mg q6h)	No adjustment	No adjustment	Safe to use usual dosage
Tetracycline	No change (250–500 mg q6h)	Best to avoid and use doxycycline instead	Best to avoid and use doxycycline instead	Avoid

Source: Adapted from Brockmann and Badr (2010), Gelot and Nakhla (2014), Munar and Singh (2007).

Q. Can penicillin be prescribed to patients with liver disease?

A. Yes.

Q. Are local anesthetics metabolized in the liver?

A. Yes. Lidocaine, mepivacaine, bupivacaine, and prilocaine are metabolized in the liver. These agents are still well tolerated by patients with mild to moderate liver disease but in severe disease, changes may be necessary. According to Little et al. (2008), three cartridges of 2% lidocaine is considered to be adequate for these patients. Consultation with the patient's physician is recommended (Pamplona et al. 2011).

Q. Which antibiotics are safe to give to patients with liver disease?

A. See Table 3.19. Penicillin V, amoxicillin, clarithromycin (Biaxin), clindamycin (OK in hepatitis but decrease dose by half in cirrhosis).

Q. Which analgesic is safe to give to patients with liver disease?

A. Acetaminophen is considered to be safe and effective overall and is the recommended analgesic for individuals with liver disease. However, avoid chronic use and only use low-dose therapy for the shortest duration possible. The maximum daily dose is <2 g (Hayward et al. 2015; Hughes et al. 2011). As mentioned earlier, the FDA has recommended that all manufacturers of combination narcotic/acetaminophen use only 325 mg of acetaminophen per dosage formulation. It can be toxic to the liver when taken in excessive doses or with alcohol. It is an absolute contraindication in alcoholic cirrhosis. It has been reported that acetaminophen is safe in patients with stable chronic alcoholic liver disease for at least a short period of time (maximum 48–72 hours) up to the maximum recommended dose (Worrlax and Flake 2007). *Therefore, it is important to not exceed recommended dosages.* It may be prudent to consult with the patient's physician before prescribing any analgesics. If a narcotic is needed, any combination narcotic with acetaminophen is safe as long as the maximum recommended dose is not exceeded. Also, hydrocodone + ibuprofen (Vicoprofen®) can be prescribed if the dentist or patient does not want to use acetaminophen.

Since the liver is the primary site for opioid metabolism, in patients with liver disease there is a risk of opioid accumulation. Codeine should be avoided because it is a prodrug which normally undergoes transformation in the liver to morphine, its active metabolite. In cases of liver damage, codeine cannot be transformed, resulting in inadequate pain relief. For moderate to severe pain, hydrocodone is recommended but with low dosage and only 2–3 days of use. Decrease dose by 50% of usual dose; prescribe one tab q6h or q8h (Gelot and Nakhla 2014).

NSAIDs should be avoided in patients with cirrhosis because of the risk of acute renal failure as a result of prostaglandin inhibition (Imani et al. 2014). Opioids should be avoided or used at the lowest dose for the least amount of time (Imani et al. 2014)

3.7 Patients with History of Bariatric Surgery

Q. If a patient has undergone bariatric (weight reduction) surgery, does drug dosing need to be adjusted?

A. Yes. Altered drug absorption may occur after the Roux-en-Y gastric bypass surgical weight reduction procedure, which is a restrictive–malabsorptive procedure (the most commonly performed surgical procedure in obese people). This can be a concern post surgery because there is less surface area of the small intestine for drug absorption. For this reason, many patients may develop nutritional deficiencies especially in fat-soluble vitamins E and D and also iron and vitamin B12. Drugs with long absorptive phases that remain in the intestine for extended periods are likely to exhibit decreased bioavailability in these patients (Miller and Smith 2006; Padwal et al. 2010). If you are concerned about altered drug absorption, it is recommended to use a drug that releases its active ingredient over an extended time (Seaman et al. 2005). Also, since individual dose adjustments may be needed, it is recommended to consult the patient's physician. These drugs include the following formulations: extended release (ER), sustained release (SR), delayed release or long-acting (LA). Antibiotics supplied as delayed release include the following.

- Doxycycline delayed-release
  - Supplied: 75 mg, 100 mg cap, tab.
  - Adults: 100 mg every 12 hours followed by a maintenance dose of 100 mg/day. The maintenance dose may be administered as a single dose or as 50 mg every 12 hours.
  - Children: the recommended dosage for children weighing 4.5 kg (100 lb) or less is 2 mg/0.5 kg body weight divided into two doses on the first day of treatment, followed by 1 mg/0.5 kg body weight given as a single daily dose or divided into two doses on subsequent days. For more severe infections, up to 2 mg/0.5 kg body weight may be used. For children over 4.5 kg (100 lb), the usual adult dose should be used (www.rxlist.com/doryx-drug.htm).
  - Taken without regard to meals.
  - Take with full glass of water.
  - Do not take concurrently with antacids.
  - If the capsule cannot be swallowed whole, it may be opened and the contents sprinkled over a spoonful of applesauce.
- ERYC® (erythromycin) delayed-release capsules
  - Supplied: 250 mg cap.
  - Adults: the usual dose is 250 mg every six hours taken one hour before meals. If twice-a-day dosage is desired, the recommended dose is 500 mg every 12 hours. Dosage may be increased up to 4 g/day, according to the severity of the infection.
  - Children: the usual dosage is 30–50 mg/kg/day in divided doses.

Additionally, it is best to use tablets that are enteric coated to protect the small stomach. It must be kept in mind that tablets must break down or disintegrate and capsules must open up before they can be absorbed. Tablets can be crushed if desired or a chewable tablet prescribed. A solution/suspension is already in an easily absorbable liquid form.

When prescribing for dental indications, the following antibiotics and analgesics can be prescribed in a liquid or suspension formulation (remember to confirm if there are any precautions or contraindications for any of the following drugs before prescribing).

1) Antibiotics available in liquid formulation for adult dosing are given in Table 3.20.
2) Analgesics available in liquid form are given in Table 3.21.

Q. Are there any over-the-counter analgesic liquid formulations?
A. Yes, acetaminophen and ibuprofen.

Table 3.20 Antibiotics available in liquid formulation for adult dosing

Rx amoxicillin suspension (250 mg/5 mL)

Disp: 100 mL bottle

Sig: Take 4 teaspoonfuls po stat, followed by 2 teaspoonfuls q8h

Note: amoxicillin is also available as extended-release tablets and chewable tablets which can be given to this patient.

Rx amoxicillin/clavulanic acid (Augmentin) 250/62.5/5 mL

Disp: 100 mL bottle

Sig: Take 4 teaspoonfuls po stat, followed by 2 teaspoonfuls q8h

Rx penicillin V 250 mg/5 mL

Disp: 100 mL bottle

Sig: Take 4 teaspoonfuls po stat, followed by 2 teaspoonfuls q6h

Rx clindamycin oral solution 75 mg/5 mL

Disp: 100 mL bottle

Sig: Take 2–4 teaspoonfuls po q8h

Rx azithromycin oral suspension

Disp: one single dose packet[a]

Sig: Empty the entire contents of the packet into a glass of water (2 oz) and mix. After swallowing, add another 2 oz of water to the glass and mix and drink. This suspension should be consumed immediately.

[a] One packet contains 1 g or 1000 mg of azithromycin.

Table 3.21 Analgesics available in liquid form

Rx acetaminophen/codeine suspension (Schedule V) (120 mg acetaminophen +12 mg codeine/5 mL)

Disp: 8 fl. oz

Sig: Take one tablespoonful (15 mL) q4h as needed

Rx acetaminophen/hydrocodone oral solution (Lortab Elixir®) (hydrocodone bitartrate 7.5 mg and acetaminophen 500 mg/15 mL) (Schedule II)

Disp: 8 fl. oz (Note: do not write for 1 bottle because it is supplied as 1 pint)

Sig: Take one tablespoonful q4–6h as needed for pain

(The total daily dosage for adults should not exceed 6 tablespoonfuls)

Source: Miller and Smith (2006).

Q. Are there problems with drug absorption in patients who have had other types of bariatric surgery such as vertical-banded (stapled) gastroplasty and adjustable gastric banding?

A. Vertical-banded (stapled) gastroplasty and adjustable gastric banding are types of bariatric surgery that allow for weight loss by reducing stomach volume (restrictive procedures) and cause malabsorption, as does the Roux-en-Y gastric bypass. In restrictive procedures, the smaller volume of the stomach can prevent adequate disintegration of the dosage formulation (tablet/capsule) needed for drug bioavailability. The suggestions for the patient with a Roux-en-Y gastric bypass also apply for the restrictive surgical procedure (Weinberg and Segelnick 2009).

References

Brockmann, W. and Badr, M. (2010). Chronic kidney disease. Pharmacological considerations for the dentist. *Journal of the American Dental Association* 141: 1330–1339.

Fayans, E.P., Stuart, H.R., Carsten, D. et al. (2010). Local anesthetic use in the pregnant and postpartum patient. *Dental Clinics of North America* 54: 697–713.

Gelot, S. and Nakhla, E. (2014). Opioid dosing in renal and hepatic impairment. *US Pharmacist* 3 (8): 34–38.

Hassan, Y., Al Ramahi, R.J., Abd Aziz, N. et al. (2009). Drug use and dosing in chronic kidney disease. *Annals of the Academy of Medicine Singapore* 38: 1095–1103.

Hayward, K.L., Powell, E.E., Irvine, K.M., and Martin, J.H. (2015). Can paracetamol (acetaminophen) be administered to patients with liver impairment? *British Journal of Clinical Pharmacology* 81 (2): 210–222.

Hughes, G.J., Patel, P., and Saxena, N. (2011). Effect of acetaminophen on international normalized ratio: clinician awareness and patient education. *Pharmacotherapy* 31 (6): 591–597.

Imani, F., Motavaf, M., Safari, S., and Alavian, S.M. (2014). The therapeutic use of analgesics in patients with liver cirrhosis: a literature review and evidence-based recommendations. *Hepatitis Monthly* 14 (10): e23539.

Kuperman, A.A. and Koren, O. (2016). Antibiotic use during pregnancy: how bad is it? *BMC Medicine* 14 (1): 91.

Little, J.W., Falace, D.A., Miller, C.S. et al. (2008). Liver disease. In: *Dental Management of the Medically Compromised Patient*, 7e (eds. J.W. Little, D.A. Falace, C.S. Miller, et al.), 140–161. St Louis, MO: Mosby Elsevier.

Lomaestro, B.M. (2009). Do antibiotics interact with combination oral contraceptives? www.medscape.com/viewarticle/707926.

Lynch, C., Sinnott, I.V.J., Holt, D.A. et al. (1991). Use of antibiotics during pregnancy. *American Family Physician* 43: 1365–1368.

Miller, C.S. and McGarity, G.J. (2009). Tetracycline-induced renal failure after dental treatment. *Journal of the American Dental Association* 140: 56–60.

Miller, A.D. and Smith, K.M. (2006). Medication and nutrient administration after bariatric surgery. *American Journal of Health-System Pharmacy* 63: 1852–1857.

Moore, P.A. (1998). Selecting drugs for the pregnant dental patient. *Journal of the American Dental Association* 129: 1281–1286.

Munar, M.Y. and Singh, H. (2007). Drug dosing adjustments in patients with chronic kidney disease. *American Family Physician* 75 (10): 1487–1496.

Munckoff, W. (2005). Antibiotics for surgical prophylaxis. *Australian Prescriber* 28: 38–40.

Padwal, R., Brocks, D., and Sharma, A.M. (2010). Systematic review of drug absorption following bariatric surgery and its theoretical implications. *Obesity Reviews* 11: 41–50.

Pamplona, M.C., Muñoz, M.M., and Pérez, M.G.S. (2011). Dental considerations in patients with liver disease. *Journal of Clinical and Experimental Dentistry* 3: e127–e134.

Paterson, I.K., Hoyle, A., Ochoa, G. et al. (2016). Optimising antibiotic usage to treat bacterial infections. *Scientific Reports* 6: article number 37853.

Seaman, J.S., Bowers, S.P., Dixon, P. et al. (2005). Dissolution of common psychiatric medications in a roux-en-Y gastric bypass model. *Psychosomatics* 46: 250–253.

Turner, M.D., Singh, F., and Glickman, R.S. (2006). Dental management of the gravid patient. *New York State Dental Journal* 72: 22–27.

Walker, M. (2018). Removal of FDA pregnancy drug categories: more harm than good? www.medpagetoday.com/meetingcoverage/acog/72592.

Weinberg, M.A. and Segelnick, S.L. (2009). Surgical procedures for weight loss. *US Pharmacist* 34 (12): HS-2–HS-10.

Worrlax, J.D. and Flake, D. (2007). Alcoholic liver disease: is acetaminophen safe? *Family Practice* 56: 673–674.

Additional Resources

www.fdalawblog.net/fda_law_blog_hyman_phelps/2009/05/fda-petition-response-reaffirms-fda-orange-book-dosage-form-nomenclature-policy.html

www.drugguide.com/ddo/ub/view/Davis-Drug-Guide/109514/0/Pediatric_Dosage_Calculations

USP DI (2005). *Drug Information for the Health Care Professional*, 25e, vol. 1. Greenwood Village, CO: Thomson Micromedex.

4

Dental Formularies

Drugs Prescribed in Dentistry

4.1 Antimicrobials, Systemic

4.1.1 General Considerations

Q. What is the difference between an antibiotic and chemotherapeutic agent?

A. An antibiotic is a substance that is of biological origin whereas a chemotherapeutic agent is a chemical made synthetically. The name "antimicrobial" agent is an inclusive term referring to either an antibiotic or chemotherapeutic agent.

Q. What factors are important in the choice of a suitable antibiotic for dental infections?

A. Before selecting an antibiotic for the treatment of an infection, the dentist must first consider two major factors: the patient and the susceptibility of the bacteria. Factors related to the patient that must be considered when selecting the appropriate antibiotic include:

- history of allergy to antibiotics
- renal and hepatic function
- host resistance to infection (e.g., whether a compromised host)
- ability to tolerate oral drugs
- severity of the infection
- age
- if female, whether pregnant, nursing or taking an oral contraceptive.

Q. For how long should an antibiotic be prescribed?

A. Duration of therapy depends on the nature of the infection and the response to treatment. Courses should not be unjustifiably prolonged because this is wasteful and may lead to adverse effects, including antibiotic resistance. If the patient has not clinically improved by the third day, then the drug should be stopped and another antibiotic started.

Q. What is the difference between bactericidal and bacteriostatic antibiotics?

A. First, an antibiotic must enter the bacterium in order to be effective. *Bactericidal* antibiotics kill the bacteria by inhibiting bacterial cell wall synthesis or interfering with bacterial DNA. Bacterial cells must be multiplying for a bactericidal antibiotic to be effective. A *bacteriostatic* antibiotic weakens, disables, and reversibly inhibits the growth and replication of bacteria, thereby giving the body's natural defense mechanisms time to overcome an infection. If an infection is quiet without multiplying and forming new protein, the bacteriostatic antibiotic

The Dentist's Drug and Prescription Guide, Second Edition. Mea A. Weinberg, Stuart J. Froum and Stuart L. Segelnick.
© 2020 John Wiley & Sons, Inc. Published 2020 by John Wiley & Sons, Inc.

will not work. There are no clinical data supporting the use of bacteriostatic versus bactericidal antibiotics (Nemeth et al. 2015).

Q. Does this difference affect the choice of appropriate antibiotic?
A. Yes. In the majority of cases, and particularly in patients whose natural resistance is lowered by disorders of the immune system (e.g., HIV/AIDS, diabetes), it is preferable to choose a bactericidal agent, resulting in a decrease in the number of bacteria, rather than simply preventing an increase with bacteriostatic agents. When a bacteriostatic antibiotic is used, the duration of therapy must be sufficient to allow cellular and humoral host defense mechanisms to eradicate the bacteria. Bactericidal drugs are effective during the log phase of bacterial growth. If growth is slowed or stopped, then bactericidal drugs will not have such an effect. As a result, combination therapy with a bactericidal and a bacteriostatic should not be used (Chambers 2003).

With bacteriostatic antibiotics, it is important to maintain minimum inhibitory concentrations (MICs) of the antibiotic during treatment.

Q. What are the MIC and minimum bactericidal concentration (MBC) and what is their importance in choosing an antibiotic?
A. MIC indicates the sensitivity of an antibiotic; it is the lowest concentration of an antibiotic that results in inhibition of visible bacterial growth on a plate or culture. The MBC is the lowest concentration of an antibiotic that kills 99.9% of the original inoculum (pool of bacteria). For an antibiotic to be effective, the MIC or MBC must be achieved at the site of the infection. The MIC and MBC are important in laboratories to verify the resistance of bacteria to an antimicrobial agent. In simple terms, the MIC is a basic laboratory measurement of the activity of an antimicrobial agent against a bacterium. The MIC is determined *in vitro* and uses a standardized inoculum of about 10^5 cells/mL. For example, an MIC_{50} of 16 indicates that a concentration of 16 μg/mL of antibiotic is required to inhibit 50% of the bacterial strains. A MIC_{90} of 128 indicates a concentration of 128 μg/mL is required to inhibit 90% of the bacterial strains.

Q. Can a bacteriostatic antibiotic become bactericidal?
A. Yes, by either increasing the dose of the bacteriostatic antibiotic past a certain point or combining it with another bacteriostatic antibiotic.

Q. Which antibiotics are bacteriostatic and which are bactericidal?
A. *Bacteriostatic*: tetracyclines, macrolides (erythromycin), azilides (azithromycin, clarithromycin), clindamycin.
Bactericidal: penicillins, cephalosporins, quinolones, metronidazole.

Q. What is the difference between a narrow-spectrum and a broad-spectrum antibiotic?
A. Narrow-spectrum antibiotics are effective against only a limited range or organisms, such as Gram-negative or Gram-positive bacteria. Broad-spectrum antibiotics affect a wider range of Gram-negative and Gram-positive bacteria. *It is recommended to choose a narrow-spectrum antibiotic when treating nonlife-threatening dental infections.* The primary indication for use of broad-spectrum antibiotics is in severe life-threatening dental infections where the causative agent is unknown. Every time bacteria are exposed to antibiotics, there is an opportunity for development of resistant strains. If narrow-spectrum antibiotics are used, fewer bacteria have the opportunity to develop resistance. Also, specific narrow-spectrum antibiotics usually are more effective against specific susceptible bacteria than broad-spectrum antibiotics. Extended-spectrum antibiotics have bacterial activity in between a narrow-spectrum and a broad-spectrum agent.

Q. Which antibiotics are considered to be narrow spectrum and which are broad spectrum?

A. *Narrow spectrum*: penicillin V, erythromycin, azithromycin, clarithromycin, clindamycin.
Extended spectrum: amoxicillin, amoxicillin/clavulanate (Augmentin®).
Broad spectrum: tetracyclines (doxycycline, minocycline), ciprofloxacin (Cipro®).

Q. How do you know that an antibiotic is not working?

A. The patient has not clinically responded within about three days and the infection is not clearing up. Resistance may develop, in which case culture and sensitivity testing may be necessary. In this case, change the antibiotic or add another antibiotic. For example, if no clinical improvement is seen in a patient taking penicillin V in 48–72 hours, then metronidazole (both are bactericidal) should be added.

Q. Why is combination antibiotic therapy sometimes better than mono drug therapy?

A. Combination therapy with two or more antibiotics is used in special cases to prevent the emergence of resistant strains; treat emergency cases during the period when an etiological diagnosis is still in progress; and take advantage of antibiotic synergism, which is when the effect of a combination of antibiotics is greater than the sum of the effects of the individual antibiotics. Sometimes when using combination drugs, a lower dose of one or both can be administered.

Q. How are antibiotics distributed in the body?

A. Through the plasma. Most antibiotics are well distributed in soft tissues.

Q. What adverse effects can occur with antibiotics that you need to warn the patient about and how are they managed?

A. Antibiotics, especially broad spectrum, alter the microflora of the stomach, resulting in diarrhea and fungal infections. To help avoid this problem, it is beneficial to take probiotics with antibiotics (Rodgers et al. 2013).

- *Superinfections*: fungal infections (e.g., vaginal) and infections by other bacteria, including enteric rods, pseudomonads, and staphylococci, are more likely with broad-spectrum antibiotics but can occur with any. The narrow-spectrum antibiotic will not kill as many of the normal microorganisms in the body as the broad-spectrum antibiotic so narrow-spectrum antibiotics have less ability to cause superinfection. This occurs because the bacteria are targeted which allow for growth of *Candida* spp. To help avoid this, it is recommended to all patients, especially females, to eat yogurt containing live and active cultures. To prevent antibiotic-related superinfections, about 5 oz of yogurt should be taken twice daily while on the antibiotic. An alternative method is to take acidophilus supplementation (capsule). As long as the product is made by a reliable manufacturer, most acidophilus supplements are relatively equal and should not cause unpleasant side effects; some cause slight bloating for the first few days or weeks, but this does not usually last. *Lactobacillus acidophilus* is one of the bacteria found in these supplements, but the term "acidophilus" usually refers to a combination of *L. acidophilus* with other beneficial bacteria.
- *Gastrointestinal problems (nausea, vomiting, and diarrhea)*: to help avoid antibiotic-related diarrhea, it is recommended that all patients eat yogurt containing live and active cultures. Approximately 4–8 oz of yogurt should be taken twice daily while on the antibiotic. Yogurt should be taken at least two hours before or two hours after the antibiotic. However, antibiotic-associated diarrhea (new onset of >3 partially formed or watery stools per 24-hour period) can be caused by toxins released from *Clostridium difficile* resulting in pseudomembranous colitis or *C. difficile*-associated diarrhea (CDAD). *C. difficile* is the leading known cause of nosocomial

intestinal infections (Ofosu 2016). If this happens, the patient should discontinue the antibiotic and call emergency services. The patient should not take antidiarrheal medications because it is advantageous to eliminate the bacterial toxins. *Pseudomembranous colitis symptoms could appear at any time while taking the antibiotic or even months after the start of antibiotic therapy.* Unless the patient has a tendency toward pseudomembranous colitis, it is not known if the patient will develop it. In reality, any antibiotic can cause pseudomembranous colitis but if used appropriately there is a lower incidence.

- *Antibiotic resistance*: a narrow-spectrum antibiotic will cause less bacterial resistance as it will deal with only specific bacteria. This is the reason for initially choosing a narrow-spectrum antibiotic. Antibiotic resistance is an increasing problem worldwide.
- *Allergic reactions*: allergic reactions range from a mild rash to wheezing and anaphylaxis. The antibiotic should be discontinued immediately.
- *Photosensitivity*: exaggerated sunburn when taking doxycycline. Avoid sunlight.

Q. How long after an antibiotic is taken can an allergic reaction occur?

A. Allergic reactions are classified based on the time of onset. Type I acute (anaphylactic) reactions can occur within minutes of taking the antibiotic and can be life-threatening. Accelerated reactions can occur between 30 minutes and 72 hours and are usually not life-threatening. Delayed allergic reactions can be seen up to two or more days later.

Q. What conditions may increase the risk of infection with antibiotic-resistant bacteria?

A. Indiscriminate use of antibiotics; recent (within six weeks) use of antibiotics for other conditions; previous antibiotic treatment that was not successful; and being in close contact with someone who recently was treated with an antibiotic. Patients must be compliant (adherent) with dosage regimen and avoid missing doses.

Q. What are the definition and symptoms of gastrointestinal distress?

A. Gastrointestinal (GI) distress is a term used to describe a variety of symptoms that arise from disturbances in the stomach/lower intestinal tract. Symptoms include nausea, vomiting, cramping and diarrhea. Most of the time, GI symptoms are caused by the irritative properties of the antibiotic and can be minimized by taking it with food.

Q. What is the cause of gastrointestinal distress while taking antibiotics?

A. Gastrointestinal disturbances occur due to an alteration in the normal GI flora.

Q. What is the treatment of CDAD?

A. Metronidazole used to be the drug of choice for *C. difficile* infection but as of 2018, it it is not recommended. Currently, oral vancomycin is the recommended drug (125 mg, four times a day) and is effective in the majority of cases (McDonald et al. 2018). Some patients will have episodes of diarrhea or colitis up to 28 days after the antibiotic has been discontinued. The patient can have repeated episodes of the disease for several years thereafter.

Q. Can combination antibiotics be used in dentistry?

A. Yes, because multiple pathogens are present in a dental infection. Two of the same category of antibiotics can be used. For example, you can prescribe two bactericidal antibiotics but not a bactericidal and a bacteriostatic together. Often amoxicillin and metronidazole are prescribed for aggressive periodontitis. Both are bactericidal antibiotics and the combination of metronidazole with penicillin V or amoxicillin increases the bacterial susceptibility.

Q. Is the mouth sterile?

A. No. There are many bacteria present in the oral cavity, both beneficial and pathogenic (disease producing). It is clear that anaerobic bacteria, both facultative and obligate, are involved in the two major oral diseases, dental caries and periodontitis.

Q. Which oral bacteria are facultative (can live with or without oxygen) anaerobes?

A. Gram-positive facultative cocci: *Streptococcus sanguis, S. mitis, S. salvarius, Staphylococcus aureus.*
Gram-positive facultative rods: *Actinomyces* (including *A. viscosus, A. naeslundii*).
Gram-negative facultative rods: *Eikenella corrodens, Capnocytophaga* spp., *Aggregatibacter actinomycetemcomitans.*

Q. Which oral bacteria are obligate or strict anaerobes?

A. Gram-positive obligate anaerobic coccus: *Peptostreptococcus* spp.
Gram-positive obligate anaerobic rod: *Eubacterium* spp.
Gram-negative obligate anaerobic rods: *Porphyromonus gingivalis, Prevotella intermedia, Tannerella forsynthensis, Fusobacterium nucleatum.*
Gram-negative anaerobic spirochete: *Treponema* spp.

Q. Which bacteria are obligate aerobes?

A. Obligate aerobic: *Mycobacterium tuberculosis, Pseudomonas aeruginosa.*

Q. How is an antibiotic chosen for prophylaxis?

A. The choice of antibiotic for prophylaxis is based on several factors. The antibiotic should be active against the bacteria most likely to cause an infection related to the dental procedure. Second, the patient must not be allergic to the antibiotic and it must not interact with the patient's other medications.

4.1.2 Antibiotics

4.1.2.1 Beta-Lactam Antibiotics

Q. What is the mechanism of action of the penicillins?

A. Penicillins cause bacterial lysis (breaking up) by interfering with the synthesis of peptidoglycan that is necessary for formation of the bacterial cell wall. This results in lysis of the cell wall and death of the bacteria. Therefore, penicillin is most active against rapidly dividing bacteria and has no effect on nonmultiplying organisms.

Q. What is the spectrum of bacterial activity of penicillin?

A. Even though narrow-spectrum penicillin V inhibits both Gram-negative and Gram-positive organisms, the cell wall of Gram-negative bacteria is more complex, therefore these bacteria are more resistant to the lytic effects of penicillin. Some bacteria effective against penicillin include the following.
Gram-positive coccus: *Streptococcus* spp. (penicillin is the traditional drug of choice for treatment of streptococcal infections).
Gram-negative anaerobes associated with dental infections: *Fusobacterium*, peptostreptocci, spirochetes, *Actinomyces*, and some *Bacteroides*.
Spirochete: *Treponema pallidum.*

Q. Why is penicillin G never prescribed in dentistry?

A. Penicillin G is completely destroyed by acid in the stomach. Therefore, it is only available for parenteral administration.

Q. How is penicillin made?

A. An antibiotic is a natural substance produced by a microorganism that will kill or stop growth of another microorganism. Penicillin, discovered by Alexander Fleming in 1929, is made by the mold *Penicillium chrysogenum*. The mold forms the beta-lactam ring. Amoxicillin and ampicillin are semisynthetic antibiotics, consisting of a mixture of natural and synthetic substances; a substance produced by microorganisms that is subsequently chemically modified to achieve desired properties. Some "antibiotics" such as fluoroquinolones are totally synthetically produced and are not really considered to be antibiotics by the true definition.

Q. What does the "V" in penicillin V stand for?

A. Penicillin V is also known as phenoxymethyl penicillin and is the orally active form of penicillin (penicillin G is not orally active). The "V" stands for the Latin word *vesco/vescor* meaning "to eat." Sometimes it is written penicillin VK where the "K" stands for potassium.

Q. What is amoxicillin?

A. Amoxicillin is a semisynthetic analog of penicillin with a broader spectrum of antibacterial activity.

Q. What are other drug names for amoxicillin?

A. Amoxil®, Trimox®.

Q. What is the spectrum of bacterial activity of amoxicillin?

A. Amoxicillin is an extended-spectrum analog of penicillin V. However, it has limited activity against streptococci or oral anaerobes compared to penicillin V. It has a broader spectrum against bacteria not in the oral cavity (e.g., *Haemophilus influenzae*, *Streptococcus pneumoniae*, *Escherichia coli*, *Salmonella*). Thus, it is no more effective in oral odontogenic/periodontal infections than penicillin V and actually since it is a broad-spectrum antibiotic, it can cause many more adverse effects, including superinfection. Penicillin V is the drug of choice for odontogenic infections because of its superior bioavailability.

Q. What is the difference between penicillin and amoxicillin?

A. Amoxicillin has a broader spectrum of bacterial activity and is completely absorbed (about 90% of an oral dose is absorbed) so that there is less gastrointestinal distress (e.g., diarrhea) because it does not stay in the intestine that long and it produces higher plasma and tissue concentrations. Also, absorption is not affected by food.

Q. How are penicillins excreted?

A. Penicillin is actively excreted via the kidneys in the urine and about 80% of a penicillin dose is cleared from the body within 3–4 hours of administration.

Q. Can penicillin or amoxicillin be given to a patient with renal impairment?

A. Yes. No dosage adjustment is necessary for penicillin V. Amoxicillin requires a reduction of dosing *interval*, not dosage, based on the patient's glomerular filtration rate (GFR) which is a blood value. If GFR is >50 mL/min, usually dose 250–500 mg q8h; GFR 10–50 mL/min, dose 250–500 mg q8-12h; GFR <10 mL/min, dose 250–500 mg q24h (http://med.stanford.edu/ bugsanddrugs/dosing-protocols/_jcr_content/main/panel_builder/panel_0/download/file. res/2017%20SHC%20ABX%20Dosing%20Guide%202017-08-08.pdf).

Q. What are the adverse effects of penicillins?

A. Hypersensitivity (anaphylactic reaction), gastrointestinal distress, nausea, vomiting, superinfections (fungal infections), and CDAD, which has been reported with use of nearly all antibacterial agents and not just penicillins.

Q. Why are individuals allergic to penicillin?

A. Approximately 5% of individuals are hypersensitive to penicillins. The breakdown products of the penicillin molecule act as the sensitizing agent for allergic reactions (Albin and Agarwal 2014). If the reaction is mild (rash), the penicillin should be discontinued and an antihistamine such as diphenhydramine (Benadryl®,) may be administered orally. This does not necessarily occur in a patient with a previous history of a reaction to penicillin. For more severe anaphylactic reaction emergency services should be contacted immediately (Fairbanks 2007).

Q. Is the incidence of developing a hypersensitive reaction to penicillin and amoxicillin the same?

A. No. Almost 7% of individuals can develop a rash-type reaction to aminopenicillins (e.g., amoxicillin) rather than the other penicillins (Fairbanks 2007).

Q. If someone is allergic to penicillin V, are they also allergic to amoxicillin and ampicillin?

A. Yes. The penicillin nucleus is the same in all penicillins including amoxicillin and ampicillin.

Q. What drug interactions occur with the penicillins?

A. • Probenecid (antigout medication): decreases renal tubular secretion of penicillin leading to higher and more prolonged serum concentrations.
   • Bacteriostatic antibiotics (e.g., tetracyclines, erythromycins): penicillin, a bactericidal antibiotic, requires the bacteria to be multiplying. If a bacteriostatic antibiotic, which stops multiplication of bacteria, is taken concomitantly with penicillin, the penicillin will not be effective. To manage this interaction, wait a few hours before taking one or the other antibiotic.
   • Oral contraceptives: penicillin interferes with oral contraceptive efficacy.

Q. Do penicillin and amoxicillin interfere with oral contraceptive efficacy?

A. This is very controversial according to clinical studies which were mostly published many years ago. Today, most products are combined estrogen-progestin oral contraceptives (COCs) which have reduced estrogen and progestin levels compared to 10 years ago, resulting in fewer side effects and presumably fewer interactions with antibiotics (Martin et al. 2018). It is best to ask a woman if she is taking an oral contraceptive before prescribing antibiotics and to advise to either practice abstinence or choose another method of birth control.

Q. Can bacteria become resistant to penicillin?

A. Yes. Certain Gram-negative bacteria produce and secrete enzymes called beta-lactamases which break down the beta-lactam ring on the penicillin (including amoxicillin) and cephalosporin molecule. Penicillinase, a type of beta-lactamase, especially breaks down the beta-lactam ring on the penicillin molecule, rendering the penicillin or amoxicillin inactive and leading to treatment failure.

Q. What can be given to a patient if penicillin or amoxicillin does not work?

A. Usually, after three days, if the patient is not clinically improving, a different antibiotic in a different classification should be given. Penicillin can be destroyed by beta-lactamases (penicillinases) produced by certain resistant bacteria. The enzyme attaches to the beta-lactam ring and breaks it up. This renders the penicillin ineffective and is a reason for the patient not getting clinically better. To prevent this type of resistance from occurring, Augmentin®, a combination of amoxicillin and clavulanate, is prescribed (the generic is usually prescribed). Clavulanate is an inert ingredient that also has a beta-lactam ring like penicillin, which strongly and irreversibly binds to the penicillinase, blocking the actions of penicillinase from breaking down the amoxicillin molecule and restoring the antimicrobial activity to amoxicillin. It is an acid (clavulanic acid) and can cause gastrointestinal irritation (e.g., nausea, vomiting, and diarrhea). It is usually prescribed in refractory cases when no other antibiotic has been clinically successful.

Q. How can the GI adverse effects be minimized when taking amoxicillin and clavulanic acid?

A. It is recommended to take amoxicillin/clavulanic acid with meals and probiotics or yogurt with active cultures, which should be taken two hours before or two hours after the antibiotic.

Q. Does penicillin V have a wide margin of safety?

A. Yes, penicillin has a very wide margin of safety. This means that a drug's usual effective dose is not toxic and if a little more of the drug is given, it still is not toxic. This is in contrast to antibiotics called aminoglycosides, which are not used in dental infections and have a narrow margin of safety (narrow therapeutic index) so that even usual doses can be toxic.

Q. What is the usual dose of penicillin V?

A. *Supplied*: tablet 250, 500 mg.
Dose: loading dose (LD) 1000 mg (two 500 mg tablet) stat on day 1, followed by 500 mg (one 500 mg tablet) q6h after the LD, up to day 7–10.

Q. What is the usual dose of amoxicillin trihydrate?

A. *Supplied*: capsules, oral suspension, and chewable tablets.
   Tablet: 500 mg, 875 mg.
   Chewable tablet: 125 mg, 400 mg.
   Capsule: 250 mg, 500 mg.
   Oral suspension: 125 mg/5 mL, 250 mg/5 mL, 400 mg/5 mL.
Dose: LD 1000 mg (two 500 mg capsules) stat, followed by 500 mg (one 500 mg capsule) q8h × 7 days.

Q. Why is the dosing interval of amoxicillin q8h and that of penicillin q6h?

A. The half-life ($t_{1/2}$) of amoxicillin is 1–1.3 hours and of penicillin 30 minutes. Dosing is less frequent with amoxicillin as it has a longer $t_{1/2}$ and stays in the body longer than penicillin with a shorter half-life.

Q. What is the adult dosing for amoxicillin chewable tablet?

A. A LD of 1000 mg on day 1 is acceptable followed by 250–500 mg three times a day (every eight hours) after the LD up to day 7–10.

Q. What is the usual dose of amoxicillin/clavulanate?

A. *Supplied*: all tabs have 125 mg clavulanic acid.

Tablet: 250 mg, 500 mg, 875 mg.

Chewable tablet: 125 mg, 200 mg, 400 mg.

Dose: (can give a LD of 1000 mg) 250–500 mg q8h depending upon the severity of the infection. When writing the prescription, only the strength (500 mg) needs to be designated because all dosage forms come with 125 mg clavulanate.

Q. Are two tablets of 250 mg amoxicillin/clavulanate equivalent to one 500 mg tablet?

A. No. Two amoxicillin/clavulanate 250 mg tablets are not equivalent to one 500 mg tablet and should not be substituted for one 500 mg tablet.

4.1.2.2 Cephalosporins

Q. Why are cephalosporins not a drug of choice in dental infections?

A. Cephalosporins are structurally related to penicillins with a similar mechanism of action. However, because most cephalosporins are poorly absorbed orally and display poor permeability into bacteria, routine use for dental infections is precluded. Additionally, cephalosporins' broader spectrum does not provide any advantage over penicillin V against principal odontogenic pathogens.

Q. Why is a cephalosporin indicated for total joint replacement prophylaxis?

A. Cephalosporins have very good bone penetration and increased activity against *S. aureus*. Cephalexin is the first drug of choice along with amoxicillin for antibiotic prophylaxis for total joint replacement.

Q. Can a cephalosporin be given to a patient allergic to penicillin?

A. No. Cephalosporins should not be prescribed to patients allergic to penicillin since there is a 10% cross-reactivity with the cephalosporins. Penicillins share a common beta-lactam ring (Herbert et al. 2000).

4.1.2.3 Erythromycins

4.1.2.3.1 Erythromycin

Q. Erythromycins belong to which classification of drugs?

A. Macrolides

Q. How is erythromycin produced?

A. Erythromycin is produced from a bacterial strain of *Streptomyces erythreus*. It is very difficult to produce erythromycin synthetically.

Q. What is the mechanism of action of erythromycins?

A. Erythromycins are bacteriostatic antibiotics that inhibit bacterial protein synthesis by binding to the 50S subunit of bacterial ribosomes.

Q. What is the spectrum of activity of erythromycins?

A. Erythromycins are primarily active against Gram-positive facultative anaerobic and strict anaerobic bacteria.

Q. Are erythromycins bacteriostatic or bactericidal?

A. Erythromycin is usually bacteriostatic, especially at standard low doses (e.g., doses prescribed in dentistry; about 1500 mg) and bactericidal at high doses (e.g., intravenous) (Engelkirk and Duben-Engelkirk 2010).

Q. What is the spectrum of microbial activity of erythromycins?

A. Most erythromycins are primarily effective against Gram-positive bacteria and some Gram-negative bacteria.

Q. Does bacterial resistance develop to erythromycin?

A. Yes. Bacteria can become resistant, especially group A streptococci. Most Gram-negative bacteria are resistant to macrolides. Also, cross-resistance can occur between erythromycin and clindamycin.

Q. Can an individual be allergic to erythromycins?

A. Yes. Allergic reactions, ranging from mild skin reactions to anaphylaxis, can occur with erythromycins. If an allergic reaction occurs, the drug should be discontinued and the reaction managed either with an antihistamine such as diphenhydramine (Benadryl) for mild reactions or epinephrine and calling for emergency services for severe anaphylactic reactions.

Q. Is there cross-over allergy between penicillins and erythromycins?

A. No. If an individual is allergic to penicillin, any erythromycin is acceptable to prescribe without any cross-over allergenicity.

Q. What are the different kinds of macrolides?

A. Erythromycin base (Ery-Tab®, Eryc®, E-Mycin®), erythromycin ethylsuccinate (EES), and erythromycin stearate (Erythrocin®). The different salts of erythromycin have been developed in order to compensate for the poor bioavailability (absorption). The base and stearate forms are acid labile (susceptible to breakdown and inactivation by stomach acid) so in order for them to be protected, they are formulated as film tabs (enteric coating). The ethylsuccinate form is absorbed first and then hydrolyzed in the blood to free erythromycin.

Q. Why is erythromycin not a preferred antibiotic in anaerobic odontogenic infections?

A. Erythromycin is usually bacteriostatic, and resistance can develop very rapidly. Since erythromycins are bacteriostatic, the minimum inhibitory concentration (MIC) must be maintained by diligently following the dosage regimen and not missing doses. Additionally, since erythromycin does not penetrate the cell wall of Gram-negative bacteria, the antibiotic will be ineffective because it needs to enter the bacteria to have an effect.

Q. What precautions are used when prescribing erythromycins?

A. Gastrointestinal distress occurs for most patients not following the entire course of therapy. Also, all members of the erythromycins prolong the electrocardiographic QT interval, resulting in the development of ventricular arrhythmias, including torsade de pointes which can be fatal. Erythromycins should be used with caution in patients with cardiac arrhythmias, uncorrected hypokalemia and with other drugs used in the management of arrhythmias that could prolong the QT interval, including quinidine, sotalol or procainamide (Fairbanks 2007). These antibiotics should *not* be prescribed in patients with preexisting heart disease, history of ventricular arrhythmias or metabolic abnormalities such as hypokalemia (Nachimuthu et al. 2012).

Additionally, caution should be used in patients with severe liver disease because of high risk of hepatotoxicity.

Q. Are there any drug interactions with erythromycins?

A. Yes. Erythromycins are metabolized in the liver via cytochrome P450 enzymes to form a stable metabolite complex that inhibits the metabolism of other drugs that are metabolized by these enzymes, including the cholesterol-lowering drugs lovastatin (Mevacor®), simvastatin (Zocor®), and atorvastatin (Lipitor®), the antiorgan rejection drug cyclosporine, the antiasthma drug theophylline, and sildenafil (Viagra®) (Fairbanks 2007).

4.1.2.3.2 *Azithromycin and Clarithromycin*

Q. What are azithromycin and clarithromycin?

A. Both are classified as azalides, which are second-generation macrolides. Azithromycin is a macrolide derivative and the first of the 15-membered ring azalide class of antimicrobials. Although its mechanism of action and susceptibility to resistance are similar to those of the macrolide antibiotics, azithromycin's extended spectrum of activity includes Gram-positive and Gram-negative organisms. Azithromycin is stable at gastric pH and has a bioavailability of about 37% following oral administration. Although its serum concentrations are typically low, the drug concentrates to a high degree in tissues, including periodontal tissues. Azithromycin is cleared primarily by the biliary and fecal routes; its serum half-life is in excess of 60 hours. Azithromycin and clarithromycin are more completely absorbed than erythromycin with less gastrointestinal distress (Ballow and Amsden 1992).

Q. What are the advantages of prescribing azithromycin or clarithromycin?

A. Azithromycin and clarithromycin are more acid stable than erythromycin, which means that they are not broken down in the acidity of the stomach before they reach the intestines where absorption occurs. There are few bacteria in the stomach because the high acidity inhibits bacterial growth. Both azalides have structural modifications, which result in better gastrointestinal tolerability and tissue penetration than erythromycin.

Additionally, azithromycin reaches higher concentrations in host (phagocytes) cells (e.g., polymorphonuclear leukocytes or PMNs) and in the periodontal tissues (gingiva) (Sefton et al. 1996). Because of its high concentration in PMNs, azithromycin is actively transported to the site of infection. During active phagocytosis, azithromycin is released in the tissues. Azithromycin has a postantibiotic effect which means that it concentrates in the gingiva (about 50 times higher in the tissues than plasma) for days after the antibiotic is stopped, providing microbial inhibition after the drug concentration has decreased below the MIC. This is a good feature when prescribing for aggressive periodontitis where bacteria have been found in the gingival connective tissue. This high tissue concentration has been thought to overcome the high incidence of resistance seen with certain bacteria (Sefton et al. 1996).

Q. Is azithromycin adequate to prescribe in oral infections?

A. Yes. Azithromycin has activity against many Gram-positive and Gram-negative bacteria and anaerobic bacteria and in a good choice for mild infections when the patient is allergic to penicillin.

Q. What precautions should be taken when prescribing azithromycin or clarithromycin?

A. Azithromycin or clarithromycin should not be prescribed to patients with severe liver disease (e.g., hepatic failure, cirrhosis), severe kidney disease (e.g., renal failure, pyelonephritis, glomerulonephritis), severe cardiovascular disease, pregnancy, breast feeding, and myasthenia gravis).

Q. What is the usual dose of azithromycin?

A. *Supplied*:

    Capsule: 250 mg

    Tablet: 250 mg, 500 mg, 600 mg

Dose: Since azithromycin has a long $t_{1/2}$ of 60–70 hours, the dose is only once a day. LD: 500 mg on day 1, then 250 mg for four days.

Q. Is there an oral suspension available?

A. Yes. Oral suspension: 100 mg/5 mL (15 mL); 200 mg/5 mL (15 mL, 22.5 mL, 30 mL). Also available in a single dose packet: 1 g (1000 mg). For the single dose packet, the entire contents are mixed with 2 oz (60 mL) of water and drunk. Then add 2 oz more water to the glass and drink to make sure the entire dose was taken. It can be taken with or without food. Do not use the packet for children.

Q. Can I prescribe a Z-Pak®?

A. Yes. The 250 mg tablets are dispensed in blister packs of six, commonly referred to as a Z-Pak (Zithromax®), whereas the 500 mg tablets are available in a blister pack of three tablets, or Tri-Pak, which has a three-day supply.

Q. When would I prescribe clarithromycin versus azithromycin?

A. Both clarithromycin and azithromycin can be prescribed when a patient is allergic to penicillin. Compared with clarithromycin, azithromycin has increased activity against Gram-negative bacilli. So, essentially, either one can be prescribed for dental infections. The bioavailability of clarithromycin is more than twice that of erythromycin and azithromycin is 1.5 times that of erythromycin. Azithromycin has a longer half-life than clarithromycin, so the dosing interval is less. As mentioned in an earlier question, azithromycin also has better uptake from the circulation into intracellular compartments (better tissue and cell penetration) followed by a slow release. For example, if azithromycin is prescribed for five days, it still has active therapeutic levels in the body at day 10. Thus, azithromycin may be superior to clarithromycin.

Q. What is the usual dose of clarithromycin?

A. *Supplied*:

    Tablet: 250 mg, 500 mg

    Extended-release tablet: Biaxin® XL® 500 mg.

    Granules for oral suspension: Biaxin 125 mg/5 mL, 250 mg/5 mL.

Dose: Since the $t\frac{1}{2}$ is 3–7 hours, dosing is 250–500 mg q12h. The extended-release formulation is given as two 500 mg extended-release tablets once daily.

Q. What are some common adverse effects of azithromycin and clarithromycin?

A. Common adverse effects include diarrhea, nausea, vomiting, dyspepsia, rash, pruritus, and abdominal pain.

Q. Are there clinically significant drug interactions with azithromycin and clarithromycin?

A. Clarithromycin and erythromycin are metabolized by the cytochrome P450 system in the liver, resulting in many drug interactions. Clarithromycin is a CYP3A4 substrate (metabolized by this isoenzyme) and a strong inhibitor of 3A4. See Chapter 5 for more detailed information about drug interactions. However, azithromycin is unlikely to interact with drugs metabolized via the hepatic cytochrome P450 enzyme system, and few interactions have been reported clinically (Shakeri-Nejad and Stahlmann 2006). There is an interaction between clarithromycin and calcium channel blockers resulting in hypotension (Horn and Hansten 2011).

Q. Can clarithromycin and azithromycin also cause QT prolongation and drug-induced torsades de pointes (TdP)?

A. Yes. As mentioned above with erythromycin, clarithromycin and azithromcyin have been documented to cause prolongation of the QT interval and TdP which is a potentially deadly cardiac rhythm. These antibiotics should *not* be prescribed in patients with preexisting heart disease, history of ventricular arrhythmias or metabolic abnormalities such as hypokalemia (Hancox et al. 2013; Nachimuthu et al. 2012).

Q. What are some drug interactions with azithromycin?

A. See Table 5.5.

Q. Is there a potential interaction of azithromycin with warfarin?

A. Yes. In 2009, the FDA revised the label for azithromycin, warning of a potential interaction with warfarin resulting in elevated international normalized ratio (INR) values. There is a risk that the patient can become overanticoagulated. If azithromycin is given, then the patient should be monitored or treatment modified. Consult with the patient's physician (Glasheen et al. 2005; Schrader et al. 2004; Waknine 2009).

4.1.2.4 Lincomycins

Q. What is the mechanism of action of clindamycin?

A. Clindamycin is bacteriostatic at low doses but can be bactericidal at usual doses (600 mg) and extended-interval dosing (Klepser et al. 1997). It inhibits bacterial protein synthesis by binding to the 50S ribosomal subunit.

Q. What is the spectrum of activity of clindamycin?

A. Clindamycin is a narrow-spectrum antibiotic effective against most Gram-positive organisms including group A streptococci, staphylococci, and pneumococci. Gram-negative aerobic microbes are resistant because clindamycin is poorly permeable to the outer membrane, but most anaerobes (*Prevotella*, *Peptostreptococcus*, *Fusobacterium*) are sensitive.

Q. Is clindamycin a good choice for odontogenic infections?

A. Yes. Clindamycin is superior to other antibiotics against anaerobes (chronic infection), making it a good choice in anaerobic infections, especially if refractory to other antibiotics. It shows good distribution in soft tissues as well as penetration into bone. Clindamycin also shows high plasma concentrations.

Q. What are some common adverse effects of clindamycin?

A. Diarrhea, nausea, vomiting, abdominal pain, and rash. Serious reactions include CDAD, Stevens Johnson syndrome, granulocytopenia (low concentration of white blood cells), and esophagitis.

Q. Is clindamycin the only antibiotic that causes *C. difficile* colitis or pseudomembranous colitis?

A. No. Almost any antibiotic can cause pseudomembranous colitis, especially if two or more antibiotics are used together. Clindamycin was the first antibiotic reported to cause pseudomembranous colitis and that is why it is always associated with this condition.

Q. Is clindamycin contraindicated in any patients?

A. Yes, patients with inflammatory bowel disease, ulcerative colitis, and pseudomembranous colitis.

Q. If a patient is allergic to erythromycin, can clindamycin be prescribed?

A. Yes. The mechanism of action of both antibiotics is similar but they are two different antibiotics.

Q. What is the dose of clindamycin?

A. *Supplied*:

Capsule: 75 mg, 150 mg, 300 mg.

Oral solution: 75 mg/5 mL (note that this is a solution, not a suspension as most other antibiotics).

Dose: LD 600 mg stat, followed by 150–450 mg q6–8h.

4.1.2.5 Metronidazole

Q. What is the spectrum of antibacterial action for metronidazole?

A. Metronidazole is effective against Gram-negative obligate (strict) anaerobes such as *P. intermedia*, *Porphyromonas gingivalis*, *Bacteroides*, and *Fusobacterium*.

Q. What is the mechanism of action of metronidazole?

A. Metronidazole is taken up into the bacteria where it produces toxic products which accumulate in the anaerobes and interact with DNA to cause a loss of the helical structure.

Q. Does metronidazole concentrate in the gingival crevicular fluid (GCF)?

A. The GCF is a serum transudate that originates in the gingival connective tissue. Irritation and inflammation of the gingival tissue increase the flow of GCF from the connective tissue into the gingival crevice. Metronidazole concentrates equally in the crevicular fluid and serum as well as in the gingival tissue.

Q. Why is metronidazole not recommended for the treatment of odontogenic infections?

A. Metronidazole alone is mainly effective against Gram-negative anaerobic rods and is not effective against *Streptococcus viridans*, which is primarily isolated in odontogenic infections. However, when used together with amoxicillin, there is an additive effectiveness against Gram-negative anaerobic rods.

Q. Is bacterial resistance to metronidazole common?

A. No. Metronidazole resistance is relatively uncommon.

Q. Does the ingestion of alcohol cause adverse effects when taking metronidazole?

A. Yes, but this is controversial. Ingestion of alcohol when taking metronidazole and for one week after metronidazole is stopped can result in a disulfiram-like reaction. Disulfiram (Antabuse®) is a medication used to wean individuals off alcohol. Chronic alcoholics are treated with disulfiram. If alcohol is ingested while on disulfiram, acute psychoses (hallucinations) and confusion, abdominal cramps, nausea, facial flushing, and headache can occur. This is a similar reaction with metronidazole. However, some studies found no disulfiram-like reaction with alcohol (Visapää et al. 2002).

Q. What is a commonly encountered oral adverse effect of metronidazole?

A. Metallic taste.

Q. Is there an interaction if metronidazole is taken with warfarin (Coumadin®), an anticoagulant?

A. Yes. Metronidazole can decrease the metabolism of warfarin, resulting in bleeding. Dosage reduction of warfarin is necessary. Warfarin is metabolized by cytochromes 2C and 3A4 and metronidazole is a potent inhibitor of CYP2C and 3A4, resulting in decreased metabolism of warfarin (Hersh 1999). Consultation with the patient's physician is necessary.

Q. What is the dose of metronidazole?

A. *Supplied*:
   Tablet: 250 mg, 500 mg.
   Capsule: 375 mg.
Dose: 500 mg q6–8 h × 7–14 days. For severe infections, give a LD of 1000 mg on day 1 followed by 500 mg q6–8h after the LD on day 1 up to 5–7 or 10 days if needed.

4.1.2.6 Tetracyclines

Q. What is the microbial spectrum of activity of the tetracyclines?

A. Effective against many Gram-positive and Gram-negative bacteria.

Q. What is the mechanism of action of the tetracyclines?

A. Tetracyclines are broad-spectrum bacteriostatic antibiotics that inhibit bacterial protein synthesis by binding to the 30S ribosomal subunit.

Q. What are doxycycline and minocycline?

A. Doxycycline and minocycline are semisynthetic members of the tetracycline group that are classified as longer acting tetracyclines with greater half-lives than the parent compound tetracycline HCl.

Q. Is doxycycline the same as the drug used in the treatment of acne?

A. No. Doxycycline is available in two different salts: hydrate and monohydrate, which is the form prescribed for acne.

Q. Why should doxycycline be prescribed rather than tetracycline?

A. Doxycycline has a longer half-life so that dosing is much less frequent than with tetracycline, which increases patient adherence.

Q. Why have tetracycline and its analogs doxycycline and minocycline gained so much attention and popularity in the last two decades?

A. Tetracycline concentrations were found to be higher in GCF than in serum. When tetracycline is administered orally, high levels are found in the gingival crevice or periodontal pocket where it is desirable to have the antibiotic when treating periodontal diseases.

Q. Why is tetracycline prescribed for periodontal diseases?

A. A unique mechanism of action of the tetracyclines is inhibition of the synthesis and release of collagenase (anticollagenase) from human PMNs. This collagenase is destructive and breaks down collagen present in the periodontium (gingiva, bone, periodontal ligament). Doxycycline has the greatest anticollagenase activity. A subantimicrobial dose (20 mg) of doxycycline is used in the management of generalized chronic periodontitis in conjunction with scaling and root planing. It is prescribed to take one tablet twice a day (q12h) for up to nine months.

Q. Do the same adverse effects, precautions, and contraindications follow with a subantimicrobial dose of doxycycline 20 mg?

A. Yes. It is still a tetracycline, so it is contraindicated in pregnant women and children less than 8 years of age. Give the same instructions to the patient as with an antibiotic strength dose of doxycycline.

Q. Can doxycycline be taken at bedtime?

A. Doxycycline should not be taken at bedtime. Numerous reports have documented an increased incidence of esophageal erosions (ulcers). It is best to tell the patient to drink a full glass of water and not to lie down directly afterward (Segelnick and Weinberg 2008).

Q. Can dairy products, iron, and antacids be taken together with tetracycline?

A. Not at the same time. Divalent or trivalent cations including antacids containing aluminum (Amphojel®), aluminum and magnesium combinations (Gelusil®, Maalox®, Mylanta®), calcium including antacids (Tums®, Citracal®, Caltrate®, Os-Cal®) and dairy products (milk), iron and magnesium (Milk of Magnesia®) reduce the absorption of tetracycline when taken concurrently by forming insoluble complexes or chelates with tetracycline, resulting in a reduction of the amount of tetracycline. Note: the amount of tetracycline is reduced, not the time of absorption. The tetracycline that is not absorbed into the bloodstream is eliminated in the feces. To manage this interaction, wait one hour before or two hours after taking the dairy product before taking tetracycline.

Q. Can food and dairy products be taken with doxycycline?

A. It depends on the brand of doxycycline. With most brands, there is only about a 30% decrease in bioavailability (absorption). The effects of dairy products, including milk, on doxycycline absorption are less than observed with other tetracycline derivatives, including tetracycline and minocycline.

Q. Can antacids and iron be taken with doxycycline?

A. No. Antacids, zinc, and iron should not be taken at the same time as doxycycline, minocycline or tetracycline. Antacids (containing calcium, aluminum, magnesium) and iron markedly reduce absorption of tetracycline. Space the antacid apart about one or two hours after taking doxycycline.

Q. Why is it contraindicated to prescribe tetracyclines, including doxycycline and minocycline, to a pregnant woman and children less than 8 years of age (children who do not have all permanent teeth)?

A. Tetracyclines are readily deposited into bone and teeth during calcification, which can cause a yellow-gray-brown discoloration/fluorescence and inhibit bone growth. The color of staining is dependent on which tetracycline was used, the dosage and the length of time. The tetracycline binds or chelates to calcium ions present on the hydroxyapatite crystals in the dentin, forming a stable calcium orthophosphate complex (ADA 2010).

Q. Can individuals taking tetracycline be exposed to sunlight?

A. Photosensitivity or a phototoxic reaction can occur when taking any tetracycline, especially doxycycline. Phototoxic reactions occur due to the damaging effects of light-activated compounds on cell membranes and DNA.

Q. Is dizziness an adverse effect of tetracycline?

A. Yes, especially with doxycycline (Segelnick and Weinberg 2010). Care must be taken to avoid falls when taking doxycycline.

Q. Is there a problem if an expired tetracycline product is systemically taken?

A. Yes. Expired tetracyclines can become nephrotoxic at a pH less than 2 due to the formation of anhydro-4-epitetracycline, which can cause acquired Fanconi syndrome, a disorder with clinical features of polyuria, polydipsia, and dehydration (Fathallah-Shaykh 2011; Ubara et al. 2005).

Q. What is the dose of doxycycline?

A. *Supplied*: 50 mg, 100 mg capsule; 20 mg, 50 mg, 100 mg tablet.
Dose: LD 100 mg q12h on day 1, followed by a maintenance dose of 100 mg once daily.

4.1.2.7 Fluoroquinolones

Q. What are fluoroquinolones?

A. Fluoroquinolones are not really considered to be antibiotics because they are entirely synthetic, but they are still classified as broad-spectrum antibiotics.

Q. What is the mechanism of action of fluoroquinolones?

A. Fluoroquinolones are bactericidal and block bacterial nucleic acid synthesis by inhibiting DNA gyrase.

Q. What is the microbial spectrum of activity of fluoroquinolones?

A. They are broad-spectrum drugs active against aerobic Gram-negative bacteria and many Gram-positive microorganisms. Anaerobes are usually resistant.

Q. If a patient is allergic to penicillin, can a fluoroquinolone be prescribed?

A. Yes.

Q. Is there cross-resistance between a fluoroquinolone and other antibiotics such as penicillins?
A. No. Since fluoroquinolones have a different mechanism of action, bacteria resistant to other antibiotics may be susceptible to fluoroquinolones.

Q. Why are fluoroquinolones useful for the treatment of pneumonia?
A. Because tissue and fluid concentrations exceed the serum drug concentration.

Q. When are fluoroquinolones prescribed in dentistry?
A. Fluoroquinolones are prescribed in dentistry if a patient is allergic to penicillin and/or has substantial gastrointestinal upset with erythromycins and clindamycin.

Q. What are some common fluoroquinolones used in dentistry?
A. Ciprofloxacin (Cipro®) and levofloxacin (Levaquin®).

Q. What are the adverse effects of fluoroquinolones?
A. Nausea, vomiting, diarrhea, headache, dizziness, phototoxicity (exaggerated sun reaction when exposed to the sun), insomnia, abnormal liver function tests, tendonitis and Achilles tendon rupture (especially in children and the elderly). Do not prescribe in patients younger than 18 years of age.

Q. Can fluoroquinolones be prescribed in pregnant patients?
A. Ciprofloxacin and levofloxacin are assigned a pregnancy category C. It is recommended not to prescribe either drug to pregnant or nursing women.

Q. Is there a **Black Box Warning** with fluoroquinolones?
A. Yes there are two **Black Box Warning**s.

1) March 2011: fluoroquinolone antibiotics including levofloxacin (Levaquin) can exacerbate muscle weakness in persons with myasthenia gravis. Fluoroquinolones have neuromuscular blocking activity.
2) July 2008: fluoroquinolone antibiotics (ciprofloxacin [Cipro], levofloxacin [Levaquin]) have an increased risk of tendonitis and tendon rupture that could cause permanent injury. This risk is further increased in patients over 60 years of age, in patients taking corticosteroid drugs, and in those with kidney, heart or lung transplants.

Q. Does pseudomembranous colitis occur with fluoroquinolones?
A. Yes. There is a high association between fluoroquinolones and *C. difficile*.

Q. Should fluoroquinolones be prescribed to a patient who is athletic and does a lot of running?
A. No. Fluoroquinolones can cause tendonitis and tendon rupture. The patient should be informed about this adverse effect and stop running while taking the medication.

Q. Can divalent and trivalent cations be taken concurrently with fluoroquinolone?
A. No. Similar to tetracyclines, divalent and trivalent cations (e.g., antacids containing aluminum and magnesium alone or in combination, iron and calcium [calcium supplements such as Caltrate, Citracal, Os-Cal, Tums] or dairy products) form insoluble complexes in the gut if they are taken concurrently with fluoroquinolones, resulting in lower amounts of the antibiotic being absorbed. Management of this drug interaction involves spacing the antibiotic apart from the divalent or trivalent cation product by about 1–2 hours.

Q. Can a fluoroquinolone be prescribed to someone taking warfarin?

A. There is a drug interaction between levofloxacin and warfarin which may cause the patient to be overanticoagulated with elevated INR values. If a fluoroquinolone is prescribed to a patient taking warfarin, the frequency of INR monitoring needs to be increased. Consult with the patient's physician.

Q. What is the dosing for ciprofloxacin?

A. *Supplied*:
　　Tablet: 250 mg, 500 mg.
　　Dose: 250–500 mg q12h for 7–10 days.
　　Renal dosing: CrCL >30: no changes.
　　　CrCL 5–30 : 250 mg q12h or 250–500 mg q18–24h.

Q. What is the dosing for levofloxacin?

A. *Supplied*:
　　Tablet: 250 mg, 500 mg 750 mg.
　　Dose: 500 mg q24h for 7–10 days.
　　Renal dosing: CrCL >50: no change.
　　　CrCL 20–49: 500 mg once, then 250 mg q24h.
　　　CrCL 10–19 and <10: 500 mg once, then 250 mg q48h.

4.1.3　Specific Instructions for Taking Antibiotics

Q. Does dosing "every six-hour interval" for penicillin need to be strictly followed?

A. Bactericidal agents such as penicillins that inhibit bacterial cell wall synthesis *do not* require constant blood levels to be maintained because at or above the minimal lethal concentration for susceptible bacteria, permanent damage to the cell wall occurs in growing bacteria, resulting in the lysis (break down) of bacterial cells. Thus, pulse dosing, where the dose is given as four doses in 24 hours, is adequate to be taken as "every six hours while awake." The patient does not need to follow the "every 6 hours, day and night" schedule and get up in the middle of the night. The dosing for bacteriostatic agents does need to be exactly followed as "every six hours." The same follows for amoxicillin.

Q. Does the dosing interval need to be strictly followed for bacteriostatic antibiotics?

A. Yes. In contrast to bactericidal antibiotics, bacteriostatic antibiotics require constant blood levels, which need to be above the MIC for the pathogen to be affected. That means that the patient must follow the prescribed dosing interval strictly even if it means getting up in the middle of the night. Prescribing azalides such as azithromycin or clarithromycin is best for the easiest dosing interval.

Q. If a patient is taking a bacteriostatic antibiotic such as azithromycin for a medical condition and a bactericidal antibiotic needs to be prescribed (e.g., amoxicillin for antibiotic prophylaxis or bactericidal doses of clindamycin), how far apart should the antibiotics be given?

A. Allow at least a six-hour interval between the bacteriostatic antibiotic and the bactericidal drug because if the two are given together, a drug–drug interaction occurs whereby the bactericidal drug will not be effective because it requires active, multiplying bacteria (Ganda 2008).

Q. Which antibiotics can cause dysgeusia (taste disturbances)?

A. Patients with dysgeusia have an alteration in the four taste sensations, including excessively sweet, bitter, salty or metallic taste while eating. Some antibiotics that can cause dysgeusia are metronidazole, tetracycline, and clarithromycin.

Q. How is antibiotic-associated diarrhea best prevented?

A. To help prevent diarrhea resulting from antibiotics, it is recommended that patients eat 4 oz of yogurt containing live and active cultures twice a day or take probiotics while taking the antibiotic. It has been suggested to take the yogurt at least two hours before or two hours after the antibiotic.

Q. How should the patient be warned about pseudomembranous colitis?

A. If the patient experiences watery or bloody diarrhea in addition to fever and abdominal cramps, the antibiotic should be immediately stopped and medical attention sought. Dehydration, low blood pressure, and low levels of potassium can occur due to significant loss of fluids and electrolytes resulting from diarrhea. Symptoms are caused by the bacterium *C. difficile* releasing a powerful toxin. If it is truly pseudomembranous colitis, it is life-threatening. The patient should not take an antidiarrheal medication such as Lomotil® or Imodium® because the treatment objective is to rid the body of the toxins and antidiarrheal medications would only reduce the chances of eliminating the toxins. Treatment involves discontinuing the offending antibiotic which may be enough to stop the diarrhea.

Q. Should caution be used when prescribing antibiotics to women on oral contraceptives?

A. This is still a debated issue. All women of child-bearing age should be asked if they are taking an oral contraceptive before prescribing an antibiotic. Even though there are limited case reports regarding this interaction, it is still considered to be a potential drug interaction. Ethinyl estradiol, an estrogen present in oral contraceptives, is only about 40% absorbed systemically in an inactive form. The remainder undergoes extensive first-pass metabolism. Inactive ethinyl estradiol is activated in the gut by bacterial gut flora, which releases active ethinyl estradiol which is then reabsorbed in the small intestine. Thus, there is a concern when taking antibiotics, especially broad spectrum, because bacteria are needed to activate ethinyl estradiol for the oral contraceptive to be effective. Antibiotics destroy the bacteria which dihydrolyze sulfate and glucuronide conjugates (metabolites of ethinyl estradiol) (Gibson and McGowan 1994). Thus, the enterohepatic recirculation of ethinyl estradiol that usually occurs is blocked.

There are conflicting reports on which antibiotics are the offending agents. Additionally, drug interactions may be more common with the low-dose estrogen oral contraceptives (Gibson and McGowan 1994). However, the American College of Obstetricians and Gynecologists concluded that tetracycline, doxycycline, ampicillin, and metronidazole do not affect oral contraceptive levels (Archer and Archer 2002; Lomaestro 2009). However, this activation by bacterial gut flora does not occur with progestins, the other component of oral contraceptives. The first reported published link between oral contraceptives and antibiotics occurred with rifampin, an antituberculosis drug, in 1971 (Gibson and McGowan 1994). Since it cannot be predicted which women will be at greater risk for this drug interaction, it has been suggested that women use an additional contraceptive method while taking the antibiotic and for at least one week after completing it (Hoffmann et al. 2015; Osborne 2004). It is plausible that some women may have low levels of ethinyl estradiol due to differences in the pharmacokinetics of the drug which would result in oral contraceptive failure when taking antibiotics (Bauer and Wolf 2005).

In 2004, the World Health Organization (WHO) reported that there were uncertainties that broad-spectrum antibiotics lowered oral contraceptive effectiveness; however, pregnancy rates are similar in women taking oral contraceptives with or without antibiotics (WHO 2004).

Q. What specific instructions should be given to the patient on how to take antibiotics?
A. Table 4.1 reviews patient counseling on how to take antibiotics.

Table 4.1 Patient counseling on how to take antibiotics

Antibiotic	Patient instructions	Common adverse effects
Amoxicillin	Taken without regard to meals (with or without food). Advise patient to take with some kind of probiotic (e.g., yogurt or acidophilus supplement) to help prevent superinfections and gastrointestinal distress	Gastrointestinal distress (watery diarrhea could be pseudomembranous colitis), allergic reactions (e.g., rash, difficulty breathing, swelling of face, lips, tongue, or throat), black hairy tongue. Do not take concurrently with a bacteriostatic antibiotic (wait a few hours in between)
Amoxicillin/ clavulanate (Augmentin)	Because potassium clavulanate is an acid (also referred as clavulanic acid), it is best to take with food to avoid gastrointestinal distress. Advise patient to take with some kind of probiotic (e.g., yogurt or acidophilus supplement)	Most common adverse effect is diarrhea (watery diarrhea could be a sign of pseudomembranous colitis), allergic reactions (e.g., rash, difficulty breathing, swelling of face, lips, tongue, or throat), black hairy tongue. Do not take concurrently with a bacteriostatic antibiotic
Azithromycin (Zithromax)	Food delays absorption of azithromycin capsules, however tablets may be taken without regard to food. Take capsules with a full glass of water on an empty stomach (one hour before or two hours after meals) for best absorption. Oral suspension (single dose packet) can be taken without regard to meals	Diarrhea, nausea, and abdominal pain. Most of these events are mild or moderate in severity. Azithromycin is unlikely to interact with drugs metabolized via the hepatic cytochrome P450 enzyme system, and few interactions have been reported clinically. Do not take antacids that contain aluminum or magnesium within two hours before or after you take azithromycin. These antacids can cause decreased absorption of azithromycin
Ciprofloxacin (Cipro)	Can be taken with food to minimize stomach upset	Stay out of the sun; photosensitivity reaction. Avoid caffeine. Do not take concurrently with di- and trivalent cations (e.g., antacids, iron, calcium, zinc). Interaction with warfarin. Report any tendon pain or inflammation
Clarithromycin (Biaxin)	Acid stable and well absorbed from the gastrointestinal tract, irrespective of the presence of food	Fewer gastrointestinal adverse effects than erythromycin. The most frequent side effects with clarithromycin are diarrhea, nausea, abnormal taste, dyspepsia, abdominal discomfort, and headache. Because clarithromycin is metabolized by hepatic cytochrome P450 microsomal enzymes, it, like erythromycin, has the potential to interact with other drugs. However, clarithromycin is a less potent P450 inhibitor than erythromycin. Associated with QT prolongation and ventricular arrhythmias, including ventricular tachycardia and torsade de pointes

(Continued)

Table 4.1 (Continued)

Antibiotic	Patient instructions	Common adverse effects
Clindamycin (Cleocin)	Take with a full glass of water. Given without regard to meals (food may delay, but not decrease, absorption)	Nausea, diarrhea, skin rashes, pseudomembranous colitis, allergic reactions
Doxycycline (Vibramycin®, Doryx®)	Take with a full glass of water (to prevent esophageal ulceration) on an empty stomach (one hour before or two hours after meals). It can be taken with food if GI upset occurs	Causes fewer alterations of intestinal flora than the other tetracyclines. Esophageal erosions and dizziness. Can cause sore throat. Binds to calcium in teeth and bones which may cause discoloration of teeth in children <8 years of age. OK to give in renal impairment. Do not take concurrently with antacids containing di- or trivalent cations, bismuth salts, iron, or zinc salts since these products cause a reduction in doxycycline absorption. Do not prescribe to pregnant women. Do not take concurrently with bactericidal antibiotics such as penicillin which may decrease antibiotic activity
Erythromycin	Take with a full glass of water on an empty stomach (one hour before or two hours after meals) for best absorption	Gastrointestinal and dose related. They include nausea, vomiting, abdominal pain, diarrhea, and anorexia. Onset of pseudomembranous colitis symptoms may occur during or after antibacterial treatment. Symptoms of hepatitis, hepatic dysfunction, and/or abnormal liver function test results may occur. Erythromycin has been associated with QT prolongation and ventricular arrhythmias, including ventricular tachycardia and torsades de pointes. Allergic reactions with rash and eosinophilia can occur rarely. A less well-known but nonetheless significant adverse reaction to erythromycin, especially after intravenous administration, is ototoxicity, manifest as tinnitus and/or deafness.Erythromycin inhibits CYP3A4 enzymes resulting in many drug interactions and reducing metabolism of the following drugs: triazolam, warfarin, and cyclosporine.
Metronidazole (Flagyl®)	Given without regard to meals. However, taking with meals may minimize gastrointestinal distress	Diarrhea, loss of appetite, nausea, abdominal cramps, vomiting, metallic taste, dry mouth; alcohol and warfarin (increase anticoagulation effect) interactions
Penicillin V	Take with a full glass of water on an empty stomach (one hour before or two hours after meals) for best absorption	In excessive doses, seizures are common. Do not take concurrently with a bacteriostatic antibiotic
Tetracycline	Take with a full glass of water (to prevent esophageal ulceration) on an empty stomach (one hour before or two hours after meals). It can be taken with food if GI upset occurs	Nausea, diarrhea, esophageal erosions, dizziness (doxycycline), photosensitivity. Do not take concurrently with antacids containing di- or trivalent cations, bismuth salts, iron, or zinc salts since these products cause a reduction in tetracycline absorption. Do not prescribe to pregnant women. Do not take concurrently with bactericidal antibiotics such as penicillins

4.2 Antimicrobials, Local

4.2.1 Chlorhexidine Gluconate

Q. What is the difference between first-generation and second-generation oral rinses?

A. First-generation mouth rinses have a high substantivity whereby the agent binds to oral structures and is slowly released over time and remains active. Chlorhexidine gluconate is an example of a first-generation mouth rinse. The extended binding to oral soft tissues and tooth structure and slow release reduce bacterial recolonization for approximately 8–12 hours afterward. Second-generation agents have low substantivity and are not as therapeutically effective as first-generation agents. Examples of second-generation agents include Listerine®, Scope®, and Cepacol®.

Q. What is the alcohol content of chlorhexidine gluconate?

A. Chlorhexidine gluconate 0.12% contains 11.6% alcohol. The alcohol present in oral rinses is ethyl alcohol. Isopropyl alcohol is present in the skin cleanser (Medical Economics Staff 2000).

Q. Is chlorhexidine gluconate 0.12% available alcohol free?

A. Yes. GUM® chlorhexidine gluconate oral rinse 0.12%.

Q. What is the alcohol content of Listerine?

A. Listerine 26.9% and Listerine Cool Mint or Fresh Burst: 21.6%

Q. What type of alcohol is present in oral rinses?

A. Ethanol.

Q. Does the alcohol in mouth rinses cause dry mouth?

A. Yes. The alcohol is a drying agent and can cause xerostomia.

Q. What is the mechanism of action of chlorhexidine?

A. Chlorhexidine is a cationic (positively charged) bisbiguanide. Chlorhexidine binds to the negatively charged bacterial cell surface, causing a disruption of the cytoplasmic membrane, allowing the chlorhexidine to enter the bacterial cytoplasm and kill the bacteria.

Q. What is the spectrum of antibacterial activity?

A. Chlorhexidine is active against Gram-positive and Gram-negative, facultative aerobic and anaerobic bacteria.

Q. What are the indications for chlorhexidine?

A. Chlorhexidine gluconate 0.12% is a prescription medication for gingivitis, not periodontitis.

Q. How should the patient use chlorhexidine?

A. Rinse bid with 15 mL of solution which is measured in the bottle cap. Rinse for 30 seconds and expectorate. The patient should not eat or drink for at least 30 minutes after rinsing.

Q. How is a prescription for chlorhexidine written?

A. See Figure 4.1.

Rx chlorhexidine aluconate oral rinse
Disp: 1 bottle
Sig: Rinse with 15 mL (capful) of solution for 30 seconds, twice a day. The solution Should be swished through the mouth and then expectorate. Do not swallow.

Figure 4.1 How to write a prescription for chlorhexidine.

Q. Can fluoride-containing toothpaste be used directly before or after rinsing with chlorhexidine?

A. No. Fluoride toothpaste that contains sodium lauryl sulfate should be spaced at least 30 minutes apart before using chlorhexidine. The positively charged chlorhexidine causes it to bind to the negatively charged sodium lauryl sulfate (a detergent), leading to inactivation.

Q. What are some adverse effects of chlorhexidine that the patient should be warned about?

A. Brown staining of dorsum of tongue, teeth, and restorations, increased supragingival calculus formation, and temporary alteration in taste perception.

Q. What can be done to minimize the brown staining?

A. The patient should routinely brush and floss. If this is inadequate, interproximal staining may be removed when the patient returns to the office, though staining of restorations may be permanent.

4.2.2 Other Mouth Rinses and Periodontal Health Products

Q. Is Scope clinically effective as an antimicrobial mouth rinse?

A. Quaternary ammonium compounds (e.g., Scope, Cepacol) bind to oral tissues but substantivity is only about three hours. There are inconclusive data as an antiplaque/antigingivitis rinse. The active ingredient in these rinses is cetylpyridinium chloride.

Q. Is the use of iodine efficacious?

A. Povidone-iodine has been advocated as a topical antiseptic that has been used as an irrigant in periodontal pockets. Povidone-iodine 7.5–10% (Betadine®) is a combination of polyvinylpyrrolidone and iodine and is used as a surgical scrub and for the prevention of skin infections. Mixed results have been published concerning the reduction of periodontal pathogens with povidone-iodine. Some clinical studies have shown that irrigation with povidone-iodine in conjunction with mechanical debridement may improve the percent of total microbial counts (Hoang et al. 2003). Other studies have shown no additional benefit when compared with ultrasonic debridement or scaling and root planing (Leonhardt et al. 2007). A main disadvantage is staining of clothes and tissues, and irritation.

Q. Is it safe to recommend hydrogen peroxide rinses?

A. 3% hydrogen peroxide has been used as an oxygenating rinse for inflamed oral tissues. Hydrogen peroxide liberates gaseous oxygen, providing a cleansing action and effervescence for oral wounds. It also has been used as an antimicrobial agent (rinse or irrigant diluted with water). However, antiplaque/antigingivitis claims are not well supported. Hydrogen peroxide may cause irritation and delayed wound healing, so it is not advocated to be used as an oral antimicrobial agent. When hydrogen peroxide is used undiluted, it causes burning of the oral mucosa.

Q. Is Gly-Oxide® or Peroxyl® recommended for oral wounds?

A. Gly-Oxide or Peroxyl is approved as a temporary debriding agent in the oral cavity. It is composed of peroxide. It is an oxygenating agent whereby oxygen is released, providing a cleansing action and gentle effervescence for oral wounds.

4.3 Controlled-Release Drug Delivery

Q. What does controlled-release drug delivery mean?

A. When a drug is released from a device beyond 24 hours. For example, doxycycline in Atridox® is reportedly released for a period of 21 days (American Academy of Periodontology 2006).

Q. Which controlled-release drug delivery systems are used in the treatment of periodontal disease?

A. Atridox, Arestin®, and PerioChip®. All products are bioabsorbable and do not need to be removed.

Q. What are the major ingredients in Arestin, Atridox, and PerioChip?

A. Arestin: 1 mg minocycline hydrochloride microspheres; Atridox: 10% (42.5) doxycycline hyclate in a gel formulation; and PerioChip: 2.5 mg chlorhexidine gluconate.

Q. When is it indicated to use one of these products?

A. As an adjunct to scaling and root planing for the reduction of pocket depth, gain of clinical attachment and reduction of bleeding in patients with localized chronic periodontitis with recurrent pockets of ≥5 mm that continue to bleed on probing.

Q. Can Atridox and Arestin be administered to a patient who is pregnant?

A. No. Since these products are analogs of tetracyclin,e the same contraindications/precautions used with systemic tetracycline must be followed with locally applied tetracyclines.

Q. How many applications must be done with Arestin?

A. Administration of Arestin does not require local anesthesia. Up to three treatments, at three-month intervals, are recommended. No periodontal packing is required after application.

Q. What are important postapplication patient instructions?

A. Avoid tooth brushing and flossing for seven days.

Q. Do Arestin, Atridox, and PerioChip need to be refrigerated?

A. No. They do not need to be refrigerated and should be stored at room temperature.

4.4 Antivirals/Antifungal Agents

4.4.1 Antiviral Agents

Q. For which common oral conditions is antiviral therapy appropriate?

A. Herpes simplex virus (HSV) infections.

Q. What is the incidence of herpes infection?

A. HSV (type 1, herpes-1or HSV-1) causes about 80% of cases of oral herpes infections and 20% of genital lesions. In adolescents, about 30–40% of genital herpes is caused by HSV-1. About 80% of genital herpes is due to HSV-2 and 20% of oral lesions (Sharma and Dronen 2011).

Q. What are the different types of oral herpes infections?

A. The first infection with HSV-1 usually causes primary herpetic gingivostomatitis and is most common in children under 5 years of age. Prodromal symptoms include fatigue, malaise, anorexia, muscle aches, irritability, fever, and chills. A few days later, vesicles appear which rupture, leaving painful ulcers. The gingiva, lips, palate, buccal mucosa, and throat are also affected. Eating and drinking are difficult, and patients quickly become dehydrated. Signs and symptoms of dehydration usually warrant going to a hospital's emergency department, especially in infants under 6 weeks of age. After the primary infection or exposure to herpes virus, individuals can develop recurrent HSV infections. This infection, which occurs around the vermilion border of the lips and in the mouth, is referred to as recurrent herpes labialis, cold sores or fever blisters. Lesions develop from stress, sunlight, fever, trauma (e.g., after a dental procedure) or in immunocompromised patients. Cold sores or herpes labialis is caused by the HSV-1 strain. Even though the preference of the HSV-2 strain is for the genital region, it is sometimes transmitted to the oral region. Both are contagious when the virus is producing and shedding.

Q. What is the management of primary herpetic gingivostomatitis?

A. Fluids, bed rest, acetaminophen or ibuprofen (aspirin is contraindicated in viral infections in children because of the risk of developing Reye syndrome), and topical application of a local anesthetic containing lidocaine or benzocaine such as Anbesol®, Orabase® with benzocaine 20%, Zilactin L®, and Xylocaine® 2% viscous. Do not give ibuprofen to children who are asthmatic or have a hypersensitivity to aspirin. Topical antiviral medications are generally not highly effective.

Q. What is herpes labialis?

A. Herpes labialis (known as fever blisters or cold sores) occurs after an individual has had a first experience with herpes simplex infection. HSV-1, a DNA virus, causes primarily oral lesions with a small percent of genital lesions. HSV-2 causes primarily genital lesions and a small percent of oral lesions.

Typically, an individual will have prodromal symptoms of pain, tingling, burning or itching before eruption of the lesions. Healing of ulcers occurs over a few weeks. Herpes labialis presents at the commissure of the lips.

Q. Can herpes occur intraorally?

A. Yes. Herpes infection can occur anywhere intraorally. Sometimes after a dental procedure is completed, the patient will have intraoral lesions on the attached gingival due to stress or trauma.

Q. How should herpes labialis be managed?

A. Intraoral herpes infections should be treated with antiviral agents and palliative care. The mechanism of action of the antiviral drugs is to inhibit viral DNA synthesis/replication. Unfortunately, HSV remains latent in sensory ganglia so that there is a high incidence of recurrence or relapse even after the lesions are treated. The goal of using antiviral drugs is to shorten

Table 4.2 Antiviral agents

Drug	Supplied	Dosing
Acyclovir (Zovirax)	Tabs: 400, 800 mg; Caps: 200 mg Cream or ointment: 5% (15 g tube) Suspension: 40 mg/mL	Apply thin layers of ointment with a finger cot or latex glove to affected area every 3 hours up to 6 times a day for 7 days. Take 200–400 mg po 5 times a day. Administer within 1–2 hours of prodromal symptoms such as tingling, itching, burning, pain, or lesion
Penciclovir (Denavir®)	Cream 1% (2 g tube)	Apply five times a day at first sign of cold sore. Use until lesion is healed
Famciclovir (Famvir)	Tabs: 125, 250, 500 mg	1500 mg as a single dose or 500 mg every 12 hours (recurrent infection) (administer within 1–2 hours of prodromal symptoms)
Valacyclovir (Valtrex)	Tabs: 500 mg, 1000 mg	2 g twice a day at a 12-hour interval for 1 day only
Docosanol (Abreva)	Cream: 10% (OTC)	Apply 5 times a day at first sign of cold sore. Use until lesion is healed

Source: Medical Economics Staff (2000).

the clinical course, prevent complications, prevent future recurrences, and decrease transmission. Antiviral agents are listed in Table 4.2.

Q. Should antibiotics be used in the management of recurrent herpes labialis?

A. No. Antibiotics further suppress the immune system and could prolong the duration of the infection.

Q. Why is it important to administer acyclovir early?

A. Acyclovir binds viral DNA polymerase, ending viral replication. Its mechanism of action necessitates early administration because replication may end as soon as 48 hours after a recurrence (Emmert 2000). Acyclovir reduces the pain and duration of symptomatic lesions.

Q. Can acyclovir be prescribed to children?

A. Acyclovir is recommended in individuals older than 12 years of age.

Q. What are some other features of acyclovir?

A. It is a safe and well-tolerated drug with only about 15–30% bioavailability after oral administration. Its half-life is 2.5 hours and adjustment is necessary in renal impairment. It has a pregnancy category of C.

Q. When should systemic acyclovir with or without topical agents be prescribed?

A. Systemic acyclovir is widely used off-label in the treatment of recurrent herpes labialis which means that it is used in the treatment but it is not FDA approved. Administering systemic antiviral medications such as acyclovir can reduce the duration of pain, decrease the size and duration of lesions, and may decrease the recurrence rate (but this is controversial). Additionally, systemic antiviral drugs can be prescribed.

1) Oral lesions which are severe and secondarily infected or may become infected.
2) Systemic involvement (e.g., fever).
3) Immunocompromised patients (e.g., HIV/AIDS).

Q. Is there systemic absorption after taking acyclovir cream?

A. Yes, but it is minimal in adults. The systemic absorption of acyclovir following topical administration of cream has not been documented in patients <18 years of age.

Q. Does acyclovir come in an oral suspension?

A. Yes. It can be prescribed for intraoral herpes infection. Acyclovir oral suspension 200 mg per 5 mL. So, if the dose is 200 mg then only 5 mL needs to be taken. One teaspoonful equals 5 mL. This medicine should be shaken well before use and taken with water. It does not require refrigeration. Acyclovir can be taken with or without food. The suspension should be taken with plenty of water (www.drugs.com/pro/zovirax-cream.html).

Q. What other systemic agents are FDA approved for the management of recurrent herpes labialis?

A. Valacyclovir, the prodrug of acyclovir (valacyclovir is rapidly converted to acyclovir before having any antiviral effects), is FDA approved for use in recurrent herpes labialis in patients ≥12 years of age. The efficacy of Valtrex® initiated after the development of clinical signs of a cold sore (e.g., papule, vesicle, or ulcer) has not been established. Although it is more expensive than acyclovir, it has a more convenient dosing (Sharma and Dronen 2011).

Q. What agent is FDA approved in immunocompromised patients?

A. The oral prodrug of penciclovir, famciclovir, is FDA approved for recurrent herpes labialis (RHL) in immunosuppressed patients; it demonstrates efficacy in addition to a more convenient dosing regimen. It should not be used in patients under 18 years of age.

Q. What should be done if it is too late after the first symptoms appear to apply an antiviral agent?

A. Apply a topical anesthetic agent containing benzocaine such as Anbesol, Orabase with benzocaine 20%, or lidocaine such as Zilactin L®. Patients who are allergic to *para*-aminobenzoic acid (PABA) may also be allergic to benzocaine and tetracaine, so it is best to recommend Zilactin L.

Q. What is the active ingredient in OTC topical anesthetics used in the management of oral ulcer pain?

A. See Table 4.3.

Table 4.3 Active ingredients in OTC topical anesthetics

Benzocaine: Anbesol, Orabase with benzocaine 20%
Benzyl alcohol: Zilactin
Camphor and phenol: Campho-phenique®, Blistex®, Carmex®, ChapStick Medicated®
Lidocaine: Zilactin L

Q. Is there any reported clinical toxicity related to topical local anesthetics?

A. Yes. Topical anesthetics including lidocaine and benzocaine can cause seizures, bradycardia, and methemoglobinemia (Barash et al. 2015). Methemoglobinemia is a condition characterized by high levels of methemoglobin, an oxidized metabolite of hemoglobin, in the blood. The main problem is that methemoglobin does not bind to oxygen, as does hemoglobin, which leads to an anemia. Symptoms include bluish coloring of the skin, headache, fatigue, and shortness of breath. Mild cases can go unrecognized. Treatment of severe methemoglobinemia is with methylene blue, or ascorbic acid is also useful.

Q. Which is the most recommended systemic antiviral agent for the treatment of oral herpes?

A. Acyclovir (Zovirax) is the most commonly prescribed antiviral agent for the management of herpes labialis. Famciclovir (Famvir®) and valacyclovir (Valtrex) are also effective with convenient dosing but are often more expensive than acyclovir. Both also have higher bioavailability than acyclovir.

Q. Are there any reactions to applying topical acyclovir?

A. Yes. It can be very painful.

Q. What are the adverse effects of systemic acyclovir?

A. Headache, seizure, nausea, vomiting, diarrhea, skin rash.

Q. Which antiviral drug is available OTC?

A. Docosanol (Abreva®). Abreva prevents viral entry and replication at the cellular level.

Q. What are the instructions on how to apply Abreva?

A. Apply a thin layer of medication to completely cover the area of the cold sore or the area of tingling/itching/redness/swelling and rub in gently, usually five times a day every 3–4 hours.

Q. Should a patient with active herpes labialis be treated in the dental chair?

A. No. The viral lesions are highly infectious during the first two days of appearance of the vesicles; the crusted lesions also have high viral titers and are infectious during this time.

Q. What are the potential adverse effects of systemic acyclovir?

A. Some adverse effects of systemic acyclovir include nausea, vomiting, itching, hypotension, diarrhea, dizziness, fever, and renal failure.

4.4.2 Antifungal Agents

Q. What types of oral fungal infections do dentists encounter?

A. Oral candidiasis involving the oropharyngeal area.

1) Acute pseudomembranous candidiasis also referred to as oral thrush.
2) Chronic atrophic candidiasis is known as denture sore mouth.
3) Angular cheilosis or angular cheilitis.

Q. What is oral thrush?

A. Oral thrush usually develops suddenly rather than taking a long time (chronic). Oral thrush causes slightly raised, creamy white, curd-like patches on the oral soft tissues or tongue. The affected site may bleed if the lesion is wiped. The lesions can spread to the esophagus.

Q. What are some causes of oral thrush?

A. Corticosteroids (asthmatics who use a corticosteroid inhaler must rinse the mouth and brush teeth after every use of the inhaler), antibiotics (due to suppression of normal bacterial flora), diabetes, HIV infection, cancer, dry mouth, oral contraceptives (due to increased estrogen levels).

Q. What is chronic atrophic candidiasis?

A. Chronic atrophic candidiasis is known as denture stomatitis. The lesion characteristically appears as a reddish outline on mucosal tissue seen under a denture. Usually it occurs when a denture is not removed for daily cleansing by the patient. Treatment options are listed in Table 4.4.

Table 4.4 Topical antifungal agent prescription

Drug	Prescription
Clotrimazole (Mycelex®) Supplied: troche 10 mg, cream 2% (Lotrimin®), vaginal suppositories (100 and 200 mg)	*For denture sore mouth or oral thrush* Rx clotrimazole troche 10 mg Disp: #60 troches Sig: Dissolve in the mouth slowly (over 15–30 min) one lozenge five times a day (every 3 hours) for 14 days. (Note: remove dentures if necessary) *For angular cheilitis or denture sore mouth (on inside lining of denture)* Rx clotrimazole cream 1% is available OTC without a prescription
Miconazole (Monistat®) Supplied: cream 2%, ointment 2%, solution, powder, spray, buccal 50 mg tablet (Oravig)	Rx Oravig 50 mg tablet Disp: #14 buccal tabs Sig: Apply one buccal tablet to the gum region once daily for 14 consecutive days. (Note: the tablet is flat on one side [marked with the letter "L"] and rounded on the other. The rounded side is applied to the gingiva in the depressed area above the lateral incisor. Once in place, use slight pressure on the outside of the lip for 30 seconds. The tablet will slowly dissolve throughout the day. It is used only once a day. Use alternating sides each time)
Nystatin (Mycostatin) Supplied: oral suspension (100 000 USP nystatin U/mL, ready to use suspension in 2 fl oz (60 mL) bottles with 0.5 mL, 1 mL, 1.5 mL, 2 mL calibrated dropper), pastilles (lozenge), vaginal tabs, cream, ointment, powder	*For denture oral mouth or oral thrush* Rx nystatin oral suspension 100 000 units/mL Disp: 1 bottle Sig: Take 1–2 mL dropped into the mouth and held for some time before swallowing. Note: this dose may be increased to 4–6 mL (400 000–600 000 units) four times daily for more severe infections. In infants and children, the dosage is 2 mL four times a day. Shake the bottle well before each use. Dentures should be removed before using the suspension. The liquid is directly measured and used with the dropper. Place half of the dose in each side of the mouth and hold it there or swish it around for a few minutes before swallowing. It can also be spit out. Do not eat or drink for 30 minutes after using the oral suspension. Rx nystatin pastille 200 000 units Disp: #60 pastilles Sig: Remove the dentures. Dissolve slowly and completely in the mouth one pastille five times a day for 14 days. (This can take up to 15–30 minutes. Do not chew or swallow pastilles whole. Continue to use pastilles for at least 48 hours after symptoms disappear. Store in the refrigerator.) *For angular cheilitis or denture sore mouth (on inside of denture)* Rx nystatin ointment Disp: 30 g tube Sig: Apply to affected area two times daily. Rx nystatin cream Disp: 30 g tube Sig: Apply to affected area two times daily.

Source: Medical Economics Staff (2000).

Q. What is angular cheilitis?

A. Angular cheilitis or angular cheilosis features sore red splits at each side of the mouth (commissures of the lip). Angular cheilitis used to be thought to be caused by vitamin B deficiency but it is actually due to a fungal infection (*Candida*). It is seen in patients without teeth or with ill-fitting dentures who have a loss of vertical dimension causing accumulation of saliva at the commissures of the lip (increased moisture).

Q. What treatment is there for angular cheilitis?

A. Elimination of the moisture should be the first step. Application of an antifungal topical ointment or cream is recommended. See Table 4.4.

Q. How is oral candidiasis treated?

A. The first step is to correct predisposing factors if possible. It is easier to treat oral thrush in healthy patients than immunocompromised patients. Antifungal agents must be taken for about two days after oral lesions disappear to avoid recurrence of lesions. Treatment usually lasts for 7–14 days. For the treatment of oral fungal infections, there are choices of different formulations including suspension, troche/pastille, creams and ointment, or vaginal tablets (used as a lozenge). See Table 4.4.

Q. Why prescribe a cream or ointment?

A. An ointment is a semisolid emulsion or suspension that is viscous and greasy. A cream is a semisolid emulsion that is viscous and nongreasy to mildly greasy but not as thick as an ointment. The cream or ointment is applied by the patient inside the denture and on the palate. This procedure will help the antifungal ointment/cream to stay in contact with the lesion. *Remember when writing a prescription for an ointment or cream for oral use, a pharmacist may not dispense that prescription if that product says "external use only."*

Q. Can all formulations be given to patients with a high-risk for dental caries?

A. No. The suspension and troches/pastille formulations contain sugar (sucrose) and should not be given to patients with high-risk caries because these formulations remain in the mouth for prolonged periods of time. The oral suspension also contains saccharin sodium. Have the patient suck on vaginal tablets such as nystatin vaginal tablets.

Q. What is Oravig®?

A. Oravig is miconazole buccal tablets 50 mg. It is the first product available as a once-daily dosing for oral thrush. It is also orally dissolving.

Q. How is Oravig applied?

A. Oravig is supplied as a 50 mg tablet. The tablet is flat on one side (marked with the letter "L") and rounded on the other. The rounded side is applied to the gingiva in the depressed area above the lateral incisor. Once in place, use slight pressure on the outside of the lip for 30 seconds. The tablet will slowly dissolve throughout the day. It is used only once a day. Use alternating sides each time (www.oravig.com).

Q. What is Mycostatin®?

A. Mycostatin is the brand name for nystatin. It is acceptable to prescribe nystatin, the generic substitute. When prescribing for an oral fungal lesion, the oral suspension can be prescribed for the patient to swish in the mouth and then swallow. The oral suspension contains 100 000 units of nystatin per mL. The inactive ingredients include artificial flavoring, FD&C yellow #10, alcohol, sucrose, purified water, glycerin, sodium citrate, magnesium aluminum silicate, saccharin sodium, xanthan gum, benzaldehyde, edetate calcium disodium, polysorbate 80, methylparaben, and propylparaben. The bottles come in 24, 48, and 100 mL volumes.

Q. What are some common adverse effects of oral nystatin?
A. Diarrhea, nausea, vomiting, and rash.

Q. What are some antifungal drugs that can be prescribed to patients?
A. For a patient with denture sore mouth, a recommendation would be to prescribe nystatin oral suspension, nystatin pastille, or clotrimazole troche if there are no contraindications (e.g., high risk for caries) and then to prescribe an ointment to be applied to the denture base and placed in the mouth. See Table 4.4.

Q. Which antifungal agent should be used initially in the treatment of oral candidiasis?
A. Clotrimazole troches or nystatin oral suspension, pastilles or vaginal tablets should be used before an azole such as fluconazole (Diflucan®) because these agents are as effective and less expensive than the azoles.

Q. When should a systemic antifungal drug be used to treat oral candidiasis?
A. Systemic antifungal agents should be prescribed in severe cases that do not respond to topical treatment for at least seven days or if relapse occurs after topical treatment, especially in immunocompromised patients.

Q. What systemic antifungal drug can be prescribed to the above patient?
A. Ketoconazole (Nizoral®) or fluconazole (Diflucan) tablets. With ketoconazole, it is important to monitor liver function because hepatotoxicity is one of its adverse effects. Fluconazole is probably more suitable.

Q. What is the adult dose for fluconazole for oropharyngeal candidiasis?
A. *Supplied*: 50, 100, 150, and 200 mg.
Dose: LD 200 mg on the first day, followed by 100 mg once daily for 14 days.

Q. Should the dosage interval for fluconazole be adjusted in renal impairment?
A. No. Fluconazole is eliminated by renal excretion as an unchanged drug. There is no need to adjust the dosage or dosing interval in patients with renal impairment.

Q. Are there any drug interactions with fluconazole?
A. Yes, there are many. Fluconazole is a potent inhibitor of CYP P450 isoenyzmes and a moderate inhibitor of CYP3A4. The following drugs interact with fluconazole: warfarin, oral hypoglycemics, phenytoin, cyclosporine, nonsteroidal antiinflammatory drugs (NSAIDs) (ibuprofen), oral contraceptives, calcium channel blockers, azithromycin, carbamazepine, celecoxib (Celebrex®), "statin" drugs for lowering cholesterol (simvastatin [Zocor®], rosuvastatin [Crestor®], lovastatin [Mevacor®], pravastatin [Pravachol®])], and losartan (Cozaar®).

Q. Besides management of oral fungal infections, what else should be emphasized with the patient?

A. Maintenance of good oral hygiene. Inform the patient of the importance of taking out their denture at night and cleaning it.

4.5   Prescribing for Acute Dental Pain

4.5.1   General Considerations

Pain is classified as acute (short duration, easily diagnosed with a predictable prognosis, and treatment successful with analgesics) or chronic (pain lasting a long time – months to years, difficult to localize origin of pain, and treatment involves many disciplines). Dental pain is acute and nociceptive (nociceptors are nerves that sense tissue damage – not caused by injury in the nervous system). Severity of pain is classified as mild, moderate, and severe.

Q. What are the different classifications of analgesics?

A.
- Aspirin
- Acetaminophen
- NSAIDs: nonselective and selective
- Opioids

Q. What should be reviewed before prescribing an analgesic?

A. The patient's medical history/condition, vital signs, status of liver and kidneys, medication use, and assessment of the severity of pain.

Q. What is the decision-making process for prescribing for acute dental pain?

A. NSAIDs are the first-line analgesics that in optimal doses may be better than single opioids and just as effective as a combination opioid (Hersh et al. 2011).

Q. Can analgesics be prescribed before the surgical dental procedure is started?

A. It is controversial whether preemptive analgesics decrease the severity of postsurgical pain (Costa et al. 2015); however, preoperative administration of an NSAID 45 minutes before local anesthesia has been documented to obtain more profound anesthesia and the patient was more contented (Pozzi and Gallelli 2011)

4.5.2   Aspirin

Q. What is the classification of aspirin?

A. Aspirin is a salicylate and not a NSAID like ibuprofen.

Q. What is aspirin's analgesic mechanism of action?

A. Aspirin acts peripherally, not centrally, inhibiting the formation of prostaglandins by blocking the cyclooxygenase (COX) enzymes at the receptors for pain, which is the source of the pain (due to inflammation).

Q. What is low-dose aspirin?

A. Low-dose aspirin is only used in the prevention of heart attack and strokes in certain suscepti-ble individuals. It is not used as an analgesic or for the reduction of inflammation. It is dis-cussed in detail in Chapter 7.

Q. Why does aspirin cause an increased bleeding time?

A. In the gastrointestinal tract and blood, aspirin breaks down into salicylate (salicylic acid) and acetic acid. The acetic acid irreversibly binds to COX-1 within the platelets, preventing the formation of thromboxane A_2 (a potent vasoconstrictor which induces platelet aggregation), resulting in a decrease in the ability to form clots and increased bleeding time. Since platelets are nonnucleated cells and incapable of synthesizing new COX enzymes, the effect lasts for the life of the platelet which is about seven days, at which time new platelets are formed. The salicylate portion has analgesic and antiinflammatory actions. A dose of aspirin as small as 40 mg will have a strong effect on platelet function and prolong the bleeding time for up to five days (Page 2005). Thus, bleeding effects are not dose dependent as higher doses may be less effective in altering platelet function (Boss et al. 1985).

Q. What are cyclooxygenase enzymes?

A. Cyclooxygenase enzymes are endogenous enzymes normally found in most body cells and are responsible for tissue homeostasis. There are essentially two types of cyclooxygenase isoen-zymes: COX-1 and COX-2. COX-1 is considered to be the "housekeeping" or protective enzyme responsible for tissue homeostasis and serves to protect the mucosa in the gastrointestinal tract and uterus, maintain renal blood flow, and maintain normal platelet function. COX-2 is pro-duced by cells only in the presence of inflammation and is found in low amounts in the tissues (Awtry and Loscalzo 2000).

Q. What is the mechanism of action of antiinflammatory drugs?

A. Antiinflammatory drugs, including aspirin and NSAIDs, reduce inflammation which is caused by COX-2 by inhibiting the cyclooxygenase enzymes. However, the drug not only inhibits COX-2 but it also inhibits the protective COX-1, causing adverse effects of these drugs (e.g., bleeding).

Q. What is the mechanism of aspirin's effect on gastrointestinal bleeding?

A. Gastrointestinal bleeding is due to a combination of a local irritating effect on the gastric mucosa due to particles of undissolved aspirin, aspirin's antiplatelet aggregation effect and inhibition of protective function of the prostaglandins, specifically COX-1 (Cowan 1992). Aspirin-induced gas-trointestinal toxicity is dose dependent in the range of 30–1300 mg per day (Patrono et al. 2004).

Q. What is Reye syndrome?

A. Reye syndrome is a rare but serious sequela of influenza, chickenpox, and other viral infec-tions, usually in children. Symptoms include repetitive vomiting, lethargy, headache, and fever. Damage to the brain and liver occurs at later stages with organ failure and death. The cause is unknown. Aspirin has been implicated in causing Reye syndrome in children with a viral infection. Aspirin should not be given to children with a suspected viral infection.

Q. If a patient is taking low-dose aspirin, do INR values need to be determined before dental pro-cedures that cause bleeding?

A. No. INR values only need to be known for anticoagulants such as warfarin (Coumadin). Aspirin is an antiplatelet drug, not an anticoagulant.

Q. What are some adverse effects of aspirin?

A. Gastrointestinal irritation, gastrointestinal ulceration, increased bleeding time, tinnitus, hypoglycemic effect (aspirin should not be used in diabetics).

Q. What factors influence whether to stop low-dose aspirin before extractions, scaling and root planing or periodontal/implant/oral surgery?

A. Factors include the cardiovascular condition (e.g, previous stents), how long the patient has been on aspirin (e.g., <1 month or >2 years), and American Society of Anesthesiology (ASA) classification (Plümer et al. 2017). If needed, obtain a consultation from the patient's treating physician.

   Many clinical studies have concluded that patients taking aspirin to prevent blood clot formation should continue to take the aspirin during surgical procedures because there is an increased risk for emboli formation. In most cases, bleeding can be controlled by local means (Verma 2014). If required, obtain a consultation from the patient's treating physician.

Q. How much blood loss occurs in a patient taking low-dose aspirin during periodontal surgery?

A. A 2012 clinical study confirmed previous studies that blood loss during periodontal surgery is minimal. The amount of blood lost during open flap debridement and regenerative periodontal surgery is approximately 6.0–145.1 mL (overall mean of 59.47 ± 38.2 mL) which is much less than blood loss during maxillofacial surgery. Patients taking 100 mg/day of aspirin had a mean blood loss of 43.26 ± 31.5 mL which was not clinically or statistically different from patients who did not take aspirin (Zigdon et al. 2012).

4.5.3 Nonsteroidal Antiinflammatory Drugs (NSAIDs)

Q. What are the indications for use of NSAIDs?

A. NSAID indications are as an analgesic (for mild to moderate pain), an antiinflammatory, and an antipyretic (fever reducer).

Q. What is the mechanism of action of NSAIDs?

A. NSAIDs have a similar mechanism of action to aspirin. They inhibit prostaglandin synthesis by blocking the COX enzymes in the arachidonic acid pathway. Prostaglandins are fatty acids found in most tissues and organs in the body. They are produced in the cell membrane of platelets, endothelium, uterine, and mast cells. Prostaglandin (PG) E_2 is a mediator of inflammation in diseases such as rheumatoid arthritis and periodontal diseases. When released from the damaged cell membrane during mechanical/tissue trauma (e.g., dental surgery), prostaglandins act locally with a short half-life of about five minutes (Schwartz 2006). Some actions of prostaglandins include aggregation of platelets, blood pressure control, inflammation modulation, increase in GFR, increase in uterine contraction and causing fever. Prostaglandins are metabolized into many proinflammatory substances that cause pain and fever. COX-2 plays a role in inflammatory conditions. The antiinflammatory action of NSAIDs is probably due to the inhibition of COX-2. However, it is not selective in inhibiting COX-2 and also inhibits the protective actions of COX-1, leading to many adverse effects including ulcers, bleeding, and gastrointestinal distress. NSAIDs than inhibit both COX-1 and COX-2 are called nonselective NSAIDs and the prototype is ibuprofen. Celebrex is a selective COX-2 NSAID because it only inhibits COX-2 and not COX-1 (Figure 4.2).

Q. What are the different kinds of nonselective NSAIDs used in dentistry?

A. See Table 4.5.

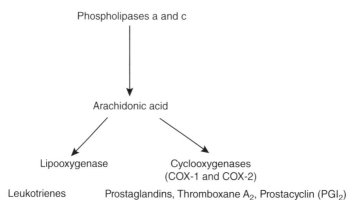

Trauma to blood vessel (platelet) wall causes:

Phospholipids (bound in cell membrane)

Phospholipases a and c

Arachidonic acid

Lipooxygenase   Cyclooxygenases
(COX-1 and COX-2)

Leukotrienes   Prostaglandins, Thromboxane A_2, Prostacyclin (PGI_2)

(involved in allergic reactions)

Figure 4.2 The sequence of prostaglandin synthesis.

Table 4.5 Common nonsteroidal antiinflammatory drugs

Drug	Supplied/dosage	OTC/Rx	Onset/duration of effect
Diflunisal (Dolobid®)	Supplied: 250 mg, 500 mg tablets Dose: 1000 mg followed by 500 mg q8–12h with meals (maximum 1500 mg/day)	Rx	Onset: 1 h Duration: 12 h
Etodolac (Lodine®)	Supplied: 400 mg, 500 mg tablets; 200 mg, 300 mg capsules Dose: 200–400 mg q6–8h with meals (maximum 1200 mg/day)	Rx	Onset: 30 minutes Duration: 4–12 h
Ibuprofen (Advil, Nuprin®, Motrin®)	Supplied: 400 mg, 600 mg, 800 mg tablets Dose: 400 mg q4h with meals. 600 mg q6h with meals (maximum 2400 mg/day)	Rx; OTC 200 mg	Onset: 1 h Duration: 6–8 h
Ketorolac tromethamine (oral: Toradol, nasal spray: Sprix®)	Supplied: 10 mg tablets 15.75/ nasal spray Dose: Oral: 10 mg q4–6h (maximum 40 mg/day). Short-term use only (≤5 days) Nasal spray: 18–65 years of age: 1 spray in each nostril ≥65 years old: 1 spray in one nostril	Rx for both tablets and nasal spray	Onset: Oral 30–60 minutes Nasal spray within 20 minutes. Maximum concentration in blood is 30–45 minutes. Duration: Oral 6–8 h Nasal spray 6–8 h

Table 4.5 (Continued)

Drug	Supplied/dosage	OTC/Rx	Onset/duration of effect
Naproxen sodium (Aleve, Anaprox®)	Supplied: Aleve: 220 mg Anaprox: 275 mg tablets Dose: Anaprox: 275–550 mg q12h or 500 mg initially, then 275 mg q6–8h Aleve: 1 tab q8–12h (maximum 1375 mg/day)	Rx; OTC: Aleve 220 mg	Onset: 30 minutes Duration: 7–12 h
Naproxen (Naprosyn®)	Supplied: 250, 375, 500 mg tablets Dose: initial dose 500 mg followed by 250 mg q12h (maximum 1250 mg/day)	Rx	Onset: 30 minutes Duration: 7–12 h

Source: Medical Economics Staff (2000).

Q. Are there differences between NSAIDs?

A. Yes. NSAIDs differ in their potency and duration of action. However, there is no evidence that any one NSAID is more effective than another. If two people take an identical drug and dose, their individual response may be considerably different. It is sometimes necessary to try one drug for a week, and then try a different one to find the optimal combination of these factors. Lower doses of NSAIDs, as recommended for use with nonprescription NSAIDs, are adequate to relieve pain in most people. To fully treat inflammation, a higher dose must be taken on a regular basis for several weeks before the full antiinflammatory benefit is realized.

If the initial dose of NSAIDs does not improve symptoms, either increase the dose gradually or switch to another NSAID. If the patient is taking one NSAID, a second NSAID should not be taken at the same time. This is a synergistic type of drug interaction where the effect of two or more drugs when taken together is greater than if given separately.

Q. What is Toradol® and can it be prescribed to a dental patient after surgery?

A. The generic name for Toradol is ketorolac and it is a NSAID which has been found to be as effective as 6–12 mg of morphine, making it more potent than other NSAIDs. It has been prescribed as an alternative to opioids for postextraction acute pain control (Abbas et al. 2004; Fricke et al. 1993; Walton et al. 1993).

Q. Is there a **Black Box Warning** for ketorolac?

A. Yes. The **Black Box Warning** is that ketorolac is indicated for moderate to severe pain that requires analgesic action on an opioid level. As with any NSAID, there is serious gastrointestinal bleeding and ulcer formation and it is contraindicated in patients with active peptic ulcer disease (PUD). As with any NSAID, there are increased cardiovascular thrombotic events, such as heart attack and stroke. Ketorolac is contraindicated in patients with advanced kidney impairment. Ketorolac should *not* be prescribed to patients already taking aspirin or another NSAID. Dosage adjustment is necessary in patients >65 years of age (www.rxlist.com).

Q. Why are ibuprofen and naproxen sodium classified as OTC medications?

A. The FDA ruled that ibuprofen 200 mg and Aleve 220 mg pain relief dose were safe for self-care. But the higher antiinflammatory doses were ruled unsafe for self-care.

Q. Are OTC analgesics as effective as the prescription-strength NSAIDs?

A. OTC medicines are intended for use for short periods of time and are usually intended for self-care, while prescription NSAIDs can be for long-term or chronic use when directed by a physician. OTC NSAIDs are usually used at a lower dose than prescription NSAIDs and are intended for self-limiting conditions and are not intended to be used for long durations.

Q. Which NSAID has a longer-lasting analgesic effect?

A. Naproxen has a longer-lasting effect than most other NSAIDs.

Q. Can Celebrex be used for dental pain?

A. It is FDA approved for acute pain. It does not replace nonselective NSAIDs for short-term acute dental pain. It is not any more effective than ibuprofen. Celebrex (celecoxib) is a selective COX-2 inhibitor, only inhibiting COX-2 and not affecting COX-1 and the associated adverse effects. It is also associated with a significantly greater number of thrombotic cardiovascular events than the other NSAIDs. There is a **Black Box Warning** stating that there "may be an increased risk of serious and potentially fatal cardiovascular thrombotic events, myocardial infarction (heart attack) and stroke; risk may increase with duration of use; possible increased risk if cardiovascular disease or cardiovascular disease risk factors are present" (Jeske 2002).

Q. Is there a difference between naproxen sodium and naproxen?

A. Sodium, a salt, is formulated with naproxen to increase the rate of absorption to reach therapeutic blood levels faster.

Q. When should an NSAID be recommended or prescribed?

A. In patients with mild to moderate pain. NSAIDs are indicated as an analgesic, antiinflammatory, and antipyretic.

Q. Why do individuals react differently to different NSAIDs?

A. Each NSAID causes a varying degree of COX-1/COX-2 inhibition. Although there is no evidence than any one NSAID is more effective than another, some are more potent than others. For example, ibuprofen may vary in effectiveness because of alterations in metabolism associated with a P450 cytochrome polymorphism, a genetic alteration (CYP2C9). If a patient does not respond to one NSAID at the maximum therapeutic level, another NSAID should be prescribed because patients may vary in their analgesic response to the different NSAIDs.

Q. How long does it take for an NSAID to take effect?

A. It takes about 30–60 minutes to achieve a profound analgesic effect of an NSAID.

Q. What is the ceiling effect of analgesia with aspirin and NSAIDs?

A. Aspirin and NSAIDs display a ceiling effect whereby a dose beyond the maximum recommended dose does not provide more analgesic effect but rather can increase the incidence of adverse effects. For example, doses above 1000 mg every six hours do not provide significantly greater analgesia than 650 mg every four hours. The duration of analgesia may be greater with

1000 mg but the amount of analgesia is not increased. If the ceiling analgesic dose of ibuprofen is 1000 mg and the pain is not relieved with that dose, then a different, more potent analgesic should be prescribed (Schwartz 2006).

Q. Can a patient with asthma or aspirin sensitivity take an NSAID?

A. NSAIDs are contraindicated in patients who have experienced bronchospasm, angioedema or allergic reactions to aspirin or other NSAIDs. Many individuals with asthma also have sensitivity to drugs such as NSAIDs and aspirin that can precipitate an asthmatic attack. A condition called Samter's triad has clinical features including asthma, aspirin sensitivity, and nasal polyps. These patients react to aspirin and NSAIDs and cannot take them. The reason for this reaction is most likely that when NSAIDs or aspirin inhibit the COX enzymes in the arachidonic acid cascade, it causes a shutdown in the other pathway whereby leukotrienes are produced which are involved in an asthmatic/allergic response.

Q. Are there any precautions when prescribing or recommending NSAIDs to a patient with cardiovascular disease, including if they are taking antihypertensive medications?

A. Yes. As mentioned above, all NSAIDs have a **Black Box Warning** for cardiovascular adverse events (Meek et al. 2010). Cardiovascular risk needs to be addressed before prescribing any NSAID. There are risks of thrombotic reactions (heart attack and stroke) that can lead to death. The chances are increased with longer use of NSAIDs and in patients who have preexisting heart disease. NSAIDs should not be prescribed before or after coronary artery bypass graft (CABG). Celebrex and nonselective NSAIDs have a **Black Box Warning** that states that there "may be an increased risk of serious and potentially fatal cardiovascular thrombotic events, myocardial infarction (heart attack) and stroke; risk may increase with duration of use; possible increased risk if cardiovascular disease or cardiovascular disease risk factors are present." There are many theories about why NSAIDs increase the cardiovascular risk and more research is needed (Elliott 2010). Other cardiovascular adverse effects include increased blood pressure, angina, and tachycardia. For nonselective NSAIDs, the risk of thrombotic cardiovascular events is also present. The least harmful of the NSAIDs is naproxen (Trelle et al. 2011).

In addition, NSAIDs prescribed or recommended in doses that are antiinflammatory and analgesic may increase blood pressure in both normotensive and hypertensive individuals (Warner and Mitchell 2008). The average rise in blood pressure varies considerably (Snowden and Nelson 2011). In addition, NSAID use may reduce the effect of all antihypertensive drugs including diuretics (e.g., hydrochlorothiazide), beta-blockers (e.g., propranolol, atenolol, metoprolol, acebutolol, timolol, nadolol), angiotensin-converting enzyme (ACE) inhibitors (e.g., enalapril, lisinopril, ramipril, quinapril, captopril) except calcium channel blockers (e.g., diltiazem, verapamil, nifedipine, felodipine, nicardipine, amlodipine) (Snowden and Nelson 2011). This effect is most likely dose dependent, which means that the higher the dose taken, the more hypertensive effect is seen. It is recommended not to prescribe NSAIDs for more than five days if patients are taking antihypertensive drugs (except calcium channel blockers) (Grover et al. 2005; Warner and Mitchell 2008). Aspirin, but not low-dose aspirin, has the same effect on blood pressure (Bautista and Vera 2010; Zanchetti et al. 2002).

Q. What is the mechanism of the hypotensive effect of NSAIDs?

A. It involves inhibition of COX-2 in the kidneys, which causes vasoconstriction and reduces sodium excretion and increases intravascular volume.

Q. What happens when NSAIDs are prescribed to a patient taking ACE inhibitors?

A. Administration of NSAIDs and ACE inhibitors in combination may cause acute renal failure and serious hyperkalemia (increased potassium blood levels) in patients with severe heart failure, preexisting renal disease, or hypovolemic states. Patients need to be closely monitored concerning their renal function and serum potassium levels.

Q. What are the different adverse effects of NSAIDs?

A. Gastrointestinal distress, platelet function inhibition, renal dysfunction (decrease blood flow), and serious gastroduodenal ulcers (Meek et al. 2010). Also, there is a **Black Box Warning** for all NSAIDs for gastrointestinal bleeding, ulceration and stomach or intestine perforation, which can be fatal; may occur at any time during use without warning; elderly patients are at greater risk for serious gastrointestinal events. It is best to limit NSAID use to the lowest effective dose and for the shortest duration (Davison 2019).

Q. Do enteric-coated aspirin or NSAIDs or buffered aspirin reduce GI toxicity and cause less GI tract bleeding?

A. Not really. It should not be assumed that enteric-coated or buffered tablets are less likely to cause GI tract bleeding than taking tablets that are not specially formulated (Patrono et al. 2004).

Q. Why do NSAIDs cause kidney damage?

A. NSAIDs cause a reduction in blood flow to the kidneys, interstitial nephritis, and papillary necrosis, especially in high-risk patients with decreased renal blood perfusion. In patients taking high doses of NSAIDs, renal failure can occur. By reducing the blood flow to the kidneys, they work more slowly so that fluid builds up, causing high blood pressure. Fluid retention is the most common NSAID-related renal complication that can occur in any healthy individual even without renal insufficiency. It is only clinically detectable in <5% of patients and is reversible when the NSAID is discontinued. The patient should be warned about this effect (Katz 2002).

   Renal failure can occur in people taking NSAIDs in large amounts and for long periods of time. NSAIDs can induce two different forms of acute kidney injury: hemodynamically mediated and acute interstitial nephritis, which is often accompanied by the nephrotic syndrome. The former and perhaps the latter are directly related to the reduction in prostaglandin synthesis induced by the NSAID. Acute kidney injury can occur with any NSAID. Although renal prostaglandins are primarily vasodilators, they do not play a major role in the regulation of renal hemodynamics in normal subjects since the basal rate of prostaglandin synthesis is relatively low. By contrast, the release of these hormones (particularly prostacyclin and PGE$_2$) is increased by underlying glomerular disease, renal insufficiency, hypercalcemia, and the vasoconstrictors angiotensin II and norepinephrine. The secretion of the latter hormones is increased in states of effective volume depletion, such as heart failure, cirrhosis, and true volume depletion due to gastrointestinal or renal salt and water losses. In these settings, vasodilator prostaglandins act to preserve renal blood flow and GFR by relaxing preglomerular resistance. This is particularly important with effective volume depletion, in which the prostaglandins antagonize the vasoconstrictor effects of angiotensin II and norepinephrine. In glomerular disease, however, the increase in prostaglandin production seems to maintain the GFR in the presence of a reduction in glomerular capillary permeability.

Q. Do NSAIDs have a long-lasting effect on bleeding?

A. No. NSAIDs do not cause bleeding but rather make the bleeding worse. They prolong bleeding time but do not alter blood clotting or platelet count. NSAIDs reversibly inhibit COX-1-mediated platelet granule release and prevent thromboxane A_2 synthesis. The effect on platelets is temporary and platelet function returns to normal in about one day after discontinuing the NSAID.

Q. Do NSAIDs have the same antiplatelet effect as aspirin?

A. Yes, NSAIDs inhibit platelet aggregation through a similar mechanism to aspirin but NSAIDs reversibly bind to the COX on platelet membranes so the antiplatelet effect does not last as long as with aspirin and is not an indication for prophylaxis against strokes, as is aspirin.

Q. Are there any contraindications with Celebrex?

A. Celebrex is contraindicated in patients hypersensitive to Celebrex and allergic to sulfa/sulfa drugs such as sulfonamides (e.g., Bactrim®).

Q. Should an NSAID be discontinued before commencing dental surgery?

A. No. In fact, ibuprofen can be taken one hour before surgery to help reduce postoperative pain.

Q. If a patient is taking an NSAID, do INR values need to be determined before dental procedures that cause bleeding?

A. No. INR values only need to be known for anticoagulants such as warfarin (Coumadin). NSAIDs affect the platelets and are not an anticoagulant.

Q. Is there a concern with bleeding during a dental procedure in a patient taking an NSAID?

A. Not significantly. Aspirin is the only analgesic that significantly prolongs bleeding time because its antiplatelet action is irreversible while NSAIDs' antiplatelet action is mild and reversible when the drug is eliminated from the body (NSAIDs bind weakly and reversibly to platelet cyclooxygenases).

Q. Are there any precautions/contraindications for NSAID use?

A. Yes. The major contraindications to NSAIDs include stomach problems (e.g., PUD), aspirin allergy (or sensitivity), bleeding problems (gastrointestinal bleeding), pregnancy, hepatic and renal disease, gastroesophageal reflux disease (GERD), chronic indigestion, cardiovascular disease, hypertension, antihypertensive drugs (except calcium channel blockers), and fluid retention.

Q. Can an NSAID be prescribed to someone who is anemic?

A. Yes, as long as the anemia is not due to bleeding from the gastrointestinal tract.

Q. Why are there so many dosages available with NSAIDs?

A. Because NSAIDs are indicated for pain relief and for antiinflammatory effects and higher doses are usually needed for antiinflammatory action.

Q. What is the maximum dose of ibuprofen?

A. The maximum dose of ibuprofen is 2400 mg in 24 hours.

Q. How should the patient be instructed to take ibuprofen?

A. Take with a full glass of water with meals and not on an empty stomach.

4.5.4 Acetaminophen

Q. What is the generic name for Tylenol®?

A. Acetaminophen or *N*-acetyl-*p*-aminophenol (APAP) in the US and paracetamol in other countries.

Q. What are the indications for the use of acetaminophen?

A. Mild to moderate dental pain and antipyretic. Acetaminophen has little peripheral antiinflammatory activity and does not inhibit platelet aggregation as do aspirin and NSAIDs.

Q. What is the safest analgesic for pregnant patients?

A. Acetaminophen.

Q. What is the mechanism of action of acetaminophen?

A. The analgesic effect is not clearly defined but acetaminophen acts centrally rather than peripherally at the nerve endings and produces its analgesic and antipyretic effect by inhibiting PGE_2 via selectively inhibiting COX-2 enzymes which are responsible for the formation of prostaglandins (Aronoff et al. 2006). Because of central nervous system (CNS) activity, acetaminophen's peripheral antiinflammatory activity is limited.

New insights have been gained into the mechanism of action of acetaminophen. Its clinical pharmacological characteristics reflect its inhibition of the two PGH_2 synthases. However, acetaminophen blocks this enzyme at its peroxidase catalytic rather than at the COX site. Therefore, the acetaminophen-mediated inhibition is sensitive to changes in the tissue peroxide levels; higher concentrations of peroxide in activated leukocytes and platelets block the effect of acetaminophen on inflammation and platelet thrombosis. Acetaminophen then can inhibit prostaglandins in the CNS, thus providing relief of pain and fever.

Q. Is there a **Black Box Warning** for acetaminophen?

A. Yes. In an attempt to reduce the risk of acetaminophen toxicity in the United States, many pharmaceutical/federal changes have been introduced since 2009. On 10 January 2011, the FDA notified healthcare professionals of a **Black Box Warning** for the potential for severe liver injury and a **Warning** highlighting the potential for allergic reactions (swelling of the face, mouth, and throat, difficulty breathing, itching or rash) will be added to the label of all prescription drug products that contain acetaminophen.

Additionally, in June 2009, the FDA recommended changing the maximum amount of OTC acetaminophen in any single dose to 325 mg. The reason for this was that severe liver damage and even death can occur due to lack of consumer awareness (www.guideline.gov/content.aspx?id=10222). The panel also recommended that the maximum single adult dose be lowered to 650 mg from 1000 mg and to lower the maximum daily dose for acetaminophen below its current 4000 mg. The maximum daily dose for extra-strength Tylenol was lowered from eight pills totaling 4 g (4000 mg) to six pills totaling 3000 mg. The patient must be aware of taking other products containing acetaminophen.

In January 2011, the FDA asked manufacturers of prescription acetaminophen/narcotic combination products to limit the amount of acetaminophen to 325 mg per unit dose. Johnson

& Johnson, manufacturers of Tylenol, already have voluntarily announced lower dosing instructions for Tylenol. A **Boxed Warning** stating that there is a potential for severe liver injury and a **Warning** highlighting the potential for allergic reactions (e.g., swelling of the face, mouth, and throat, difficulty breathing, itching, or rash) are being added to the label of all prescription drug products that contain acetaminophen (www.fda.gov/drugs/drug-safety-and-availability/fda-drug-safety-communication-prescription-acetaminophen-products-be-limited-325-mg-dosage-unit).

Q. Does acetaminophen affect bleeding?

A. No. Acetaminophen is not an antithrombotic agent, as is aspirin or NSAIDs. It is safe to give to patients with a previous history of gastric bleeding or ulcers.

Q. Why is there concern about using too much acetaminophen?

A. Acetaminophen overdose can result in severe hepatic necrosis leading to acute liver failure (ALF) and even death. Currently, the maximum amount of acetaminophen for an adult is not more than 4 g/day but there is ongoing debate to reduce the maximum amount to 3 g/day. The dose for children (<50 kg or 110 lb) is 6–12 mg/kg every four hours. The FDA revised OTC labeling as of 29 April 2010. Currently, the container must say "liver warning" with a risk of developing liver damage if the patient takes more than the maximum number of daily doses or if taken with other medications containing acetaminophen or the patient drinks three or more alcoholic beverages a day while taking acetaminophen. Not more than one product containing acetaminophen should be taken. Many OTC cold and cough medications also contain acetaminophen. It is important to warn the patient about the additive effect of acetaminophen from additional medications, including alcohol.

Q. Is there a ceiling analgesic effect for acetaminophen?

A. Yes. As with NSAIDs, acetaminophen has a ceiling analgesic effect whereby increasing the dose has no additional benefit. Doses above 1000 mg every six hours do not provide significantly greater analgesia than 650 mg every four hours and could cause more adverse effects, including liver toxicity. The duration of analgesia may be prolonged, but the amount of analgesia is not increased.

Q. What is the mechanism for liver toxicity?

A. With normal dosing, the majority of acetaminophen is metabolized in the liver to water-soluble sulfate and glucuronide conjugates which are eventually eliminated in the urine via the kidneys. A small percentage of acetaminophen also conjugates to *N*-acetyl-benzoquinoneimine (NAPQI), a potentially toxic metabolite that is excreted without consequences, which is further metabolized in the liver by glutathione. However, in an acute overdose, this pathway becomes dominant and acetaminophen-induced hepatotoxicity (liver failure) occurs when all stores of glutathione are depleted; NAPQI then binds to liver cells, causing liver necrosis. Alcohol and individuals with liver disease due to alcohol are contraindicated with acetaminophen because alcohol increases levels of NAPQI (www.medscape.com/viewarticle/410911_2). Hepatotoxicity is a leading cause of ALF. Merely taking two extra-strength Tylenol tablets more than four times a day can cause an overdose and it only takes a few days of exceeding the recommended daily dose to cause liver damage. Caution must be impressed upon the patient, including the use of other OTC products that also contain acetaminophen.

Q. Can repeated doses of slightly too much acetaminophen be toxic?

A. Yes. A clinical study in the United Kingdom reported that individuals who took repeated (more than a single dose at one time) doses of acetaminophen actually had "damage build-up" resulting in more liver damage and kidney dialysis. Repeated doses can also be more dangerous, and possibly fatal, than taking a single massive overdose. Additionally, when patients were asked why they took more than the recommended dose of acetaminophen, the answer was that they wanted more pain relief (Barclay 2011).

Q. Why are single low doses of acetaminophen not hepatotoxic?

A. Low doses of acetaminophen are not damaging because of the "threshold phenomenon." Toxicity to the liver does not occur until the glutathione content of the liver is depleted. If there is an adequate amount of glutathione, the threshold is not exceeded and there will not be any hepatotoxicity. This process, whereby more active metabolites are formed, is referred to as bioactivation (Fujimoto 1979). However, in an acute overdose or if the maximum daily dose is exceeded over a long time, metabolism by conjugation becomes saturated, and excess acetaminophen is metabolized to NAPQI, which is responsible for hepatocellular injury, death, and liver necrosis (Farrell et al. 2012).

Q. Are liver enzymes elevated while taking acetaminophen?

A. Yes. A study reported that an individual taking 4 g of acetaminophen a day for 14 days had elevated plasma alanine aminotransferase.

Q. What other condition can happen with acute liver disease?

A. The liver produces blood clotting factors so when there is liver disease, the INR is increased, resulting in decreased clotting.

Q. What are the adverse effects of acetaminophen?

A. Hepatotoxicity (either chronic use or acute overdose), less gastrointestinal distress and no platelet effect.

Q. What is the antidote for acetaminophen overdose?

A. *N*-acetylcysteine (Mucomyst®) must be administered within 12 hours of acetaminophen ingestion.

Q. Is acetaminophen as irritating to the stomach as aspirin and NSAIDs?

A. No, it does not cause gastric irritation or ulcerations.

Q. What are the different strengths of acetaminophen?

A. Regular strength: 325 mg
Extra strength (rapid release): 500 mg
Arthritis pain: 650 mg
Tylenol eight hour: 650 mg

Q. What is the usual dose for acetaminophen?

A. Regular strength: two tablets every 4–6 hours but not for more than 10 days. Maximum of 12 tablets in 24 hours.
Extra strength: two tablets, caplets or gel caps every 4–6 hours but not for more than 10 days. Maximum of eight caplets in 24 hours.

Arthritis pain: two gel caps every 8 hours but not for more than 10 days. Maximum of six gel caps in 24 hours.

Tylenol eight hour: two caplets every 8 hours but not for more than 10 days. Maximum of six caplets in 24 hours.

Q. What is the duration of action of a regular dose of acetaminophen?

A. About 4 hours.

Q. Is there a drug interaction between acetaminophen and warfarin?

A. Yes. In patients taking warfarin, the administration of acetaminophen elevates the INR, resulting in bleeding. If acetaminophen needs to be administered, it should be the lowest dose and for the shortest time. This interaction is proposed to be caused by inhibition of warfarin metabolism via hepatic cytochrome P450 enzymes (Bell 1998; Hylek et al. 1998).

4.5.5 Opioid Analgesics

Q. What is the difference, if any, between the terms "opiate," "opioid," and "narcotic"?

A. *Opiate* refers to natural substances derived from opium from the poppy plant. Morphine and codeine are examples of opiates that come from opium. More than 20 different alkaloids are obtained from the unripe seed of the opium poppy plant. The analgesic properties of opium have been known for hundreds of years. *Opioids* are substances that do not occur naturally and are manufactured and referred to as being semisynthetic or synthetic. Examples include:

- Semisynthetic: hydrocodone, oxycodone, hydromorphone
- Synthetic: meperidine, fentanyl, methadone.

  Narcotics, although a dated term, is still being used, with opiates being a subclass of narcotics.

Q. What are the different classifications of opiates/opioids?

A. Classification is based on duration of action and potency.
Short-acting: morphine (prototype), hydromorphone, oxycodone, hydrocodone, codeine, meperidine, fentanyl.
Long-acting: methadone, levorphanol, oxymorphone.

Q. What are the differences in potencies of the opioids?

A. Strong potency: morphine, methadone, meperidine, oxycodone, hydrocodone.
Moderate potency: codeine.

Q. Do opiate/opioid analgesics have a ceiling effect?

A. No. Because there is no maximum dose beyond which there is no more analgesic effect, all narcotics can supposedly provide the same amount of analgesia if administered in the same dosages and the analgesic response continues to improve as the dose is increased. The problem is that more of a narcotic is taken, increasing the risk for adverse effects and overdose (Cooper 1993).

Since there is no ceiling effect for opioids, dosage requirements vary widely among patients and opioids must be titrated to an acceptable level of analgesia or until side effects occur. Essentially, the dose must be increased until pain relief is obtained. A dosage increase of 10–20% during the first few days is appropriate with opioids. Elderly patients or those with comorbidities, such as pulmonary or CNS diseases, may require lower starting dosages. In addition, longer duration of analgesia has been reported for older patients, who commonly experience prolonged elimination of opioids (Zichterman 2007).

Q. Does tolerance develop to opioids?

A. Yes. Tolerance occurs when a constant opioid dosage produces a decreasing therapeutic response. More of the drug is necessary to produce the same effect that was obtained with the smaller dose. With the exception of constipation and miosis (constriction of the pupils), tolerance develops to opioid-induced adverse effects including respiratory depression, sedation and nausea. This means that constipation and visual changes will become bothersome for the patient. Tolerance to analgesic effects may occur within the first week or two of therapy and is usually characterized by a decrease in the duration of analgesia. After this time, tolerance to analgesia is relatively uncommon. If a patient has been stabilized on an opioid regimen and a dosage escalation is required, the development of new pathology is the most common cause.

Q. Can a patient develop physical dependence on opioids?

A. Physical dependence is an expected therapeutic drug effect that is characterized by the development of a withdrawal syndrome after therapy is rapidly stopped. Physical dependence may be expected in patients who have taken repeated doses of an opioid for more than two weeks. Withdrawal syndrome may be avoided by tapering doses by 10–20% per day.

Q. Is potency of an opioid important?

A. Yes. When comparing potency of different opioids, it is the amount of drug necessary to produce a therapeutic effect when the two drugs have the same mechanism of action and given the same route of administration. For example, when administered intramuscularly (IM), 120 mg codeine is equal to 10 mg of morphine (the prototype opioid); morphine is much more potent. Also, 30 mg codeine orally is equal to less than 2 mg IM morphine.

For example, 45 mg of codeine produces the same amount of pain relief as 5 mg oxycodone and 7.5 mg of hydrocodone.

Q. Why is morphine not as effective orally as codeine, hydrocodone, and oxycodone?

A. Morphine undergoes extensive first-pass metabolism. Before reaching the systemic circulation and brain, it goes to the liver where much is metabolized before it can reach therapeutic levels in the blood. Almost 90% of morphine is metabolized in the liver before it gets to the blood.

Q. Why is codeine not adequate for moderate to severe dental pain?

A. Codeine is a weak analgesic and should be used only for mild to moderate pain. Codeine cannot be used for severe pain because of its lack of potency; a 60 mg dose produces less analgesia than two 325 mg aspirin tablets.

Q. Which are the opioid antagonists?

A. Antagonists inhibit the effects of opioids in an overdose. Naloxone (Narcan®) is a commonly used antagonist that is administered intramuscularly, intravenously or subcutaneously. Antagonist drugs bind to the receptor but have no therapeutic action, whereas agonists bind to the receptors and have a therapeutic effect.

Q. When should a narcotic analgesic be prescribed?

A. For moderate to severe pain. A narcotic should never be prescribed alone unless it is in combination with a nonnarcotic such as acetaminophen or ibuprofen. The nonopioid plus the opioid have a greater synergistic analgesic effect.

Q. What does codeine get metabolized to?

A. Codeine is a prodrug. It is different from the other opioids in that it needs to be metabolized to morphine via the cytochrome P450 (CYP2D6) enzymes in the liver which is the active form for an analgesic effect. A problem with effective analgesic effect occurs if a patient is taking a drug that inhibits the CYP2D6 enzyme (e.g., a phenothiazine, haloperidol, fluoxetine, or paroxetine), thereby inhibiting the metabolism of codeine, resulting in reduced analgesic efficacy. Additionally, up to 10% of the population lack the CYP2D6 enzyme and may not achieve analgesia with codeine-containing products.

Q. Why is codeine alone not used for pain management?

A. About 10% of Caucasians are deficient in the cytochrome (CYP2D6) enzymes that metabolize codeine, resulting in lack of efficacy so that codeine alone is a relatively poor analgesic.

Q. What is the minimum dose of codeine that is an effect analgesic dose when used in a combination nonopioid?

A. 30 mg, but 60 mg is recommended as the initial dose. Codeine is not needed for mild pain, only moderate pain. Thus, a minimum of 60 mg is probably required for pain relief. A 60 mg dose of codeine produces less analgesia than two 325 mg aspirin tablets. That is why it is used in combination with a nonnarcotic.

Q. Does codeine dose need to be adjusted in liver and renal impairment?

A. Yes. Codeine is excreted in the urine via the kidneys and is not recommended in patients with severe renal impairment.

Q. Which opioid is best used in a patient with renal impairment?

A. Hydromorphone, due to minimal changes in kinetics (Davison 2019).

Q. What are the different available formulations and doses of codeine?

A. Codeine phosphate is usually given in combination with acetaminophen as follows.

Tylenol #1 (7.5 mg codeine/300 mg acetaminophen)
Tylenol #2 (15 mg codeine/300 mg acetaminophen)
Tylenol #3 (30 mg codeine/300 mg acetaminophen)
Tylenol #4 (60 mg codeine/300 mg acetaminophen)

Q. What is the usual dose of codeine/acetaminophen?

A. 30–60 mg (Tylenol #3 or #4), even though # 3 is mostly prescribed (one to two tabs q4–6h for dental pain; maximum dose is 12 tabs over 24 hours). It makes more sense to prescribe two tablets rather than one because two tablets equal 60 mg codeine and 600 mg acetaminophen. If Tylenol #4 were prescribed, there is 60 mg codeine but only 300 mg acetaminophen and it is best to have 600 mg acetaminophen which will provide most of the analgesic effect.

Q. What are other opioid/nonopioid combinations?

A. A combination of 400 mg ibuprofen and 15 mg hydrocodone is a better analgesic choice than 400 mg ibuprofen alone.

Q. When prescribing combination opioid analgesics, is the amount of acetaminophen as important as if it were used alone and not in combination with an opioid?

A. Yes. Remember that the maximum amount of acetaminophen is 3–4 g/day or 3000–4000 mg/day. For example, Vicodin® ES contains 7.5 mg hydrocodone and 750 mg acetaminophen so five tablets of Vicodin ES provide the maximum amount of acetaminophen per day and 37.5 mg of hydrocodone. On the other hand, Vicodin has 5 mg hydrocodone and 500 mg acetaminophen so eight tablets are the maximum amount of acetaminophen to be taken in 24 hours and 40 mg of hydrocodone. The patient can take six tablets of Vicodin HP (10 mg hydrocodone/600 mg acetaminophen) which will provide the maximum of 3960 mg acetaminophen and 60 mg hydrocodone. Therefore, it is best to prescribe Vicodin HP for moderate to severe pain (see Table 4.6).

Table 4.6 Opioid/nonopioid combination products for dental pain

	Brand name	Dosage
Hydrocodone/acetaminophen combinations (C-II)		
2.5 mg hydrocodone bitartrate/500 mg acetaminophen	Lortab® 2.5/500	1 tab q4h
5 mg hydrocodone bitartrate/500 mg acetaminophen	Vicodin C-III Lortab 5/500 Lorcet® HD	1 tab q4h
7.5 mg hydrocodone bitartrate/325 mg acetaminophen	Narco® 7.5/325	1 tab q4h
7.5 hydrocodone bitartrate/750 mg acetaminophen	Vicodin ES	1 tab q4h
7.5 mg hydrocodone bitartrate/500 mg acetaminophen	Lortab 7.5/500	1 tab q4h
7.5 mg hydrocodone bitartrate/650 mg acetaminophen	Lorcet Plus	1 tab q4h
10 mg hydrocodone bitartrate/325 mg acetaminophen	Narco 10/325	1 tab q4h
10 mg hydrocodone bitartrate/660 mg acetaminophen	Vicodin HP	1 tab q4h
10 mg hydrocodone bitartrate/500 mg acetaminophen	Lortab 10/500	1 tab q4h
7.5 mg hydrocodone/200 mg ibuprofen	Vicoprofen®	1 tab q4h

Table 4.6 (Continued)

	Brand name	Dosage
Oxycodone/acetaminophen combinations (C-II)		
1.5 mg oxycodone HCl/325 mg acetaminophen 5 mg oxycodone HCl/325 mg acetaminophen 7.5 mg oxycodone HCl/325 mg acetaminophen 10 mg oxycodone HCl/325 mg acetaminophen 7.5 mg oxycodone HCl/500 mg acetaminophen 10 oxycodone HCl/650 mg acetaminophen	Percocet (must indicate the strength prescribed)	1 tab q6h
5 mg oxycodone HCl/500 mg acetaminophen	Tylox	1 tab q6h
5 mg oxycodone HCl/400 mg ibuprofen	Combunox®	1 tab q4h
4.5 mg oxycodone HCl/0.38 mg aspirin	Percodan	1 tab q4h
16 mg dihydrocodeine/325 mg aspirin	Synalgos DC®	1 tab q4h
Controlled-release tablets: 10, 15, 20, 30, 40, 60, 80, and 160 mg (60, 80, and 160 mg are used in opioid-tolerant patients only)	OxyContin	Not recommended for dental pain. OxyContin (oxycodone HCl) is only indicated for postoperative use if the patient is already receiving the drug prior to surgery or if the postoperative pain is expected to be moderate to severe and persist for an extended period of time; around-the-clock dosing (www.rxlist.com/oxycontin-drug.htm)
Centrally acting analgesics		
50 mg tramadol (alone not recommended for acute dental pain) (C-IV)	Ultram®	Should be started at 25 mg/day and titrated in 25 mg increments as separate doses every 3 days to reach 100 mg/day (25 mg qid). Thereafter the total daily dose may be increased by 50 mg as tolerated every 3 days to reach 200 mg/day (50 mg qid). After titration, 50–100 mg can be administered as needed for pain relief every 4–6 hours not to exceed 400 mg/day (www.rxlist.com/ultram-drug.htm)

Source: Medical Economics Staff (2000).

Q. Is hydrocodone available alone and not in combination with a nonopioid?

A. No. Compared to codeine, hydrocodone gives more pain relief with a longer duration of action. Hydrocodone is a prodrug metabolized via CYP2D6 cytochromes to hydromorphone, the active metabolite.

Q. Is there any concern about overdosing on combination opioid/acetaminophen?

A. Yes. Titrating (continuously adjusting the drug dosage) the dose of a combination drug is difficult due to the acetaminophen (nonopioid) component. Most hydrocodone combination agents contain a minimum of 500 mg acetaminophen. At these dosages, the maximum 4 g dose of acetaminophen is reached after ingestion of eight tablets. When taken as usually prescribed at one or two tablets every 4–6 hours, the daily dose of acetaminophen will exceed the maximum of 4 g, which may result in liver toxicity. So care must be taken, and the patient must be instructed not to take more than the maximum 4 g of acetaminophen.

Q. Does everyone taking an opioid obtain an analgesic response?

A. No. Certain individuals (e.g., Caucasians) have a genetic predisposition whereby codeine and hydrocodone are metabolized poorly. These individuals will not develop analgesia in the same way as individuals who do not have the inherited gene for cytochrome P450 CYP2D6.

Q. What is tramadol?

A. Tramadol is a central synthetic analgesic compound that is not derived from natural sources nor is it chemically related to opiates. Tramadol is a synthetic, centrally acting pain reliever indicated for moderate to moderately severe oral pain. Its analgesic action affects both opioid receptor and serotonin uptake. It is classified as a Schedule IV controlled drug due to its abuse and dependence potential. The serious adverse effects usually seen with opioids, such as dependence, sedation, respiratory depression, and constipation, occur less often with tramadol. If it is abruptly stopped there is withdrawal. Practitioners should be cautious when prescribing this drug for patients recovering from substance abuse disorders. It is contraindicated in patients with a previous history of seizures. Essentially, when taken alone, it is not recommended for acute dental pain (Moore 1999).

There are conflicting reports on whether tramadol is indicated for management of acute dental pain in dentistry; it is used more for chronic pain. If NSAID or opioid use is contraindicated, then it is a plausible alternative analgesic. The dose of tramadol is one tab q4–6h and for tramadol/acetaminophen two tabs q4–6h for dental pain. In patients with creatinine clearances of <30 mL/min, the recommended dose and dosing interval are 2 tabs q12h.

Q. Can Talwin® be used for the management of dental pain?

A. Talwin (pentazocine) has been used in the management of acute dental pain but there are some adverse effects such as psychotic events (hallucinations) that may preclude its use. The incidence of abuse is relatively low (Swift and Hargreaves 1993). Also, when discontinued there is withdrawal. Therefore, Talwin is not an analgesic of choice for dental pain.

Q. Can I prescribe meperidine (Demerol®) for dental pain?

A. Meperidine is not such a good drug for dental pain because it undergoes extensive first-pass metabolism, reducing the amount of active drug available to produce an analgesic response, and it has a short duration of action so that constant dosing would be necessary.

Q. For how many days should a patient take an opioid?

A. Not for more than 2–3 days. After that, the patient should take a nonopioid analgesic.

Q. What is oxycodone?

A. Oxycodone, unlike codeine, is a very potent analgesic with fewer severe adverse effects such as histamine release and nausea. Oxycodone, a prodrug, is metabolized by CYP2D6 to an active metabolite, oxymorphone. However, unlike codeine and hydrocodone, oxycodone is itself a potent analgesic. It is unknown whether oxymorphone significantly contributes to the analgesic activity of oxycodone. Patients with CYP2D6 deficiencies who do not respond well to codeine or hydrocodone may achieve more pain relief using oxycodone. Oxycodone is available in combination with nonopioids or alone. In the elderly and in patients with renal impairment, less dosage adjustment is needed.

Q. How does physical dependence develop with long-term opioid use?

A. With long-term opioid use, liver enzymes enhance the metabolism of the opioid, thus requiring more drug to be stratified (tolerance develops).

Q. When is it appropriate to prescribe opioid analgesics?

A. In patients with moderate to severe dental pain such as surgical removal of impacted wisdom teeth.

Q. For which type of patients should opioids be avoided?

A. Patients taking antipsychotics or CNS depressants; acute alcoholism; patients addicted to opioids; respiratory insufficiency or depression, bronchial asthma, advanced emphysema, heart failure secondary to chronic lung disease, cardiac arrhythmias, known hypersensitivity; and pregnant women. Precautions should be taken in the elderly and in patients with undiagnosed abdominal pain, liver disease, a history of addiction to opioids, hypoxia, supraventricular tachycardia, prostatic hypertrophy, and renal or hepatic impairment. The obese must be monitored closely for respiratory depression while taking opioid analgesics. For a complete list of opioid–drug interactions, see Table 5.6.

Q. Is it OK to prescribe codeine, hydrocodone or oxycodone to patients taking fluoxetine (Prozac®) and paroxetine (Paxil®)?

A. No. Drugs that are inhibitors of CYP450 2D6 may interfere with the analgesic effect of codeine. The mechanism is decreased *in vivo* conversion of codeine to morphine, a metabolic reaction mediated by CYP450 2D6. Fluoxetine (Prozac) and paroxetine (Paxil) are selective serotonin reuptake inhibitors (SSRIs) and there is a definitive drug–drug interaction with codeine and its derivatives. These drugs can delay the metabolism of codeine, resulting in less of an analgesic response because codeine and its derivatives require metabolism to be effective. These two drugs should not be taken concurrently. There seems to be a documented response with only these two SSRIs.

Q. What is the difference in the opioids prescribed?

A. Codeine alone has not been found to be as effective as other common analgesics (acetaminophen and NSAIDs) for relief of dental pain. Oxycodone and hydrocodone are about as effective as codeine. Dihydrocodeine, pentazocine, and meperidine show no advantages over codeine orally and can even be less effective. Their effectiveness in combination therapy (combining opioids with acetaminophen and NSAIDs) is better than that in monotherapy. It is all related to the different degrees of potency.

Q. Why is it important to know the different potencies of opioids/opiates?

A. The relative potencies of opioids aid in the decision on which opioid to prescribe. The most effective analgesic effect for moderate to severe pain has been found to be with 60 mg codeine. So, if a hydrocodone/nonopioid drug is prescribed, a hydrocodone strength equivalent to 60 mg codeine is ideal.

- 30–60 mg codeine orally is equivalent to 5–10 mg hydrocodone and 5 mg oxycodone.

Q. Why can histamine-like symptoms appear after taking an opiate/opioid?

A. These drugs bind to histamine receptors, causing the release of histamine. This results in symptoms such as itching. This is not a true allergy which would be a reaction due to the drug molecule. A true allergy to opioids is very rare. Rather, itching is just an adverse effect. If the patient reports an allergy to codeine, it is important to question them as to what happened when it was taken. This will clarify if it was a true allergic reaction or merely an adverse effect of the drug. Naturally occurring and semisynthetic compounds are the most potent histamine releasers.

Q. What are other adverse effects of opiates/opioids?

A. Constipation, nausea, vomiting, dizziness, vertigo, sedation, dizziness, pruritus, urine retention, and cardiovascular and respiratory depression. All patients must be made aware of these adverse effects. However, the relative risk of opioid-like adverse effects varies with individuals. Remind patients not to drive due to sedation and dizziness.

Q. Why does constipation occur with opioids?

A. Constipation occurs when the sphincters and intestinal wall contract.

Q. Is dose adjustment needed in liver impairment?

A. Yes. The dose is reduced, and the dosing interval is increased.

Q. What should be done if a patient says they are allergic to codeine?

A. First, the patient should be questioned on what happened when the opioid was taken. A true allergy to opioids is rare. If the patient mentions itching or stomach problems, they are most likely not allergic to opioids. These are adverse effects, not anaphylaxis, relating to the release of histamine and constipation.

Q. Why has there been a lot of media attention about abuse of OxyContin®?

A. First introduced in 1995, OxyContin is a Schedule II controlled substance with an abuse potential similar to morphine. OxyContin has been used inappropriately and is easily abused for its euphoric effect. It is supplied in a controlled (slow)-release form of oxycodone. It is not available in combination with a nonopioid, as is Percodan®, Percocet®, or Tylox®. It is indicated for moderate to severe pain when continuous, around-the-clock opioid analgesic is needed. The reason for causing death is because when used as a recreational drug, it is either crushed and snorted or dissolved in water and intravenously injected. When taken in these forms, it can cause an overdose and death (American Dental Association 2010).

4.5.6 Management Plan for Acute Dental Pain

Q. What features are used to determine which analgesic should be prescribed to a patient?

A. Patient's medical condition, severity of pain (mild, moderate or severe), and medications taken by the patient.

Q. Why is the use of NSAIDs important in dental pain?

A. The major component of dental pain is inflammation and NSAIDs possess antiinflammatory properties while the opioids do not. Patients should take an NSAID on a regular, around-the-clock basis for mild to moderate pain (Becker 2010).

Q. What analgesic is acceptable to use in patients taking blood thinners such as aspirin or warfarin?

A. The only analgesics that can be used are acetaminophen or opioids. NSAIDs taken with blood thinner cause an additive effect and this is contraindicated.

Q. What is the best analgesic for a recovering substance abuser?

A. It is recommended to contact the patient's primary care physician or drug abuse physician. First, it is important to determine if the patient is a former or current substance abuser. In former abuse patients with severe acute dental pain, it is advisable not to avoid prescribing opioids because of addiction concerns. If an opioid is prescribed, it is advisable that drug users should be treated with longer-acting opioids and hydrocodone/acetaminophen and not to start with a weaker drug and wait until it fails to prescribe a stronger opioid. Only prescribe enough to last for a couple of days. Do not give the patient more than six tablets and no refills. The concern with using opioids in former or current substance abusers is the effect of euphoria from the opioid. Another obstacle in treating these patients is that most develop tolerance and physical dependence to the opioid. The patient usually will require a higher dose of the opioid at more frequent intervals to achieve adequate pain relief. To achieve adequate pain relief, the doses should be give around the clock or scheduled rather than on an "as needed" basis. Using around-the-clock dosing suppresses the pain better than dosing on an as needed basis where the pain may go up and require more medication to control it. If there are concerns with prescribing an opioid for moderate to severe pain, an NSAID (dose 400–600 mg) can be taken preoperatively and postoperatively (Denisco et al. 2011; Goureitch and Arnsten 2005; Prater et al. 2002).

Q. How much of an analgesic should initially be prescribed to any patient?

A. It is always advisable to prescribe the smallest dose that produces an acceptable analgesic response. Overprescribing of opioids happens when the dentist prescribes in excessive quantities that are needed to relieve dental pain. There is no need to prescribe an opioid for more than a few days. If severe pain persists afterward then most likely there is either poor healing or an infection which requires the patient to go immediately to the dental office or emergency department (Denisco et al. 2011).

Q. Is it acceptable to take the analgesic just when the patient has pain?

A. No. An analgesic should not be taken on a "prn" basis because therapeutic bloods levels will not be maintained. It is recommended at least for the first few days to take the analgesic on a scheduled basis to provide a fairly consistent level of pain control. The disadvantage of administering analgesics on an as needed basis is that pain must be present before it can be managed. Repeated prn dosing may result in high peaks and low troughs, causing alternating periods of uncontrolled pain and toxicity as more doses may be used to catch up with the pain.

Q. Why do individuals respond differently to the same drug?

A. Sometimes drugs, especially opioids, can cause unpredictable and inconsistent therapeutic effects because everyone differs in the way they metabolize the drug. If one drug does not produce the therapeutic effects anticipated, switch to another one.

Q. Is pretreating with a nonopiate/opioid analgesic before a painful dental procedure to reduce postsurgical pain effective?

A. Yes. The patient should take an NSAID within two hours before the dental procedure. Pretreatment with acetaminophen has not been shown to be as effective as pretreating with an

NSAID. It is most effective in managing postoperative pain when the NSAID is administered between 30 and 60 minutes before the procedure and after the procedure as well. The reasoning behind this is that trauma caused by tissue manipulation during the dental procedure releases prostaglandins within two hours and by having the analgesic already in the blood, it prevents the synthesis of inflammatory prostaglandins which are quickly released after the surgical insult (Huynh and Yagiela 2003). Giving analgesics before the procedure delays the onset of postsurgical pain and the severity is much less.

Q. Do pediatric patients require more than the strength of OTC analgesics?

A. Generally, pediatric patients do not require prescription-strength analgesics. For children, give:

- ibuprofen oral suspension (100 mg/5 mL) at a dose of 10 mg/kg every four hours with a maximum dose of 40 mg/kg/day (each 5 mL = 1 teaspoonful)
- acetaminophen oral suspension (contains 160 mg acetaminophen/5 mL) (ages 2–11) 15 mg/kg every four hours. It is recommended to consult with a pediatrician for two year olds.

Q. Which analgesic is recommended to start with for dental pain?

A. Generally, if there are no contraindications, an NSAID is the first-line drug.

Q. Can an NSAID be taken together with acetaminophen?

A. Yes. It is best to take the combination for a short time only. NSAIDs plus acetaminophen are superior to NSAIDs alone (Altman 2004; Hyllested et al. 2002). Combining acetaminophen and NSAIDs can lead to greater efficacy with fewer adverse effects (Altman 2004). However, Altman (2004) emphasizes that further clinical studies are needed to determine the clinical safety of acetaminophen/NSAID combination analgesic therapy for common conditions associated with mild to moderate pain. So, in the meantime, it is recommended to take pain medications as directed to help avoid any potential adverse effects of either medication. There are many products on the market that contain both. For example, Excedrin® Migraine contains acetaminophen, aspirin, and caffeine (caffeine has been reported to increase the analgesic effect) (Granados-Soto et al. 1993).

Q. When should opiates/opioids be prescribed for acute dental pain?

A. Effective doses of a nonopioid such as ibuprofen or acetaminophen are more efficacious than an opiate/opioid alone and almost or equally effective as an opioid/nonopioid combination product (Hersh et al. 2011). Remember to advise patients about the many adverse effects of opioids and that they should not drive while on an opioid. The general management plan is as follows.

- The ideal nonopiate/opioid to start with is 400–800 mg ibuprofen q4–6h. Can increase dosage if needed but the maximum dose is 2400 mg/day.
- If an NSAID is contraindicated, then acetaminophen 650–1000 mg is recommended. The maximum dosage is 4000 mg (4 g) per day.
- Can use acetaminophen plus an NSAID. This combination produces synergistic actions.
- Acetaminophen is recommended in patients at risk of experiencing gastrointestinal distress.
- If this regimen does not provide adequate pain relief, then 650 mg acetaminophen/10 mg hydrocodone q4–6h (following strictly the q4–6h and not just as needed) *or* Tylenol #3

(2 tablets q4–6h) (following strictly the q4–6h and not just as needed) *or* 7.5 mg hydroco-done/200 mg ibuprofen (Vicoprofen) *plus* (if needed) 200–400 mg ibuprofen.

 – Should not exceed 360 mg codeine a day.
 – Caution should be exercised because opioids do not have a ceiling effect so when used in combination with acetaminophen, increasing the dose for more profound analgesic effect will also increase the dose of acetaminophen which can result in hepatotoxicity.

Q. Can a combination of opiate/opioid and nonopioid analgesic be prescribed?

A. Yes. NSAIDs have an opioid-sparing effect of 20–30%. Combinations of NSAIDs with opioids produce a synergistic effect. Additionally, not all analgesics work the same way. Most nonopi-oids work peripherally, while opioids work centrally on brain receptors. Combining analgesics with different modes and sites of action can increase the analgesic effect and be better tolerated by the patient because lower doses are used (Hersh et al. 2011; Mehlisch 2002).

Q. Can taking two different NSAIDs or two different opioids be more beneficial in reducing pain?

A. No, because with NSAIDs, the maximum pain relief is usually reached with an effective dose of a single NSAID. Taking more than one NSAID only increases the incidence of adverse effects. There will be increased analgesic effect by taking two or more opioids but also increased adverse effects and the increased analgesic effect could also be achieved with a larger dose of just a single opioid (Huynh and Yagiela 2003).

Q. For moderate to severe pain, is it better to take a nonopioid alone or as a combined tablet with an opioid or separate nonopioid and separate opioid at the same time or a separate nonopioid plus a combination nonopioid/opioid?

A. For all severities of acute pain, it is recommended to begin management with ibuprofen or acetaminophen. Always use the lowest possible effective dose to avoid unwanted adverse effects. If either one alone does not provide profound pain relief then for moderate pain relief, add to the ibuprofen a nonopioid/opioid combination drug such as Tylenol #4 or 10 mg hydroc-odone (Vicodin HP). Remember the maximum amount of ibuprofen for profound pain relief is 2400 mg/day (Mehlisch 2002).

Q. What approach can be used to enhance the analgesic effect of oral drugs?

A. To enhance the analgesic effect, it has been recommended to combine two different drugs with different mechanisms of action – for example, ibuprofen and hydrocodone or acetaminophen and codeine.

Q. Can acetaminophen be combined with an NSAID?

A. Yes, but there is not enough literature to show if this combination produces any more pain relief than just taking acetaminophen alone because it is not exactly known if acetaminophen has the same mechanism of action as NSAIDs (Huynh and Yagiela 2003).

Q. Why is caffeine added to many OTC analgesics?

A. Caffeine does not have any analgesic action but is added to many OTC analgesics to increase the potency of the other ingredients including ibuprofen, acetaminophen and aspirin (Huynh and Yagiela 2003). Caffeine, a vasoconstrictor, is useful in these OTC analgesics to help relieve headaches.

Q. What is the best analgesic for *mild* dental pain (e.g., after scaling and root planing, restorative dentistry)?

A. • Start with the lowest dosage and then titrate higher to a safe and effective dosage (Quinlan-Colwell 2014). Use 200–400 mg ibuprofen q4–6h for dental pain when there are no contraindications such as ulcers, gastric bleeding, anticoagulant therapy, aspirin sensitivity or asthma. The maximum dose of ibuprofen is 800 mg per dose or 2400 mg/day.
- If the patient is hypertensive and taking any antihypertensive drug except for calcium channel blockers, then the duration of use should be limited to less than 7–14 days. This is due to a blood pressure destabilizing effect (Floor-Schreudering et al. 2015). Short courses of NSAIDs (of less than a week or two) will likely not cause a clinically important increase in blood pressure (Horn and Hansten 2006).
- If ibuprofen is contraindicated (see the above situations) then recommend 650–1000 mg acetaminophen alone (World Health Organization 1986). If there is not enough pain relief with 200–400 mg ibuprofen, a higher dosage can be tried; initially prescribe up to 600 mg q4–6h then reduce to 400 mg as needed.
- Note: if the patient takes Aleve (naproxen sodium 220 mg) then take 2 tabs q8h.

Q. What is the best analgesic for *moderate* dental pain (e.g., periodontal surgery, endodontic therapy)?

A. • Step 1: ibuprofen 400–600 mg for the first day, if there are no contraindications such as ulcers, gastric bleeding, aspirin sensitivity, anticoagulant therapy or asthma. The maximum dose of ibuprofen is 800 mg per dose or 2400 mg/day.
- Reduce dose after the first day to 400 mg.
- If the patient is hypertensive and taking any antihypertensive drug except for calcium channel blockers, then the duration of use should be limited to five days.
- If ibuprofen is contraindicated (see above situations) then recommend 600–1000 mg acetaminophen plus an opioid such as codeine (60 mg) or hydrocodone (10 mg) *or* 37.5 mg tramadol/325 mg acetaminophen (Ultracet®).
- Step 2: if pain relief with ibuprofen is inadequate, an opioid/nonopioid-narcotic combination is necessary. Choices include *adding* to 400 mg ibuprofen (taken two hours before surgery) then:
  – Tylenol #3 2 tabs q4–6h for dental pain (taking two #3 is equal to 600 mg acetaminophen and 60 mg codeine) *or*
  – 10 mg hydrocodone/650 mg acetaminophen (Vicodin HP) *or*
  – 7.5 mg hydrocodone/200 mg ibuprofen (Vicoprofen) *or*
  – if NSAIDs are contraindicated, just use the recommended opioid combinations without NSAID.

Q. What is the best analgesic for *severe* dental pain (e.g., extraction of impacted wisdom teeth, extensive periodontal surgery, and acute pulpitis)?

A. • To start: ibuprofen 400–600 mg, then add:
  – 10 mg hydrocodone/650 mg acetaminophen (Vicodin HP) *or*
  – 7.5 mg hydrocodone/200 mg ibuprofen (Vicoprofen) *or*
  – 10 mg oxycodone/650 mg acetaminophen (Percocet) (try hydrocodone before prescribing oxycodone) (American Association of Endodontists 1995; Hersh et al. 2011).

4.6   Prevention and Management of Opioid Prescription Drug Misuse

Q. If a patient is already taking opioids for a chronic medical condition, is it recommended to prescribe an additional opioid for severe dental pain?

A. No. If necessary, the patient's treating physician should be contacted.

Q. In recent years, there has been an increase in prescribing opioids and an increase in overdose-related deaths. What concerns are raised by this current opioid epidemic and what are specific recommendations for prescribing opioids in dentistry?

A. In many states, prescribers must access the state prescription drug monitoring program (PDMP). This has aided prescribers in identifying patient drug misuse, abuse and/or addiction (American Association of Oral and Maxillofacial Surgeons 2017).

Q. Are there concerns if an opioid has to be prescribed to a patient who is not listed in the PDMP?

A. Yes. If an opioid has to be prescribed, it is recommended to use a short-acting analgesic and to start with the lowest effective dose for the shortest time (American Association of Oral and Maxillofacial Surgeons 2017). Also, it is recommended to prescribe a combination opioid/non-opioid because less of the opioid is used when in combination with an NSAID or acetaminophen. Short-acting analgesics include hydromorphone, oxycodone (alone or in combination with acetaminophen or ibuprofen), and codeine (in combination with acetaminophen).

Q. What is the Opioid Analgesic Risk Evaluation and Mitigation Strategy (REMS)?

A. The Opioid Analgesic REMS is required by the FDA for opioids that are used in outpatient care. It is required for all healthcare providers registered with the DEA to prescribe Schedule II, III, and IV opioid analgesics. Under the terms of REMS, a healthcare provider is highly recommended to complete a REMS-compliant education program, and to counsel patients when giving a prescription about the risks, safety, adverse effects, proper storage and disposal of opioids. REMS-compliant CE is also available starting March 2019 (www.fda.gov/drugs/information-drug-class/opioid-analgesic-risk-evaluation-and-mitigation-strategy-rems).

Q. Can an individual develop tolerance to opioids?

A. Yes. Drug tolerance develops when a specific drug is used continually over time or even after a single dose, whereby the individual does not respond to the drug the way they did when the drug was first taken. Thus, higher doses of the drug are then required to obtain the intended response, which can result in overdose. Tolerance develops when there is a loss of analgesic potency (Benyamin et al. 2008) and euphoric effects (Volkow and McLellan 2016).

Patients will call the office and say that the drug prescribed is no longer helping them. This is tolerance. It develops rapidly to the analgesic effects of opioids and it will build up as long as the drug is being taken. This is why all opioids for dental pain should be prescribed on a short-term basis.

Q. How does an individual develop opioid tolerance?

A. There are many mechanisms of opioid tolerance. One type of mechanism occurs when opiates (e.g., morphine, heroin) bind to opiate receptors in the brain, inhibiting adenylate cyclase so that eventually after repeated binding to and inhibiting this enzyme, it will adapt so that the morphine effect is reduced and more morphine is needed to get the same effect that was initially felt (www.drugabuse.gov/publications/teaching-packets/neurobiology-drug-addiction/section-iii-action-heroin-morphine/8-definition-dependence) (Benyamin et al. 2008). Tolerance can also develop with opioids such as codeine, oxycodone, and hydrocodone.

Q. What is drug addiction?

A. Drug addiction occurs when an individual uses drugs consistently to excess and the drugs become a significant part of their life. Sometimes it is difficult to distinguish between tolerance and addiction. Addiction develops slowly over months of taking an opioid (Volkow and McLellan 2016). Symptoms of addiction include craving the opioid, compulsively taking the opioid, and continuously thinking about the opioid (Volkow and McLellan 2016). Addiction is not as predictable an outcome as is physical dependence and tolerance and it does not occur in the majority of opioid users (Volkow and McLellan 2016).

Q. What is dependence?

A. Dependence is the psychological and physical loss of control due to drug abuse. Dependence alone is not necessarily an addiction but it can lead to addiction. Once the opioid is stopped, most often the dependency will resolve (Volkow and McLellan 2016).

Q. What are some ways in which prescription opioids can be misused?

A. Opioid analgesics can be misused even if they are prescribed for legitimate therapeutic uses. Other sources of misuse are getting the drug from a family member or friend or using previously prescribed drugs that were not used up at the time (Denisco et al. 2011).

Q. What can the dentist do to help prevent prescription opioid abuse?

A. When opioids are prescribed for dental pain, the dentist must be cognizant about the potential for developing addiction, tolerance, and/or dependence. Guidelines the dentist can follow include those listed below.

1) Dental schools (e.g., University of Alabama at Birmingham School of Dentistry) are helping diminish the growing opioid epidemic by forming a new opioid council (Koplon 2018). This will better educate the graduating dental student and faculty on the importance of establishing guidelines and standards when prescribing opioids to patients.
2) Prevent drug diversion by hindering the illegitimate obtaining of opioids from multiple dentists/physicians, family, and friends (Volkow and McLellan 2016). Proper disposal of unused or outdated opioids is important.
3) Prescribe NSAIDs, if not contraindicated, as the first-line analgesic treatment for dental pain.

4.7 Oral Sedation

Q. Is the enteral and parenteral sedation terminology still used today?

A. "Enteral" and "parenteral" are terms used to describe the *route* of medication administration, and not the *level* of sedation. The terms used to describe the level of sedation are minimal, moderate, deep sedation, and general anesthesia. *Enteral* is defined as any technique of administration in which the agent is absorbed through the gastrointestinal tract or oral mucosa (e.g., oral, rectal, sublingual). *Parenteral* is a technique of administration in which the drug bypasses the gastrointestinal tract (e.g., IM, intravenous, intranasal, submusoal, subcutaneous, intraosseous). Thus, administration of a benzodiazepine can result in different levels of anesthesia such as minimal, moderate or even deep sedation depending on the dosage given (American Dental Association 2016).

Q. What is moderate sedation?

A. Moderate sedation is a more up-to-date term for conscious sedation. Moderate sedation is a pharmacologically induced state of depressed consciousness and analgesia where the patient's protective airway reflexes are intact and the patient can ventilate without assistance. The patient can respond purposefully to verbal stimuli or light tactile stimulation.

Q. Can moderate sedation be performed in the dental office?

A. Yes. Moderate sedation is usually administered in the dental office or hospital.

Q. What is minimal sedation?

A. Previously known as anxiolysis. Minimal sedation is primarily used in the dental office for anxious patients. It is a drug-induced state during which patients respond normally to verbal commands. Ventilatory and cardiovascular functions are not affected (www.ada.org/~/media/ADA/Education%20and%20Careers/Files/anesthesia_use_guidelines.pdf).

Q. What does moderate sedation induce?

A. Antianxiety, analgesia, and some degree of amnesia.

Q. Can moderate sedation be achieved by the oral administration of drugs?

A. Yes. Moderate sedation is administered either orally (enteral)or intravenously (parenteral). Combinations of enteral and inhalation or inhalation and parenteral can be used.

Q. How should the patient be assessed before any anesthesia is administered?

A. Patients undergoing moderate sedation in the office should have a preoperative evaluation the day of the procedure. This should include assigning them to the appropriate American Society of Anesthesiologists (ASA) classification. This is based on the patient's medical history. See Table 4.7. Only ASA I and II patients are appropriate for in-office moderate sedation. The provider should also assess the patient's nil per os (nothing by mouth) (NPO) status. See Table 4.8. The patient's body mass index (BMI) should also be evaluated. Patients with higher BMI can be at risk for adverse airway events, especially if obstructive sleep apnea is a contributing factor. Once this history and physical is completed, the patients should have baseline vital signs recorded, including blood pressure, pulse rate, respiratory rate, and oxygen saturation.

Table 4.7 Patient physical status classification

ASA I	Normal healthy patient
ASA II	Patient with mild systemic disease: type 2 diabetes, hypertension
ASA III	Patient with severe systemic disease: stable angina, type 1 diabetes, chronic obstructive pulmonary disease
ASA IV	Patient with severe systemic disease that is a constant threat to life: heart attack within six months, unstable angina, uncontrolled diabetes or uncontrolled epilepsy
ASA V	Moribund patient who is not expected to survive without the operation: patient is not expected to survive 24 hours with or without medical intervention
ASA VI	A declared brain-dead patient whose organs are being removed for donor purposes
E	Emergency operation used to modify any of the above classifications

Source: Adapted from ASA Physical Status Classification System (www.asahq.org/standards-and-guidelines/asa-physical-status-classification-system).

Table 4.8 Assessment of the patient's NPO status

Ingested material	Minimum hasting
Clear liquids	2 h
Breast milk	4 h
Infant formula	6 h
Nonhuman milk	6 h
Light meal	6 h
Fried foods, fatty foods, meat	8 h

Q. How should the patient be monitored throughout the procedure?
A. See Table 4.9.

Table 4.9 Monitoring a patient under anesthesia

Consciousness	Level of sedation (how the patient responds to commands)
Oxygenation	Continuous with pulse oximetry
Ventilation	Use of end-tidal CO_2 monitoring or precordial stethoscope
Circulation	Continual electrocardiogram monitoring

Q. What intravenous agents are commonly used for moderate sedation?
A. Propofol, midazolam, fentanyl.

Q. What is EMLA?
A. EMLA stands for eutectic mixture of local anesthetics. It is a cream that supplies effective topical analgesia to intact skin with an occlusive dressing placed at least one hour before venipuncture.

4.7.1 Benzodiazepines

Q. What are some orally administered antianxiety drugs used for patients who are anxious about dental treatment?
A. Benzodiazepines (antianxiety) are the main drugs used for minimal sedation because they produce sedation, anxiolysis, and amnesia, which are desirable attributes for minimal and sometimes moderate sedation. There is less risk for respiratory depression, as with the opioids. Table 4.10 lists the common benzodiazepines.

Q. What are common adverse effects of benzodiazepines that the patient should be advised of?
A. Sedation (do not drive), drowsiness, xerostomia, blurred vision, diarrhea, nausea, decreased respiratory rate.

Q. What is the **Black Box Warning** for midazolam?
A. Midazolam HCl syrup has been associated with respiratory depression and respiratory arrest, especially when used for sedation in noncritical care settings. Midazolam HCl syrup has been associated with reports of respiratory depression, airway obstruction, desaturation, hypoxia, and apnea, most often when used concomitantly with other central nervous system depressants (e.g., opioids). Midazolam HCl syrup should be used only in hospital or ambulatory care

Table 4.10 Common benzodiazepines used for minimal sedation/antianxiety

Drug	Dosage
Alprazolam (Xanax)	Antianxiety: Adults: 0.25–0.5 mg Child: has not be determined Supplied: tabs 0.25, 0.5, 1, 2 mg
Clorazepate (Tranxene®)	Antianxiety: Adults: 7.5–15 mg bid or tid Child: has not be determined Supplied: Tabs 3.75, 7.5, 11.25, 15, 22.5 mg Caps 3.75, 7.5, 15 mg
Diazepam (Valium®)	Antianxiety: Adults: 2–10 mg bid, tid or qid Child: 0.1–0.5 mg/kg (maximum dose 10 mg) Supplied: tabs 2, 5, 10 mg
Lorazepam (Ativan®)	Antianxiety: Adults: 1–3 mg bid or tid Child: not determined or not recommended Supplied: Tabs 0.5, 1, 2 mg Sublingual tabs 0.5, 1, 2 mg
Midazolam (Versed®)	0.5 mg/kg oral (syrup) 0.08 to 0.5 mg/kg intramuscular 0.2 to 0.3 mg/kg intranasal

settings, including physicians' and dentists' offices, which can provide for continuous cardiac and respiratory monitoring.

Q. In what conditions are benzodiazepines contraindicated?
A. Narrow angle glaucoma and severe chronic obstructive pulmonary disease.

Q. What are common drug interactions with benzodiazepines?
A. Oral contraceptives (decreased metabolism of diazepam), isoniazid (INH; for tuberculosis) (increases half-life of diazepam), valproic acid (anticonvulsant, bipolar disease) (displaces diazepam from its protein binding sites, resulting in increased blood levels), atorvastatin (increased serum concentration of midazolam)

Q. What are patient instructions for taking a benzodiazepine?
A. Avoid alcohol and other CNS depressants, avoid driving or other similar activities, can cause xerostomia. If given for sedation in the dental office, the patient must be discharged into the care of a competent adult and should be warned about not driving. Do not make important decisions on the day of procedure.

Q. Can benzodiazepines be prescribed for pregnant women?
A. Benzodiazepines should not be prescribed to pregnant women.

Q. Which benzodiazepine can be given for antianxiety in a child?
A. Young children are more sensitive to the CNS depressive effects. Diazepam dose: 0.1–0.5 mg/kg and midazolam dose: 0.5–1 mg/kg.

Q. Should the dose of a benzodiazepine be adjusted in the elderly?

A. Yes. For example, the adult dose of alprazolam (Xanax®), which is 0.25–0.5 mg, should be halved in the elderly.

Q. What is midazolam?

A. Commonly used preanesthesia medication. It will produce hypnosis, sedation, anxiolysis, anterograde amnesia, anticonvulsant effects, and centrally produced muscle relaxation. It will not provide any analgesia. It has a rapid onset and short duration. It does not cause cardiorespiratory depression. Onset of action is about 10 minutes intranasally. Midazolam should not be taken with some antiviral medications (HIV/AIDS), grapefruit juice, ketoconazole, and itraconazole.

Q. Can benzodiazepines be prescribed for the elderly?

A. Yes, but in the smallest dose necessary to produce a therapeutic response.

4.7.2 Other Agents

Q. Why are barbiturates not routinely used?

A. Barbiturates have more of an effect on the heart, CNS, and lungs than the benzodiazepines. Their popularity over the years has been reduced in favor of benzodiazepines, which have fewer adverse effects. Longer-acting barbiturates such as phenobarbital are usually used as anticonvulsants and shorter-acting barbiturates such as pentobarbital and secobarbital are used as sedative/hypnotics.

Q. What is propofol?

A. Propofol is a very potent sedative/hypnotic nonbarbiturate that is administered intravenously with minimal amnesic and analgesic properties. It readily crosses the blood–brain barrier, causing a rapid onset of moderate sedation. Recovery is quick because it is rapidly redistributed from the CNS and undergoes rapid metabolism. Caution should be taken not to use high doses which may lead to respiratory depression or arrest.

Q. What is fentanyl?

A. Fentanyl, an analgesic, has a quick onset of action (highly lipophilic) and short duration so it is frequently used for intravenous moderate sedation. It is 100 times more potent than morphine. In addition, its duration is relatively short compared to other opioids, usually lasting only 30–60 minutes. Fentanyl is safe for patients with renal failure.

4.8 Glucocorticosteroids

Q. What are common indications for the use of glucocorticosteroids in dentistry?

A. Mucocutaneous diseases (e.g., pemphigus, pemphigoid, systemic lupus erythematosus, lichen planus), erythema multiforme, aphthous ulcers (canker sores).

Q. What other conditions are glucocorticoids used for?

A. Rheumatoid arthritis, severe persistent asthma, vesicular bullous disorders. When a patient is taking a steroid, it is important to ask the indication.

4.8.1 Topical Glucocorticosteroids

Q. How are topical steroids used for oral mucocutaneous/bullous diseases?

A. Topical steroids are used for the treatment of inflammatory conditions of the skin or oral mucosa. Topical steroids do not cure the condition and when therapy is discontinued a rebound effect may occur.

Q. When topical steroids are applied in the mouth, is there any systemic absorption?

A. Any topical application of medications causes systemic absorption into the blood but only in negligible amounts.

Q. How are topical steroids applied to oral lesions?

A. Topical steroids are applied to oral lesions by using a finger cot and either dabbing or smoothing on the lesion, or a soft acrylic mouthguard is custom made from the patient's models and the steroid is applied to the inside of the splint to allow better contact of the steroid to the lesion.

Q. What is the difference between mineralocorticoids and glucocorticoids?

A. Mineralocorticoids are used to treat patients with hypoadrenalism by increasing kidney sodium retention and potassium loss. The medical use of mineralocorticoids is limited. Aldosterone is the most important naturally occurring mineralocorticoid.

   Glucocorticoids are antiinflammatory agents used in the treatment of many medical conditions. This is the steroid that is primarily used in medicine and dentistry.

Q. What is the major natural glucocorticoid produced in the human body?

A. Hydrocortisone (cortisol) is synthesized and released from the adrenal gland (adrenal cortex). Remember the adrenal medulla synthesizes catecholamines such as epinephrine. Cortisol production is controlled by adrenocorticotropic hormone (ACTH). In the healthy individual, hydrocortisone levels being to rise between 2 a.m. and 6 a.m. with peak levels occurring between 6 a.m. and 8 a.m. Cortisol levels decrease during the day until midnight when minimal levels occur. Cortisol increases available energy in the form of glucose, and causes gluconeogenesis (glucose formation).

Q. What are the synthetically manufactured glucocorticoid steroids?

A. Prednisone, beclomethasone, triamcinolone, dexamethasone.

Q. What is the mechanism of action of the antiinflammatory actions of glucocorticoids?

A. In general, glucocorticoids support cell membrane integrity which results in suppressing an increase in vascular permeability and preventing the release of damaging lysosomes from inside the cell and the release of prostaglandins. In addition, there is suppression of vasodilation.

Q. How are topical steroids classified?

A. Steroids are classified according to potency. Table 4.11 lists different topical steroids used for the management of oral lesions. Group VII have the lowest potency and Group I have the highest potency. Group I steroids are not used in dentistry.

Table 4.11 Classification of selective topical steroids used in dentistry

Lowest potency (does not penetrate mucosa well)
Hydrocortisone 2.5% cream (various brand names: Cortaid®, Cortizone® – OTC; 0.5% and 1%)
Hydrocortisone acetate in Orabase 0.5% (for oral lesions) (Orabase-HCA) (prescription only)
Low potency
Dexamethasone elixir (Decadron) F
Medium potency
Betamethasone valerate ointment (Valisone®)
Triamcinolone acetonide dental paste 0.1% (Oralone®) (prescription only)
High potency
Fluocinonide gel (Lidex®) F
Highest potency
Clobetasol propionate gel (generic, Temovate®) F

Source: Adapted from Ference and Last (2009).
F, fluoride.

Q. What corticosteroid formulations are used in dentistry for treating aphthous ulcers (canker sores), blistering mucocutaneous diseases of the oral mucosa including pemphigus, lichen planus, and mucous membrane pemphigoid?
A. Topically applied creams, dental paste, and rinses.

Q. Why do some steroids contain a fluoride atom added to the steroid molecule?
A. Some preparations of steroids are fluorinated which increases the potency and prolongs the duration of action. Also, the incidence of adverse effects is increased.

Q. How do I choose which steroid preparation to use?
A. Absorption of a steroid depends on the water and lipid solubilities of the drug. Lipid solubility is more important for topical administration where the effect is localized with slow absorption.

Q. Which preparations are used topically for intraoral lesions?
A. Topical gels, dental paste, ointments, and elixirs. Hydrocortisone and triamcinolone are specially formulated in a dental paste (Orabase) that contains cellulose gum, flavor, pectin, plasticized hydrocarbon gel, preservatives, and tragacanth gum. This product is only available with a prescription. Dexamethasone elixir and clobetasol propionate can be prescribed.

Q. When are steroid agents contraindicated?
A. Topical steroids can cause topical and systemic adverse effects. Contraindications include immunocompromised patient, fungal infection, and herpes infection. Potent topical steroids can cause purpura and ulcerations, especially in thin-mucosal areas (Cornell 1987).

Q. How is a prescription written for triamcinolone dental paste?
A. Table 4.12 lists prescription samples for various steroids.

Q. What is Orabase?
A. Orabase is the trade name (Oral Colgate Pharmaceuticals) for dental paste.

Table 4.12 Prescriptions for various steroids

How a prescription for triamcinolone dental paste is written

Rx Triamcinolone acetonide dental paste 0.1%

Disp: 5 g tube

Sig: Apply a thin film by dabbing on affected area up to three times a day, preferably after meals.

How a prescription for clobetasol propionate is written

Rx Clobetasol propionate 0.05% ointment

Disp: 15 g tube

Sig: Apply a thin layer of ointment to affected area six times a day until lesion is gone (treatment should be limited to 2 consecutive weeks and amounts greater than 50 g/week should not be used).

How a prescription for dexamethasone elixir is written for an adult

Rx Dexamethasone elixir 0.5 mg/mL

Disp: 8 oz.

Sig: Rinse with 1 tsp 4 times a day and then expectorate. Do not swallow.

How a prescription for Benadryl and Kaopectate is written

Rx diphenhydramine elixir 4 oz.

Kaopectate 4 oz.

qs 8 oz.

Disp: 8 oz.

Sig: Swish with one teaspoonful q2h.

(Note: *qs* is a Latin term meaning quantum sufficient or sufficient quantity which means to make the final product ounces.)

How a prescription for Xylocaine viscous is written

Rx lidocaine viscous 2%

Disp: 450 mL bottle

Sig: Swish with one tablespoonful qid.

Q. How should products with dental paste be applied?

A. Products with dental paste should be "dabbed" or "pressed" on rather than "rubbed" on because the product will not stay on the oral tissue well if rubbed on. Apply to the affected area two to three times daily after meals or at bedtime.

Q. What is Kenalog® in Orabase?

A. Kenalog is the brand name for triamcinolone in dental paste. It is a prescription drug.

Q. How is a prescription for clobetasol propionate written (see Table 4.12)?

A. Clobetasol topical exists as multiple brands and as a generic drug. Also, this product is not labeled for intraoral use and some pharmacists will not fill this prescription.

Q. How is a prescription for dexamethasone elixir written for an adult (see Table 4.12)?

A. Dexamethsone elixir is indicated for intraoral use.

4.8.2 Other Nonsteroidal Topical Agents Used in the Management of Oral Lesions

Q. What is Benadryl and Kaopectate and how is a prescription for Benadryl and Kaopectate written?
A. Benadryl (diphenhydramine) and Kaopectate is prescribed for aphthous ulcers. This product has to be compounded by the pharmacist (see Table 4.12).

Q. How is a prescription for Xylocaine viscous written?
A. Lidocaine (Xylocaine) viscous 2% is a topical anesthetic for relief of intraoral pain or burning (see Table 4.12).

4.8.3 Systemic Corticosteroids

Q. When is a systemic corticosteroid prescribed in dentistry?
A. Systemic corticosteroids such as methylprednisolone are indicated for sinus floor elevation surgery to minimize swelling and inflammation.

Q. What are the equivalent doses in milligrams of glucocorticoids?
A. See Table 4.13.

Table 4.13 Equivalent doses in milligrams of glucocorticoids

Corticoid drug	Equivalent dose (mg)
Cortisone	25
Dexamethasone	0.75
Hydrocortisone	20
Methylprednisolone	4
Prednisone	5
Triamcinolone	4

Q. How are systemic glucocorticoid preparations classified?
A. Systemic corticosteroids are classified as short-acting, intermediate-acting or long-acting. See Table 4.14.

Table 4.14 Systemic glucocorticosteroids classification

Short-acting (8–12 hours)
Cortisone
Hydrocortisone
Intermediate acting (12–36 hours)
Methylprednisolone (Medrol)
Prednisolone
Prednisone
Trimacinolone
Long-acting (36–54 hours)
Betamethasone (Celestone®)
Dexamethasone (Decadron)

Q. Which systemic corticosteroids are used in dental sinus surgery?

A. Usually methylprednisolone pack (Medrol®) or dexamethasone (Decadron®). The generic can be prescribed with both medications.

Q. Should patients taking steroids receive steroid supplementation before dental surgery or other dental procedures?

A. The major concern about performing dental surgery in patients taking systemic steroids on a long-term basis is the development of adrenal crisis; however, it seems to be a rare event (Khalaf et al. 2013). It is the consensus that these patients do not require supplemental steroid coverage for routine dental procedures, including periodontal scaling and root planning or minor surgery under local anesthesia (Gibson and Ferguson 2004). However, if general anesthesia is used then supplemental coverage may be indicated and a consult with the patient's physician is recommended. There are no concerns with patients taking topical steroids, including inhalers.

Q. What are common adverse effects with systemic corticosteroids?

A. Adverse effects are usually rare if used for a short time. Some adverse effects include peptic ulcers, osteoporosis (usually if takenchronically), sleep problems, nervousness, and diabetes.

Q. Are there any drug interactions with corticosteroids?

A. Yes. Insulin, oral diabetic medications, diuretics, cyclosporine, warfarin, estrogen drugs, and oral contraceptives interact with corticosteroids. Consult with the patient's physician before prescribing corticosteroids.

Q. What are patient instructions on how to take corticosteroids?

A. Take with food and a full glass of water or milk to minimize development of ulcers.

References

Abbas, S.M., Kamal, R.S., and Afshan, G. (2004). Effect of ketorolac on postoperative pain relief in dental extraction cases – a comparative study with pethidine. *Journal of the Pakistan Medical Association* 54: 319–323.

ADA Professional Product Review (2010). *Journal of the American Dental Association* 5: 3–4.

Albin, S. and Agarwal, S. (2014). Prevalence and characteristics of reported penicillin allergy in an urban outpatient adult population. *Allergy and Asthma Proceedings* 35 (6): 489–494.

Altman, R.D. (2004). A rationale for combining acetaminophen and NSAIDs for mild-to-moderate pain. *Clinical Experimental Rheumatology* 22: 110–117.

American Academy of Periodontology (2006). American Academy of Periodontology statement on local delivery of sustained or controlled release antimicrobials as adjunctive therapy in the treatment of periodontitis. *Journal of Periodontology* 77: 1458.

American Association of Endodontists (1995). Management of acute pain. *Endodontics Colleagues for Excellence* Spring/Summer: 1–4.

American Association of Oral and Maxillofacial Surgeons (AAOMS) (2017). www.aaoms.org/docs/govt_affairs/advocacy_white_papers/opioid_prescribing.pdf.

American Dental Association (2016). *Guidelines for the Use of Sedation and General Anesthesia by Dentists*. Chicago: American Dental Association.

Archer, J.S. and Archer, D.F. (2002). Oral contraceptive efficacy and antibiotic interaction: a myth debunked. *Journal of the American Academy of Dermatology* 46: 917–923.

Aronoff, D.M., Oates, J.A., and Boutaud, O. (2006). New insights into the mechanism of action of acetaminophen: its clinical pharmacologic characteristic reflect its inhibition of the two prostaglandin H2 synthases. *Clinical Pharmacology and Therapeutics* 79: 9–19.

Awtry, E.H. and Loscalzo, J. (2000). Aspirin. *Circulation* 101: 1206–1218.

Ballow, C.H. and Amsden, G.W. (1992). Azithromycin: the first azalide antibiotic. *Annals of Pharmacotherapy* 26: 1253–1261.

Barash, M., Reich, K.A., and Rademaker, D. (2015). Lidocaine-induced methemoglobinemia: a clinical reminder. *Journal of the American Osteopathic Association* 115: 94–98.

Barclay, L. (2011). Acetaminophen: repeated use of slightly too much can be fatal. *British Journal of Pharmacology* www.medscape.com/viewarticle/754104?sssdmh.73674&src=nldne.

Bauer, K.L. and Wolf, D. (2005). Do antibiotics interfere with the efficacy of oral contraceptives? *Journal of Family Practice* 54: 1079–1080.

Bautista, L.E. and Vera, L.M. (2010). Antihypertensive effects of aspirin: what is the evidence? *Current Hypertension Reports* 12: 282–289.

Becker, D.E. (2010). Pain management: part 1: managing acute and postoperative dental pain. *Anesthesia Progress* 57 (2): 67–79.

Benyamin, R., Trescot, A.M., Datta, S. et al. (2008). Opioid complications and side effects. *Pain Physician* S11: S105–S120.

Bell, W.R. (1998). Acetaminophen and warfarin. Undesirable synergy. *Journal of the American Medical Association* 279: 702–703.

Boss, H.A., Boysen, G., and Olseen, J.S. (1985). Effect of incremental doses of aspirin on bleeding time, platelet aggregation and thromboxane production in patients with cerebrovascular disease. *European Journal of Clinical Investigation* 15 (6): 412–414.

Chambers, H.F. (2003). Bactericidal vs. bacteriostatic antibiotic therapy: a clinical mini review. *Clinical Updates in Infectious Diseases* VI (4): October.

Cooper, S.A. (1993). Narcotic analgesics in dental practice. *Compendium* 14: 1061–1068.

Cornell, R. (1987). Contraindications for using topical steroids. *Western Journal of Medicine* 147: 459.

Costa, F.W.G., Esses, F.S., de Barros Silva, P.G. et al. (2015). Does the preemptive use of oral nonsteroidal anti-inflammatory drugs reduce postoperative pain in surgical removal of third molars? A meta-analysis of randomized clinical trials. *Anesthesia Progress* 62: 57–63.

Cowan, F.F. (1992). Analgesics. In: *Dental Pharmacology*, 2e (ed. F.F. Cowan), 164–203. Philadelphia, PA: Lea & Febiger.

Davison, S.N. (2019). Clinical pharmacology considerations in pain management in patients with advanced kidney failure. *Clinical Journal of the American Society of Nephrology* 14 (6): 917–931.

Denisco, R.C., Kenna, G.A., ONeil, M.G. et al. (2011). Prevention of prescription opioid abuse. The role of the dentist. *Journal of the American Dental Association* 142: 800–810.

Elliott, W.J. (2010). Do the blood pressure effects of nonsteroidal anti-inflammatory drugs influence cardiovascular morbidity and mortality? *Current Hypertension Reports* 12: 258–266.

Emmert, D.H. (2000). Treatment of common cutaneous herpes simplex virus infections. *American Family Physician* 61: 1697–1604, 1705–1706, 1708.

Engelkirk, P.G. and Duben-Engelkirk, J. (eds.) (2010). Controlling microbial growth in vivo using antimicrobial agents, Chapter 9. In: *Burton's Microbiology for the Health Sciences*, 9e, 147. Philadelphia, PA: Lippincott Williams & Wilkins.

Fairbanks, D.N.J. (2007). *Pocket Guide to Antimicrobial Therapy in Otolaryngology – Head and Neck Surgery*, 13e. Alexandria, VA: American Academy of Otolaryngology – Head & Neck Surgery Foundation, Inc.

Farrell, S.E., Tarabar, A., Burns, M.J. et al. (2012). Acetaminophen toxicity. www.emedicine.medscape. com/article/820200-overview#aw2aab6b2b2.

Fathallah-Shaykh, S. (2011). Fanconi syndrome clinical presentation. www.emedicine.medscape. com/article981774-clinical#a0218.

Ference, J.D. and Last, A.R. (2009). Choosing topical corticosteroids. *American Family Physician* 79: 135–140.

Fricke, J., Halladay, S.C., Bynum, L., and Francisco, C.A. (1993). Pain relief after dental impaction surgery using ketorolac, hydrocodone plus acetaminophen. *or placebo. Clinical Therapeutics* 15 (3): 500–509.

Floor-Schreudering, A., de Smet, P., Buurma, H. et al. (2015). NSAID – antihypertensive drug interactions: which outpatients are at risk for a rise in systolic blood pressure? *European Journal of Preventive Cardiology* 22 (1): 91–99.

Fujimoto, J.M. (1979). Pharmacokinetics and drug metabolism. In: *Practical Drug Therapy* (ed. R.J.H. Wang), 11–16. Philadelphia: J.B. Lippincott Company.

Ganda, K.M. (2008). Odontogenic infections and antibiotics commonly used in dentistry: assessment, analysis, and associated dental management guidelines. In: *Dentist's Guide to Medical Conditions and Complications* (ed. K. Ganda), 63–82. Ames, IA: Wiley Blackwell.

Gibson, N. and Ferguson, J.W. (2004). Steroid cover for dental patients on long-term steroid medication: proposed clinical guidelines based upon a critical review of the literature. *British Dental Journal* 197: 681–685.

Gibson, J. and McGowan, D.A. (1994). Oral contraceptives and antibiotics: important considerations for dental practices. *British Dental Journal* 177: 419–422.

Glasheen, J.J., Fugit, R.V., and Prochazka, A.V. (2005). The risk of overanticoagulation with antibiotic use in outpatients on stable warfarin regimens. *Journal of General Internal Medicine* 20: 653–656.

Goureitch, M.N. and Arnsten, J.H. (2005). Medical complications of drug abuse. In: *Substance Abuse. A Comprehensive Textbook* (eds. J.H. Lowinson, P. Ruiz and R.B. Millman), 840–862. Philadelphia, PA: Lippincott Williams & Wilkins.

Granados-Soto, V., López-Muñoz, F.J., Castañeda-Hernández, G. et al. (1993). Characterization of the analgesic effects of paracetamol and caffeine in the pain-induced functional impairment model in the rat. *Journal of Pharmacy and Pharmacology.* 45: 627–631.

Grover, S.A., Coupal, L., and Zowall, H. (2005). Treating osteoarthritis with cyclo-oxygenase-2-specific inhibitors: what are the benefits of avoiding blood pressure destabilization? *Hypertension* 45: 92.

Hancox, J.C., Hasnain, M., Vieweg, W.V. et al. (2013). Azithromycin, cardiovascular risks, QTc interval prolongation, torsade de pointes, and regulatory issues: a narrative review based on the study of case reports. *Therapeutic Advances in Infectious Disease* 1 (5): 155–165.

Herbert, M.E., Brewster, G.S., and Lanctot-Herbert, M. (2000). Ten percent of patients who are allergic to penicillin will have serious reactions if exposed to cephalosporins. *Western Journal of Medicine* 172: 341.

Hersh, E.V., Kane, W.T., O'Neil, M.G. et al. (2011). Prescribing recommendations for the treatment of acute pain in dentistry. *Compendium* 32 (3): 22–31.

Hersh, E.V. (1999). Adverse drug reactions in dental practice: interactions involving antibiotics. *Journal of the American Dental Association* 130: 236–251.

Hoang, T., Jorgensen, M.A.G., Kelm, R.G. et al. (2003). Povidone-iodine as a periodontal pocket disinfectant. *Journal of Periodontal Research* 38: 311–317.

Hoffmann, K., George, A., Heschl, L. et al. (2015). Oral contraceptives and antibiotics. A cross-sectional study about patients' knowledge in general practice. *Reproductive Health* 12: 43.

Horn, J.R. and Hansten, P.D. (2006). NSAIDs and antihypertensive agents. www.pharmacytimes.com/ publications/issue/2006/2006-04/2006-04-5484.

Horn, J.R. and Hansten, P.D. (2011). CCBs and CYP3A4 inhibitors: watch out for enhanced cardiovascular response. www.pharmacytimes.com/publications/issue/2011/june2011/ccbs-and-cyp3a4-inhibitors-watch-out-for-enhanced-cardiovascular-response-.

Huynh, M.P. and Yagiela, J.A. (2003). Current concepts in acute pain management. *Journal of the California Dental Association* 31: 419–427.

Hylek, E.M., Heiman, H., Skates, S.J. et al. (1998). Acetaminophen and other risk factors for excessive warfarin anticoagulation. *Journal of the American Medical Association* 279: 657–662.

Hyllested, M., Jones, S., Pedersen, J.L., and Kehlet, H. (2002). Comparative effect of paracetamol, NSAIDs or their combination in postoperative pain management: a qualitative review. *British Journal of Anaesthesia* 88: 199–214.

Jeske, A.H. (2002). Selecting new drugs for pain control: evidence-based decisions or clinical impressions? *Journal of the American Dental Association* 133: 1052–1056.

Katz, W.A. (2002). Use of nonopioid analgesics and adjunctive agents in the management of pain in rheumatic disease. *Current Opinion in Rheumatology* 14: 63–71.

Khalaf, M.W., Khader, R., Cobetto, G. et al. (2013). Risk of adrenal crisis in dental patients. *Results of a systematic search of the literature. Journal of the Dental Association* 144 (2): 152–160.

Klepser, M.E., Nicolau, D.P., Quintillian, I.R. et al. (1997). Bactericidal activity of low-dose clindamycin administered at 8- and 12-hour intervals against *Staphylococcus aureus, Streptococcus pneumoniae*, and *Bacteroides fragilis. Antimicrobial Agents and Chemotherapy* 41: 630–635.

Koplon, S. (2018). UAB School of Dentistry on front lines of combating opioid epidemic. www.uab.edu/news/health/item/9105-uab-school-of-dentistry-on-front-lines-of-combating-opioid-epidemic.

Leonhardt, A., Bergström, C., Krok, L. et al. (2007). Microbiological effect of the use of an ultrasonic device and iodine irrigation in patients with severe chronic periodontal disease: a randomized controlled clinical study. *Acta Odontologica Scandinavica* 65: 52–59.

Lomaestro, B.M. (2009). Do antibiotics interact with combination oral contraceptives? www.medscape.com/viewarticle/707926.

Martin, K., Barbieri, R., Crowley, W., Martin, K. (2018). Overview of the use of combination oral contraceptives.
www.uptodate.com/contents/overview-of-the-use-of-combination-oral-contraceptives

McDonald, L.C., Gerding, D.N., Johnson, S. et al. (2018). Clinical practice guidelines for *Clostridium difficile* infection in adults and children: 2017 update by the Infectious Diseases Society of America (IDSA) and Society for Healthcare Epidemiology of America (SHEA). *Clin Infect Disease* 66: e1–e48.

Medical Economics Staff (2000). *Advice for the Patient. USP DI*, vol. 2. Colorado: Thomson MICRONEDEX.

Meek, I.L., van de Laar, M.A., and Vonkeman, H. (2010). Non-steroidal anti-inflammatory drugs: an overview of cardiovascular risks. *Pharmaceuticals* 3 (7): 2146–2162.

Mehlisch, D.R. (2002). The efficacy of combination analgesic therapy in relieving dental pain. *Journal of the American Dental Association* 133: 861–871.

Moore, P.A. (1999). Pain management in dental practice: tramadol vs. codeine combinations. *Journal of the American Dental Association* 130: 1075–1079.

Nachimuthu, S., Assar, M.D., and Schussler, J.M. (2012). Drug-induced QT interval prolongation: mechanisms and clinical management. *Therapeutic Advances in Drug Safety* 3 (5): 241–253.

Nemeth, J., Oesch, G., and Kuster, S.P. (2015). Bacteriostatic versus bactericidal antibiotics for patients with serious bacterial infections: systematic review and meta-analysis. *Journal of Antimicrobial Chemotherapy* 70: 382–395.

Ofosu, A. (2016). Clostridium difficile infection: a review of current and emerging therapies. *Annals of Gastroenterology* 29 (2): 147–154.

Osborne, N.G. (2004). Antibiotics and oral contraceptives: potential interactions. *Journal of Gynecologic Surgery* 18: 171–172.

Page, II, R.L. (2005). Weighing the cardiovascular benefits of low-dose aspirin. ACPE Program I.D. Number 290-000-05-H01.

Patrono, C., Coller, B., FitzGerald, G.A. et al. (2004). Platelet-active drugs: the relationhips among dose, effectiveness, and side effects. The seventh ACCP conference on antithrombotic and thrombolytic therapy. *Chest* 126 (3 suppl): 234S–264S.

Plümer, L., Seiffert, M., Punke, M.A. et al. (2017). Aspirin before elective surgery – stop or continue? *Deutsches Arzteblatt International* 114 (27–28): 473–480.

Pozzi, A. and Gallelli, L. (2011). Pain management for dentists: the role of ibuprofen. *Annali di Stomatologia* 2 (3–4 Suppl): 3–24.

Prater, C.D., Zylstra, R.G., and Miller, K.E. (2002). Successful pain management for the recovering addicted patient. *Primary Care Companion to the Journal of Clinical Psychiatry* 4: 125–131.

Quinlan-Colwell, A. (2014). What you should know about first-line pain medications. *American Nurse Today* 9 (12) www.americannursetoday.com/what-you-should-know-about-first-line-pain-medications.

Rodgers, B., Kirley, K., and Mounsey, A. (2013). PURLs: prescribing an antibiotic? Pair it with probiotics. *Journal of Family Practice* 62 (3): 148–150.

Schwartz, S.R. (2006). Perioperative pain management. *Oral and Maxillofacial Surgical Clinics of North America* 18: 139–150.

Schrader, S.P., Fermo, J.D., and Dzikowski, A.L. (2004). Azithromycin and warfarin interaction. *Pharmacotherapy* 24: 945–949.

Sefton, A.M., Maskell, J.P., Beighton, D. et al. (1996). Azithromycin in the treatment of periodontal disease. Effect on microbial flora. *Journal of Clinical Periodontology* 23: 998–1003.

Segelnick, S.L. and Weinberg, M.A. (2008). Recognizing doxycycline-induced esophageal ulcers in dental practice. A case report and review. *Journal of the American Dental Association* 139: 581–585.

Segelnick, S.L. and Weinberg, M.A. (2010). Doxycycline-induced dizziness in the dental patient. *New York State Dental Journal* 76: 28–32.

Shakeri-Nejad, K. and Stahlmann, R. (2006). Drug interactions during therapy with three major groups of antimicrobial agents. *Expert Opinion on Pharmacotherapy* 7 (6): 639–651.

Sharma, R. and Dronen, S.C. (2011). Herpes simplex in emergency medicine mediation. http://emedicine.medscape.com/article/783113-medication#2.

Snowden, S. and Nelson, R. (2011). The effects of nonsteroidal anti-inflammatory drugs on blood pressure in hypertensive patients. *Cardiology in Review* 19 (4): 184–191.

Swift, J.Q. and Hargreaves, K.M. (1993). Pentazocine analgesia: is there a niche for Talwin Nx? *Compendium* 14: 1048,1050.

Trelle, S., Reichenbach, S., Wandel, S. et al. (2011). Cardiovascular safety of non-steroidal anti-inflammatory drugs: network meta-analysis. *British Medical Journal* 342: c7086.

Ubara, Y., Tagami, T., Suwabe, T. et al. (2005). A patient with symptomatic osteomalacia associated with Fanconi syndrome. *Modern Rheumatology* 15: 207–212.

Verma, G. (2014). Dental extraction can be performed safely in patients on aspirin therapy: a timely reminder. *International Scholarly Research Notices* 2014: 463684.

Visapää, J.P., Tillonen, J.S., Kaihovaara, P.S. et al. (2002). Lack of disulfiram-like reaction with metronidazole and ethanol. *Annals of Pharmacotherapy* 36 (6): 971–974.

Volkow, N.D. and McLellan, T. (2016). Opioid abuse in chronic pain – misconceptions and mitigation strategies. *New England Journal of Medicine.* 374: 1253–1263.

Waknine, Y. (2009). FDA Safety Changes: Zantac, Zithromax, Noxafil. www.medscape.com/viewarticle/701796.

Walton, G.M., Rood, R.P., Snowdon, A.T. et al. (1993). Ketorolac and diclofenac for postoperative pain relief following oral surgery. *British Journal of Oral and Maxillofacial Surgery* 31: 158–160.

Warner, T.D. and Mitchell, J.A. (2008). COX-2 selectivity alone does not define the cardiovascular risks associated with non-steroidal anti-inflammatory drugs. *Lancet* 371: 270.

World Health Organization (1986). *Cancer Pain Relief*. Geneva: WHO.

World Health Organization (2004). *Medical Eligibility Criteria for Contraceptive Use*, 3e. Geneva: Reproductive Health and Research, WHO.

Zanchetti, A., Hansson, L., Leonetti, G. et al. (2002). Low-dose aspirin does not interfere with the blood pressure-lowering effects of antihypertensive therapy. *Journal of Hypertension* 20: 1015.

Zichterman, A. (2007). Opioid pharmacology and considerations in pain management. http://sonoranhealth.org/resources/Opiod+Pharmacology+$26+Considerations+in+Pain+Managment.pdf.

Zigdon, H., Levin, L., Filatov, M. et al. (2012). Intraoperative bleeding during open flap debridement and regenerative periodontal surgery. *Journal of Periodontology* 83: 55–60.

Additional Resources

http://emedicine.medscape.com/article/1049648-overview
http://emedicine.medscape.com/article/783113-overview
http://medscape.com/viewarticle/715208

5

How to Manage Potential Drug Interactions in Dentistry

5.1 Introduction to Drug Interactions

Q. What are the different types of drug interactions?

A. Interactions between drugs usually will either increase or decrease the therapeutic effects or can result in adverse effects (Cascorbi 2012). There are two different types of drug interactions (Becker 2011).

a) *Pharmacokinetic* drug interaction: A change in the pharmacokinetics of one drug caused by the interacting drug. Examples include inhibition of absorption, cytochrome (CYP) P450 enzymes, altered renal excretion and altered plasma protein binding (Corrie and Hardman 2011).

b) *Pharmacodynamic* drug interaction: A change in the pharmacodynamics of one drug caused by the interacting drug (Dawoud et al. 2014). There are different types of pharmacodynamic drug interaction.

- Additive (same response as the sum of the two drugs individually)
- Synergistic (greater response)
- Antagonistic (less of a response)

With additive effects, two or more drugs with similar pharmacodynamic effects are given together resulting in excessive response and possible toxicity; for synergistic effects, the effect of two drugs taken together is greater than the sum of their separate effects at the same dose; and antagonistic effects occur where drugs with opposing therapeutic effects may reduce the response to one or both drugs. For instance, nonsteroidal antiinflammatory drugs (NSAIDs) that increase blood pressure may inhibit the antihypertensive effects of angiotensin-converting enzyme (ACE) inhibitors when given together (Hansten and Horn 2003).

Synergistic drug interaction: The effect of two or more drugs when administered together is greater than if the drugs were given separately; may produce responses equivalent to overdosage. For example, patients with hypertension who do not respond adequately with one drug must take combination drugs (Meredith and Elliott 1992).

The Dentist's Drug and Prescription Guide, Second Edition. Mea A. Weinberg, Stuart J. Froum and Stuart L. Segelnick.
© 2020 John Wiley & Sons, Inc. Published 2020 by John Wiley & Sons, Inc.

Q. How are drug–drug/food interactions rated according to how much of an impact they make?

A. Table 5.1 classifies the rating of drug interactions.

Table 5.1 Rating of drug interactions

Severity rating	Documentation rating
Major: Potentially life threatening or causing permanent body damage	Established: Proven with clinical studies to cause an interaction
Moderate: Could change the patient's clinical status and require hospitalization	Probable: Very likely to cause an interaction
Minor: Only mild effects are evident or no clinical changes seen	Suspected: Supposed to cause an interaction, but more clinical studies are required
	Possible: Limited data proven
	Unlikely: Not certain to cause an interaction

Q. What is the relative importance of drug interactions in dentistry?

A. Many drug interactions are harmless or go clinically unnoticed; many of those which are potentially harmful occur in only a small percentage of patients given the interacting drugs. Results of the interaction differ among individuals and may be more serious in one patient than another. The drugs most often involved in serious interactions are those with a small therapeutic index, such as phenytoin, and those where the dose must be carefully controlled according to the response, as with anticoagulants, antidiabetics, and antihypertensives. The elderly and patients with impaired renal and liver function are especially prone to drug interactions.

Q. When does a drug interaction show clinically?

A. It depends. Factors that must be considered include the drug's half-life, the dosages that are being administered and the mechanism of metabolism. For example, if the offending drug takes a long time to accumulate, the interaction may be delayed several days. However, if the patient is receiving a large dose of the drug, the interaction may occur more rapidly. Also, if the patient is not getting the expected response from the drugs then a drug–drug interaction could be suspected.

Q. Explain the cytochrome P450 enzyme interactions.

A. Few drugs are eliminated from the body unchanged in the urine. Most drugs are metabolized or chemically altered to a less lipid-soluble compound which is more easily eliminated from the body. One way of metabolizing drugs involves alteration of groups on the drug molecule via the cytochrome P450 enzymes. These enzymes are found mostly in the liver, but can also be found in the intestines, lungs, and other organs. Each enzyme is termed an isoenzyme, because each derives from a different gene. There are more than 30 cytochrome P450 enzymes present in human tissue (Hersh and Moore 2004).

Q. How does one drug interact with another drug via the cytochrome P450 enzymes?

A. The *substrate* is a drug that is metabolized by a specific CYP450 isoenzyme. An *inhibitor* is a drug that inhibits or reduces the activity of a specific CYP450 isoenzyme. An *inducer* is a drug that increases the amount and activity of that specific CYP450 isoenzyme.

Q. When does a drug interaction occur via the cytochrome P450 enzymes?

A. Drug interactions can occur when a drug that is metabolized and/or inhibited by these cytochrome enzymes is taken concurrently with a drug that decreases the activity of the same enzyme system (e.g., an inhibitor). The result is often increased concentrations of the substrate. Another scenario is when a substrate that is metabolized by a specific cytochrome enzyme is taken with a drug that increases the activity of that enzyme (e.g., an inducer). The result is often decreased concentrations of the substrate.

Some substrates are also inhibitors for the same enzyme, probably due to competitive inhibition of enzyme activity. Some inhibitors affect more than one isoenzyme and some substrates are metabolized by more than one isoenzyme.

Q. What common drug–drug interactions that occur with the cytochrome P450 isoenzymes are significant in dentistry?

A. Table 5.2 lists common drugs (related to drugs the patient is taking and dental medications prescribed to the patient) that are metabolized (substrate) by specific cytochrome P450 isoenzymes and the drugs that inhibit (inhibitor) or accelerate (inducer) the specific isoenzyme causing a drug interaction. Please note: only commonly encountered drugs in dental practice are listed in Table 5.2; there are many more drugs involved in the cytochrome P450 isoenzyme metabolism. Please refer to Hersh and Moore (2004) and Cupp and Tracey (1998) for more details.

Table 5.2 Substrates (drugs) metabolized by specific isoenzymes

Isoenzyme	Drug
CYP1A2	Amitriptyline (Elavil®)
	Clozapine (Clozaril®)
	Haloperidol (Haldol®)
	Imipramine (Tofranil®)
	Fluvoxamine (Luvox®)
	Tacrine (Cognex®)
	Theophylline
CYP2C9	Nonsteroidal antiinflammatory drugs (ibuprofen, naproxen, celecoxib [Celebrex®])
	Glipizide (Glucotrol®)
	Glyburide (Micronase®, DiaBeta®)
	Irbesartan (Avapro®)
	Losartan (Cozaar®)
	Phenytoin (Dilantin®)
	Warfarin (Coumadin®)
CYP2C19	Amitriptyline (Elavil)
	Diazepam (Valium®)
	Imipramine (Tofranil)
	Lansoprazole (Prevacid®)
	Omeprazole (Prilosec®)
	Pantopropazole (Protonix®)
CYP2D6	Amitriptyline (Elavil)
	Clomipramine (Anafranil®)
	Codeine and its derivatives (oxycodone, hydrocodone)
	Doxepin (Sinequan®)
	Fluoxetine (Prozac®)

(Continued)

Table 5.2   (Continued)

Isoenzyme	Drug
CYP2D6	Haloperidol (Haldol)
	Imipramine (Tofranil)
	Lidocaine (local) (Xylocaine®)
	Metoprolol (Lopressor®)
	Nortriptyline (Pamelor®)
	Paroxetine (Paxil®)
	Propranolol (Inderal®)
	Risperidone (Risperdal®)
	Timolol (Blocadren®)
	Tramadol (Ultram®)
	Venlafaxine (Effexor®)
CYP2E1	Acetaminophen (Tylenol®)
	Ethanol
CYP3A4	Alprazolam (Xanax)
	Amitriptyline (Elavil)
	Amlodipine (Norvasc®)
	Aripiprazole (Abilify®)
	Atorvastatin (Lipitor®)
	Citalopram (Celexa®)
	Clarithromycin (Biaxin)
	Clomipramine (Anafranil)
	Clonazepam (Klonopin®)
	Cyclosporine
	Diltiazem (Cardizem®)
	Erythromycin
	Ethinyl estradiol/progesterone (oral contraceptives)
	Fluoxetine (Prozac)
	Haloperidol (Haldol)
	Hydrocodone (Vicodin® with acetaminophen)
	Indinavir (Crixivan®)
	Ketoconazole (Nizoral®)
	Lidocaine, topical
	Lovastatin (Mevacor®)
	Methadone
	Methylprednisone
	Midazolam (Versed®)
	Nelfinavir (Viracept®)
	Nifedipine (Procardia®, Adala®t)
	Oxycodone (Percodan® with acetaminophen)
	Prednisone
	Ritonavir (Norvir®)
	Saquinavir (Invirase®)
	Sertraline (Zoloft®)
	Theophylline
	Simvastatin (Zocor®)
	Sirolimus
	Sertraline (Zoloft)
	Tacrolimus (Prograf®)
	Triazolam (Halcion®)
	Verapamil (Calan®)
	Warfarin (Coumadin)

Source: Hersh and Moore (2004).

Q. Which are the most abundant cytochrome enzymes in humans?

A. The CYP3A4 isoenzymes make up about 30% of all cytochromes in the liver.

Q. Why is it important to know about substrates and inhibitors and how are the tables used?

A. Inhibitors are drugs prescribed by the dentist that can interfere with a substrate or a drug already taken by the patient. Tables 5.3 and 5.4 are used to look up a drug that you are prescribing to see if it is an inhibitor or an inducer of an isoenzyme. If it is found in the table then determine which isoenzyme is affected and go to Table 5.2 to see if the patient is taking a drug that is metabolized by that isoenzyme.

Table 5.3 Inhibitors (drugs) of specific cytochrome P450 isoenzymes: the drugs listed on the right side inhibit the specific isoenzyme on the left side of the table

CYP1A2	**Ciprofloxacin (Cipro®)** **Fluvoxamine (Luvox)** **Grapefruit juice**
CYP2C9	Fluconazole (Diflucan®) Ketoconazole (Nizoral) Metronidazole (Flagyl®)
CYP2C19	Fluoxetine (Prozac) Ketoconazole (Diflucan) Sertraline (Zoloft) Ticlopidine (Ticlid®)
CYP2D6	Cimetidine (Tagamet®) Cocaine Fluoxetine (Prozac) Paroxetine (Paxil) Sertraline (Zoloft)
CYP2E1	Disulfiram (Antabuse®)
CYP3A4	Clarithromycin (Biaxin) Erythromycin Grapefruit juice Ketoconazole (Diflucan)

Source: Hersh and Moore (2004).

Table 5.4 Inducers (drugs) of the CYP450 isoenzymes

CYP1A2	**Charcoal-broiled meat** **Smoking**
CYP2C9	Rifampin
CYP2C19	No drugs
CYP2D6	No drugs
CYP2E1	Ethanol Isoniazid (INH)
CYP3A4	Carbamazepine (Tegretol®) Dexamethasone St John's wort

Source: Hersh and Moore (2004).

If the dentist prescribes a drug that could inhibit the metabolism of the substrate (look under the correct CYP isoenzyme) then possibly there is a drug interaction that could result in toxicity (elevated plasma levels) of the substrate. It is necessary to check on the list to avoid this problem. For example, if the patient is taking atorvastatin for cholesterol problems and an antibiotic is needed because of a dental infection and the patient is allergic to penicillin, clarithromycin (Biaxin®) should not be prescribed because according to the table, clarithromycin is a *potent* inhibitor of atorvastatin, resulting in toxic plasma levels of the statin drug. If it is appropriate, prescribe clindamycin or azithromycin (Zithromax®). Remember that azithromycin is not metabolized by the CYP isoenyzmes so that there are fewer drug interactions.

Q. What could happen if the patient is taking alprazolam (Xanax®) for anxiety and is prescribed clarithromycin or erythromycin?

A. Excessive central nervous system (CNS) depression could occur.

5.2 Antibiotic–Drug Interactions in Dentistry

Q. What common significant antibiotic drug–drug interactions are seen in the dental practice?

A. Table 5.5 lists clinically significant drug–drug/food interactions in dentistry.

Table 5.5 Clinically significant antibiotic–drug/food interactions in dentistry

Drug	Interacting drug	Effect	What to do
Doxycycline (including doxycycline 20 mg and Atridox®)	Antacids (magnesium hydroxide/aluminum hydroxide), zinc, iron (ferrous sulfate)	Decreased *amount* of doxycycline and minocycline absorption into the blood	Do not take both drugs at same time. Take these products two hours apart from the doxycycline
Minocycline (including Arestin)			
	Penicillins	Interferes with bactericidal effect of penicillins	Do not take at same time; take penicillin a few hours before doxycycline
	Warfarin	Increased anticoagulant effect	Minimal risk; monitor patients for enhanced anticoagulant effects; warfarin dosage may need adjustment
	Oral contraceptives	May interfere with contraceptive effect; altered enterohepatic recirculation	May not be clinically significant; some sources say to use alternative methods of birth control
	Phenytoin (Dilantin)	Decreased serum doxycycline levels	Either switch to another antibiotic or monitor

Table 5.5 (Continued)

Drug	Interacting drug	Effect	What to do
	Vitamin A or related compounds (e.g., retinoids – isotretinoin [Accutane®], acitretin, tretinoin)	Risk of pseudotumor cerebri or benign intracranial hypertension	Tetracyclines including doxycycline and minocycline are contraindicated; choose another antibiotic
	Methotrexate	Elevated serum methotrexate concentrations	Avoid using doxycycline in patients taking high-dose methotrexate
Tetracycline	Antacids (magnesium hydroxide/aluminum hydroxide), calcium- containing products (including calcium-containing foods such as milk), zinc, iron (ferrous sulfate)	Decreased tetracycline absorption into the blood	Do not take concurrently. Space two hours apart from these products
	Warfarin	Possible interaction: increased anticoagulant effect due to decreased production of vitamin K in the gut from inhibition of bacteria that produce the vitamin K	Minimal risk; monitor patients for enhanced anticoagulant effects
	Penicillins	Interferes with bactericidal effect of penicillins	Do not take at same time; take penicillin a few hours before tetracycline
	Digoxin	Digoxin is partially metabolized by bacteria in the intestine; increased digoxin blood levels	Either switch antibiotic or monitor for increased serum digoxin levels
	Oral contraceptives	May interfere with contraceptive effects; altered enterohepatic recirculation	May not be of clinical significance; some sources recommend the use of alternative form of birth control
	Vitamin A or related compounds (e.g., retinoids – isotretinoin [Accutane], acitretin)	Risk of pseudotumor cerebri or benign intracranial hypertension	Tetracyclines including doxycycline and minocycline are contraindicated; choose another antibiotic
	Methotrexate	Elevated serum methotrexate concentrations	Avoid using doxycycline in patients taking high-dose methotrexate
Penicillins (amoxicillin)	Erythromycin, tetracyclines	Decreased effectiveness of penicillin	Do not take at same time; give the penicillin a few hours before the tetracycline

(Continued)

Table 5.5 (Continued)

Drug	Interacting drug	Effect	What to do
	Probenecid (Benemid®): drug for gout	Inhibits penicillin excretion	Can take together; make sure penicillin levels are not excessive
	Oral contraceptives	May interfere with contraceptive effects	May not be clinically significant; some say to use alternative birth control methods
	Methotrexate	Reduced clearance with high doses of penicillins	Only seen in a small group; not enough evidence to avoid. Monitor and consult with physician
Erythromycins Erythromycin and clarithromycin	Theophylline	Increased theophylline levels	Avoid together; consult with physician; reduce theophylline dosage to avoid toxicity
	Advir Diskus®, HFA	Increase levels of salmeterol, increasing risk of ventricular arrhythmias and increases levels of fluticasone	Avoid coadministration
	Carbamazepine (Tegretol)	Increased carbamazepine levels seen as ataxia, vertigo, drowsiness	Avoid concurrent use
	Statins: atorvastatin (Lipitor), simvastatin (Zocor), lovastatin (Mevacor), including combination drugs (amlodipine/atorvastatin)	Increases statin levels (increased myopathy, including muscle pain)	Either switch to azithromycin or to another statin drug like lovastatin (Mevacor) or pravastatin (Pravachol®)
	Oral contraceptives	Interfere with contraceptive effects; altered enterohepatic recirculation	Some sources recommend alternative birth control
	Digoxin	Increased digoxin levels (see increased salivation and visual disturbances)	Switch antibiotic to penicillin. Monitor for signs of digoxin toxicity or switch antibiotic
	Cyclosporine	Cyclosporine toxicity	Cyclosporine doses may need reduction
	Ergot alkaloids (e.g., ergotamine [Bellergal-S®, Cafergot®]) (for migraine headache)	Toxic ergot levels (ergotism; pain, tenderness, and low skin temperature of extremities)	Use azithromycin or another antibiotic
	Benzodiaepines: including alprazolam (Xanax), midazolam (Versed), triazolam (Halcion)	Increased sedation	Avoid combination; use alternative drugs

Table 5.5 (Continued)

Drug	Interacting drug	Effect	What to do
	Citalopram (Celexa)	Dose-dependent prolongation of the QT interval with increased risk of ventricular arrhythmias	Avoid concurrent use
	Calcium channel blocker: disopyramide (Norpace®)	Prolongation of QTc interval	Switch to another antibiotic or monitor for development of arrhythmias
	Class 1A (disopyramide, quinidine, procainamide) and Class III antiarrhythmia drugs (amiodarone, dofetilide, sotalol)	Causes dose-related prolongation of the QT interval with increased risk of ventricular arrhythmias	Avoid concurrent use
	Warfarin (Coumadin)	Increases anticoagulant (bleeding) effect	Switch to another antibiotic such as clindamycin or penicillin or monitor for INR values; contact physician
	Haloperidol (Haldol)	Causes dose-related prolongation of the QT interval with increased risk of ventricular arrhythmias	Avoid concurrent use
	Methadone	Increased risk of QT prolongation with increased risk of ventricular arrhythmias due to an additive effect	Avoid using both drugs together; use alternative
Azithromycin	Food delays absorption of azithromycin capsules, however tablets may be taken without regard to food	Decreased absorption resulting in a major reduction in bioavailability	Take on an empty stomach (1 hour before or 2 hours after meals)
	Aluminum and magnesium antacids	Decrease the rate but not the extent of azithromycin absorption	Take antacid 1 hour before or 2 hours after azithromycin
	Warfarin	Increases bleeding	Contact physician; monitor INR values or switch to another antibiotic that does not interact with warfarin
	Pimozide (Orap®): typical antipsychotic to control repeated movement caused by Tourette's disorder	Increased risk of QT prolongation with increased risk of ventricular arrhythmias due to an additive effect	Contraindicated to use both drugs together

(Continued)

Table 5.5 (Continued)

Drug	Interacting drug	Effect	What to do
	Dronedarone (Multaq®): for atrial fibrillation	Increased risk of QT prolongation with increased risk of ventricular arrhythmias due to an additive effect	Contraindicated to use both drugs together
	Phenothiazine antipsychotics (e.g., chlorpromazine, fluphenazine, promethazine, thioridazine)	Increased risk of QT prolongation with increased risk of ventricular arrhythmias due to an additive effect	Contraindicated to use both drugs together
	Class 1A (disopyramide, quinidine, procainamide) and Class III antiarrhythmia drugs (amiodarone, dofetilide, sotalol)	Causes dose-related prolongation of the QT interval with increased risk of ventricular arrhythmias	Avoid concurrent use; use alternative antibiotic
	Haloperidol (Haldol)	Causes dose-related prolongation of the QT interval with increased risk of ventricular arrhythmias	Avoid concurrent use
	Methadone	Increased risk of QT prolongation with increased risk of ventricular arrhythmias due to an additive effect	Avoid using both drugs together; use alternative
Fluoroquinolones (ciprofloxacin [Cipro], levofloxacin [Levaquin®])	Di- and trivalent cations (e.g., antacids, iron, calcium, zinc)	Decreases fluoroquinolone effect because of decreased absorption	Do not take together; space dose apart either 4 hours before or 2 hours after fluoroquinolone dose
	Caffeine	Increases caffeine effects	Do not take together
	Warfarin	Increases anticoagulant effect	Monitor INR more frequently; consult with patient's physician
	Steroids (e.g., prednisone)	Increased risk of tendinitis and tendon rupture (Achilles tendon)	Caution is recommended when fluoroquinolones are taken at same time as steroid. Best to avoid
	Pimozide (Orap): typical antipsychotic to control repeated movement caused by Tourette's disorder	Increased risk of QT prolongation with increased risk of ventricular arrhythmias due to an additive effect	Contraindicated to use both drugs together
	Pimozide (Orap): typical antipsychotic to control repeated movement caused by Tourette's disorder	Increased risk of QT prolongation with increased risk of ventricular arrhythmias due to an additive effect	Contraindicated to use both drugs together
Clindamycin (Cleocin®)	Neuromuscular blockers (succinylcholine)	Increased neuromuscular blocking effect	Since most dental patients are not taking these drugs, there are no special precautions
	Oral contraceptives	Reduced efficacy of oral contraceptive	Caution advised; limited evidence with clindamycin

Table 5.5 (Continued)

Drug	Interacting drug	Effect	What to do
Metronidazole (Flagyl)	Alcohol (drinking alcohol, using alcohol mouth rinse, alcohol in foods)	Severe disulfiram-like reaction with headache, flushing, and nausea	Avoid alcohol until at least 3 days after discontinuing metronidazole
	Warfarin	Inhibits warfarin metabolism; increased anticoagulant effect	High risk: contact physician; adjustment of warfarin dosage or select different antibiotic
	Lithium	Lithium excretion inhibited, resulting in toxic levels	Contact physician
	Phenytoin	Increased phenytoin levels	Contact physician

Note: Most drug–drug or drug–food interactions occur when two or more drugs are taken at the same time. To avoid these interactions, most drug dosing is spaced so as not to administer them concurrently. If in doubt, the patient's physician should be contacted. www.drugs.com.

Q. Is there a drug interaction between alcohol and metronidazole?

A. Yes. Ingestion of alcohol when taking metronidazole and for one week after metronidazole is stopped can result in a disulfiram-like reaction. Disulfiram (Antabuse) is a medication used to wean individuals off alcohol. Chronic alcoholics are treated with disulfiram. If alcohol is ingested while on disulfiram, acute psychoses (hallucinations) and confusion, abdominal cramps, nausea, facial flushing, and headache can occur. These are similar reactions that also occur with metronidazole.

Q. Can alcohol-containing mouth rinses be used while taking metronidazole?

A. No. Any product containing alcohol is contraindicated. This includes alcohol-containing mouth rinses, foods with alcohol, and skin-to-skin contact with perfumes.

Q. How long after finishing the course of metronidazole can alcohol be started?

A. About three days after the metronidazole is finished.

Q. Is there a drug interaction if antibiotics are initiated in patients taking warfarin?

A. Yes. There is an increase in both the incidence and degree of overanticoagulation with certain antibiotic use in patients taking warfarin. In these cases, there is an elevation of international normalized ratio (INR) associated with a change in bleeding events. It is suggested that all antibiotics should have warning labels about an increased warfarin effect. The most common antibiotics/antifungal agents causing this drug interaction include metronidazole, tetracyclines, trimethoprim/sulfamethoxazole (Bactrim®), ciprofloxacin (Cipro) azithromycin (Zithromax), and fluconazole (Diflucan). In 2009, the FDA approved label revisions for azithromycin, warning of a potential interaction with warfarin. The exact cause of this interaction is not clear. However, there are a few proposed mechanisms: (i) these antibiotics can decrease the metabolism of warfarin (warfarin is metabolized in the liver by CYP2C9), primarily inhibitors of CYP2C9, resulting in bleeding or (ii) antibiotics inhibit gastrointestinal flora which produce vitamin K2, which is associated with the body's natural clotting factors. With less absorption of vitamin K due to the antibiotic, there can be an increase in anticoagulation when warfarin is administered concurrently. Signs of this interaction include increased bruising and bleeding. Even a modest inhibition in warfarin metabolism could lead to a considerable risk of bleeding. Dosage reduction of warfarin may be necessary. Consultation with the patient's physician is necessary (Glasheen et al. 2005; Rice et al. 2003; Sims and Sims 2007).

Q. Is there a drug interaction between antibiotics and oral contraceptives (OCs)?

A. Historically, the first case involving an interaction between OCs and antibiotics was with rifampin, an antituberculosis drug (Skolnick et al. 1976). OCs available in the United States include estrogen–progestin monophasic, biphasic, or triphasic combination products and progestin-only products. Reports and concerns exist regarding the hypothesis that oral antibiotics can reduce the efficacy of combination OCs. One of many proposed mechanisms is that about 50% of ethinylestradiol, the estrogen component in OC, needs to be activated by intestinal bacteria and undergo enterohepatic circulation (Hansten and Horn 2003). Once activated, it is then reabsorbed as active drug. Antibiotics affect intestinal bacteria so that estrogen cannot be activated. The American College of Obstetricians and Gynecologists concluded that tetracycline (Sumycin®), doxycycline (Vibramycin®, Doryx®), metronidazole (Flagyl), and quinolones do not affect OC steroid levels in women taking combination OCs (American College of Obstetricians and Gynecologists 2006). However, dental literature has implicated amoxicillin, metronidazole, and tetracycline in reducing the effectiveness of OCs (ADA Council on Scientific Affairs 2002; Hersh 1999). The World Health Organization (WHO) (2004) states that there have been suspicions that broad-spectrum antibiotics may lower OC effectiveness based on case reports, but that pregnancy rates are similar among women on OCs and women on both OCs and antibiotics. Essentially, it is a rare interaction but can occur (DeRossi and Hersh 2002). Today's concentration of estrogen is much lower than years ago. However, a small decrease in efficacy, especially in the "low-dose" (<35 μg estrogen) combination OCs when taken with an antibiotic, has been documented (Burroughs and Chambliss 2000).

The ADA Council on Scientific Affairs recommends advising patients of the potential risk of the antibiotic reducing the effectiveness of the OC and advising the patient to discuss with her physician the use of an additional nonhormonal type of contraception and to continue compliance with OCs while on antibiotics (ADA Council on Scientific Affairs 2002). In any case, it is best to advise the female patient taking OCs to select a nonhormonal back-up birth control for at least two weeks after discontinuation of the antibiotic or through the end of the current cycle, whichever is longer, switch to an OC with a higher dose of estrogen and progestin for one cycle or to abstain from sexual activity (Hansten and Horn 2003; Osborne 2002).

Q. What is the mechanism of the drug interaction between metronidazole and lithium?

A. It is a pharmacokinetic interaction whereby metronidazole decreases the renal clearance of lithium, resulting in elevated lithium plasma levels. Since lithium has a relatively narrow therapeutic index, there is a risk of toxicity.

Q. Are clarithromycin and azithromycin both inhibitors of the cytochrome P450 enyzmes?

A. Clarithromycin is a potent inhibitor, but azithromycin inhibits CYP enzymes to a lesser degree, resulting in less drug–drug interaction (Schrader et al. 2004).

5.3 Analgesic–Drug Interactions in Dentistry

Q. What common significant analgesic drug–drug interactions can be seen in the dental practice?

A. Table 5.6 lists common analgesic drug–drug interactions.

Table 5.6 Analgesic drug–drug interactions

Drug	Interacting drug	Effect	What to do?
Aspirin and nonsteroidal antiinflammatory drugs (NSAIDs) (ibuprofen, naproxen)	Warfarin	Synergistic anticoagulant effects with aspirin and NSAIDs (increased bleeding)	Avoid concurrent use/contact patient's physician
	Angiotensin-converting enzyme (ACE) inhibitors (e.g., enalapril, captopril); beta-blockers, angiotensin II receptor blockers (ARBs)	With NSAIDs: decrease antihypertensive response (lowers blood pressure). Short-term course (5 days) may not significantly increase blood pressure. This drug interaction does not occur with aspirin or low-dose aspirin	Interaction causes lowering of blood pressure. Monitor blood pressure. Use alternative analgesic such as acetaminophen or narcotic after 5 days or more of use of NSAIDs
	Lithium	NSAIDs inhibit renal clearance of lithium	Decrease lithium dosage. Best to use diflunisal (Dolobid)
	Oral antidiabetic drugs (occurs with aspirin)	Aspirin and NSAIDs increase hypoglycemic effects	Limited importance
	Furosemide (Lasix®)	Decreased diuretic effect	Monitor patient
	Venlafaxine (Effexor®)	Possible serotonin syndrome	Avoid concurrent use
	Phenytoin (Dilantin)	Decreased hepatic phenytoin metabolism (increased serum levels)	No special precautions
	Aspirin or NSAID	Synergistic effect (increased bleeding)	Contraindicated
	Low-dose aspirin + ibuprofen	Ibuprofen may inhibit cardioprotective effect of low-dose aspirin	Avoid concurrent use
Acetaminophen	Alcohol	Increased incidence of hepatotoxicity (liver disease)	Contraindicated in alcoholics; avoid taking together
	Carbamazepine (Tegretol)	Increased risk of acetaminophen toxicity	Avoid concurrent use or maximum amount of acetaminophen use <2 g/day
	Warfarin	Increased anticoagulant effect	Avoid concurrent use. May require adjustment of warfarin dosage. Contact physician

(Continued)

Table 5.6 (Continued)

Drug	Interacting drug	Effect	What to do?
Narcotics (codeine, hydrocodone, oxycodone, meperidine)	Fluoxetine (Prozac), sertraline (Zoloft) and paroxetine (Paxil)	These selective serotonin reuptake inhibitors (SSRIs) are potent inhibitors of CYP2D6 and can delay the metabolism of codeine resulting in less of an analgesic response because codeine and its derivatives require metabolism to be effective	Do not take together; an increase in the codeine dosage or a different analgesic agent may be necessary in patients requiring therapy with CYP450 2D6 inhibitors. Or space doses apart or prescribe the parent compound such as hydromorphone
	Other depressants such as alcohol or drugs (e.g., benzodiazepines, CNS depressants)	Increase sedative properties	Do not take together or limit the amount of alcohol
	Amiodarone (Cordarone®) and quinidine (medicines for cardiac arrhythmias)	These medications are potent inhibitors of CYP2D6. Pain relief would not occur, but there will be unpleasant side effects	Do not take together; an increase in the codeine dosage or a different analgesic agent may be necessary in patients requiring therapy with CYP450 2D6 inhibitors. Or space doses apart or prescribe the parent compound such as hydromorphone
	Haloperidol (Haldol)	This typical antipsychotic is a potent inhibitor of CYP2D6	Do not take together; an increase in the codeine dosage or a different analgesic agent may be necessary in patients requiring therapy with CYP450 2D6 inhibitors. Or space doses apart or prescribe the parent compound such as hydromorphone
	Indinavir (Crixivan) (an HIV protease inhibitor for HIV/AIDS)	Potent inhibitor of CYP2D6	Do not take together; an increase in the codeine dosage or a different analgesic agent may be necessary in patients requiring therapy with CYP450 2D6 inhibitors. Or space doses apart or prescribe the parent compound such as hydromorphone

Q. If a patient is taking warfarin, is it safe to give ibuprofen as an analgesic after a dental procedure?

A. No. This is a synergistic drug–drug interaction where both the warfarin and ibuprofen increase the risk for bleeding. Warfarin is an anticoagulant that inhibits the vitamin K-dependent clotting factors and ibuprofen and aspirin are antiplatelet drugs that inhibit the formation of thromboxane A_2 by inhibiting the cyclooxygenase enzyme. The better choice for an analgesic for a patient taking warfarin would be acetaminophen alone or in combination with a narcotic such as acetaminophen with codeine or acetaminophen with hydrocodone. However, there is also a drug–drug interaction between warfarin and acetaminophen. If a patient is taking warfarin, then acetaminophen is recommended. The prothrombin time should be measured once or twice a week and should not exceed an INR of 4.0, beyond which there is an increased incidence of bleeding. So, if acetaminophen is recommended in a patient taking warfarin, notifying the patient's physician with careful patient monitoring is necessary. Additionally, the lowest dose for the shortest duration is advised (Bell 1998; Hylek et al. 1998).

Q. What is the mechanism of the interaction between an NSAID such as ibuprofen and warfarin?

A. When an NSAID and warfarin are taken together, the NSAID decreases plasma protein binding of warfarin, resulting in an increase in the circulation or plasma levels of warfarin because the NSAID displaces warfarin from the proteins in the plasma.

Q. Is there a drug interaction between ibuprofen and antihypertensive medications such as diuretics, ACE inhibitors, and beta-blockers?

A. Yes. NSAIDs such as ibuprofen and naproxen (Aleve) alter the effectiveness of certain antihypertensive medications including diuretics, ACE inhibitors, and beta-blockers, but not calcium channel blockers (e.g., nifedipine, amlodipine, diltiazem, verapamil). NSAIDs inhibit renal prostaglandin synthesis, thus blocking the antihypertensive's mechanism of action. It is recommended that NSAIDs be used only short term (not for more than 7–14 days) if taking the offending antihypertensive drug but are contraindicated in patients with heart failure. In these cases, it is best to use acetaminophen (Haas 1999). On the other hand, aspirin does not alter the effectiveness of antihypertensive medications (Bautista and Vera 2010).

Q. If a patient is taking ibuprofen but finds it ineffective in reducing the pain, can another NSAID or acetaminophen be taken to increase the analgesic effectiveness?

A. No. The addition of another NSAID or acetaminophen if you are already taking an NSAID may increase the chance of developing renal damage in long-term use. A short duration using this combination is less likely to cause kidney damage. It is recommended that acetaminophen or another NSAID not be taken within three days of another NSAID (Haas 1999; Henrich et al. 1996).

5.4 Sympathomimetic Agents and Drug Interactions in Dentistry

Q. What common significant vasoconstrictor/drug interactions can occur in dental practice?

A. Table 5.7 lists common sympathomimetic (in local anesthetics)–drug interactions.

Table 5.7 Sympathomimetic drug–drug interactions

Drug	Interacting drug	Effect	What to do?
Epinephrine (contained in local anesthetics)	Nonselective (beta-1, beta-2) beta-blockers such as propranolol (Inderal), nadolol (Corgard®), timolol (Blocadren), and sotalol (Betapace®)	Elevated blood pressure and heart rate because these drugs block both beta receptors, allowing epinephrine to bind to alpha receptors which causes vasoconstriction of skin and mucous membranes. Care must be taken when injecting to avoid intravascular administration. The patient's vital signs should be recorded before the injection and five minutes afterward. If there are no cardiac changes, additional local anesthetic can be administered	Epinephrine should be used cautiously. Limit the amount used to 0.04 mg (two cartridges of a local anesthetic with 1 : 100000 epinephrine)
	Selective beta-blockers (beta-1) such as atenolol (Tenormin®), metoprolol (Lopressor), acebutolol (Sectral®), and betaxolol (Kerlone®)	No elevation in blood pressure because these drugs bind only to the beta-1 receptors	No concerns, especially in the controlled hypertensive
	Tricyclic antidepressants (e.g., amitriptyline [Elavil])	Hypertension (enhances sympathomimetic effects)	Treat similar to the cardiac patient; maximum amount is two cartridges of a local anesthetic containing epinephrine 1 : 100000
	Typical phenothiazidine antipsychotics (alpha receptor blockers) such as haloperidol and chlorpromazine (Thorazine).	"Older" typical antipsychotic blocks alpha-1 receptors, resulting in orthostatic hypotension. Epinephrine in low doses causes beta-2 stimulation which may worsen the hypotension. This interaction is rare but if accidental intravascular injection, there is a possibility for a hypotension episode.	Use epinephrine cautiously; use as low a dose as possible especially with the typical antipsychotics because of its actions on alpha receptors
	The "newer" atypical antipsychotics (e.g., risperidone [Risperdal], olanzapine [Zyprexa], quetiapine [Seroquel], aripiprazole [Abilify] and ziprasidone [Geodon])	The "newer" atypical antipsychotics have much less alpha receptor blocking action and thus less incidence of orthostatic hypotension. These atypical antipsychotics are more prescribed today because of fewer adverse effects from binding to the different receptors	
	Cocaine	Increased heart contraction leading to death	Do not use epinephrine if the patient used cocaine within 24 hours
	Marijuana (cannabis)	Seriously prolongs tachycardia in an intoxicated patient. Peak blood levels occur within 10 minutes	Best to use a local anesthetic without vasoconstrictor if you suspect the patient has just used marijuana
	Methamphetamine	Methamphetamine is an amphetamine which is an adrenergic receptor agonist which increases norepinephrine release. Duration of action can be from 8 to 12 hours	Avoid using epinephrine which can result in a severe myocardial infarction. Use a local anesthetic without a vasoconstrictor

Note: these are the more commonly severe drug interactions. www.drugs.com.

Q. What are the effects of epinephrine on the sympathetic receptors in the body?

A. Theoretically, epinephrine binds to all sympathetic receptors (alpha-1, alpha-2, beta-1, beta-2) in the body. Epinephrine in low concentrations (two to three cartridges) achieved systemically after anesthetic injections in dentistry is fairly selective for beta receptors rather than alpha receptors. The beta-2 receptors, when activated, cause peripheral vasodilation in skeletal muscle blood vessels, thus lowering total peripheral resistance and therefore diastolic blood pressure which is governed by peripheral vascular resistance. At the same time, the beta-1 (and beta-2) receptors in the heart are activated to increase cardiac output and therefore systolic blood pressure; this is influenced by peripheral vascular resistance as well, but is also heavily influenced by the cardiac output, which epinephreine increases strongly. With an increase in systolic blood pressure and a decrease in diastolic blood pressure (BP), there is no real change in mean blood pressure; these two influences cancel each other out regarding mean blood pressure. A couple of cartidges (two or three) typically will cause a slight or no rise in systolic BP and a slight fall in diastolic BP.

However, in higher doses (more than three or four cartridges), alpha-1 receptors are also stimulated. Since there are more of them, the net effect is vasoconstriction throughout the body, and an increase in peripheral resistance. This results in an increase in both systolic and diastolic blood pressure, and a possible reflex slowing of the heart mediated by the vagus nerve releasing acetylcholine onto the sinoatrial node (Hersh and Giannakopoulos 2010; Yagiela 1999).

Q. Is there an interaction between epinephrine and noncardioselective beta-blockers such as propranolol and timolol?

A. Yes. Although rare, it can happen. The interaction is due to the nonselective blocking of both beta-1 and beta-2 adrenoceptors (named after the adrenergic nerves that innervate them) allowing the binding of epinephrine to alpha-1 receptors, which results in vasoconstriction and possible increase in blood pressure and hypertension. It is important to avoid intravascular injection of the local anesthetic (Hersh and Giannakopoulos 2010).

Q. What is the mechanism of interaction between epinephrine in a local anesthetic and a tricyclic antidepressant?

A. The hypothesis of depression is that there is a decrease in the amount of norepinephrine and serotonin in the brain. Tricyclic antidepressants, such as amitriptyline (Elavil) and clomipramine (Anafranil), work by inhibiting the reuptake of norepinephrine from the synapse by blocking the noradrenergic reuptake pump, allowing more of norepinephrine to stay in the neuronal synapse. Injected epinephrine can be terminated in two ways: metabolized by catechol-*O*-methyltransferase (COMT) and neuronal reuptake by the noradrenergic reuptake pump, the same pump that takes up norepinephrine. Thus, if the pump is not removing epinephrine from the synapse, it will accumulate. Accumulation of epinephrine from the local anesthetic could essentially cause cardiac arrhythmias and hypertension in a patient taking a tricyclic antidepressant. The amount of epinephrine should be limited to two cartridges of 1 : 100 000 (Goulet et al. 1992).

Q. Is there an interaction between epinephrine and other antidepressants such as selective serotonin reuptake inhibitors such as Zoloft or Lexapro®?

A. No. The same is not true for SSRIs such as fluoxetine (Prozac), fluvoxamine (Luvox), citalopram (Celexa), escitalopram (Lexapro), paroxetine (Paxil), and sertraline (Zoloft), because SSRIs stop the movement of serotonin back into neurons by inhibiting the serotonin reuptake pump and not the noradrenergic reuptake pump so that SSRIs have no effect on epinephrine.

Q. Is epinephrine contraindicated in patients taking monoamine oxidase (MAO) inhibitors?

A. No. Theoretically, there are no restrictions for using epinephrine in patients taking MAO inhibitors such as isocarboxazid (Marplan®), phenelzine (Nardil®), tranylcypromine (Parnate®), and selegiline (Eldepryl®). MAO inhibitors do not affect the noradrenergic reuptake pump.

Q. Are there any interactions with lidocaine?

A. Yes. Lidocaine is contraindicated in patients with known hypersensitivity to amide local anesthetics, a severe degree of SA, AV or intraventricular heart block (if not with pacemaker), or Adams–Stokes syndrome. There is controversy regarding Wolff–Parkinson–White syndrome.

Q. Can epinephrine be used safely in patients taking antipsychotics?

A. First, there are two types of antipsychotics indicated for the treatment of schizophrenia: "older" typical antipsychotics and the "newer" atypical antipsychotics. The typical antipsychotics include phenothiazines such as chlorpromazine (Thorazine®) and other neuroleptic drugs such as haloperidol (Haldol) and trifluoperazine (Stelazine®) which control the acute symptoms but not the emotional response.

The typical "older" antipsychotics such as haloperidol have high affinity with alpha-1 receptors, which causes the adverse effect of orthostatic hypotension. Theoretically, epinephrine stimulates beta-2 receptors causing vasodilation and hypotension, although this is a rare event. The "newer" atypical antipsychotics include:

- Risperidone (Risperdal)
- Olanzapine (Zyprexa®)
- Quetiapine (Seroquel®)
- Aripiprazole (Abilify)
- Ziprasidone (Geodon®)
- Lurasidone (Latuda®).

Introduced since 1990, some atypicals have much less alpha-1 and alpha-2 receptor blocking action and thus fewer incidences of orthostatic hypotension, and work primarily by blocking serotonin 5-HT receptors and dopamine receptors. No two atypical antipsychotics have the same binding affinities to the receptors. For instance, risperidone binds much less to alpha receptors than olanzapine and quetiapine (Goulet et al. 1992; Yagiela 1999).

There are numerous annoying adverse effects because typical and atypical antipsychotics bind to many different receptors. See Table 5.8.

Table 5.8 Adverse effects

- Alpha-adrenergic receptor blockade: orthostatic hypotension, reflex tachycardia (body responds to a decrease in blood pressure by increasing heart rate in an attempt to raise blood pressure) and sexual dysfunction
- Muscarinic receptor blockade: xerostomia, confusion
- Histamine receptor blockade: sedation/drowsiness, weight gain
- Serotonin receptor blockade: weight gain
- Dopamine blockade: extrapyramidal side effects

Epinephrine has a paradoxical hypotensive effect in persons taking typical antipsychotics. The typical antipsychotics may inhibit or reverse the vasopressor (vasocontrictor) effect of epinephrine. Many of these agents, including the atypical antipsychotics, exhibit alpha-1 adrenergic blocking activity and produce hypotension as an adverse effect. Use of epinephrine in patients receiving neuroleptic therapy may cause a paradoxical further lowering of blood pressure, since beta stimulation (due to epinephrine in low doses) may worsen hypotension in the setting of alpha blockade. There may be less of an interaction between the atypical antipsychotics because some cause less alpha receptor blockage because of less binding affinity (e.g., risperidone and less affinity than clozapine, quetiapine, and olanzapine). However, it is best to avoid or use a low dose of epinephrine in these patients (www.drugs.com/drug-interactions/epinephrine-with-phenergan-989-0-1949-1259.html).

Q. Is there an interaction between epinephrine and drugs for attention deficit hyperactivity disorder (ADHD)?

A. Even though some drugs such as atomoxetine (Strattera®) inhibit the noradrenergic reuptake pump similarly to tricyclic antidepressants, there have not been any adverse reports with the use of injected epinephrine. Other drugs used for ADHD include amphetamine or amphetamine-like stimulants which could increase the risk of cardiovascular events in children and adults with preexisting cardiovascular disease. It is recommended to monitor blood pressure and heart rate in these patients and limit the use of epinephrine to 0.4–0.54 mg (Hersh and Moore 2008).

Q. Is epinephrine contraindicated in patients with a true sulfite allergy?

A. Yes. If a patient has a true sulfite allergic, another local anesthetic without epinephrine should be used.

5.5 Antianxiety Drug Interactions in Dentistry

Q. What common significant antianxiety (benzodiazepine) drug–drug/food interactions can be seen in the dental practice?

A. Table 5.9 lists common antianxiety drug–drug/food interactions.

Q. Does grapefruit juice alter the metabolism of drugs?

A. Yes. Furanocoumarin compounds found in grapefruit interfere with liver and intestinal cytochrome P450 isoenzymes by inhibiting CYP3A4. Any drug metabolized by CYP3A4 will have a decreased breakdown if taken with grapefruit juice which can result in increased plasma levels of the drug (toxicity). Grapefruit juice is also a P-glucoprotein inhibitor. The management of these drug interactions is basically to avoid having grapefruit when taking any medication. The only dental drugs that can be affected by grapefruit juice are hydrocodone, oxycodone, carbamazepine (Tegretol), and benzodiazepines (diazepam, triazolam, midazolam, alprazolam) (Stump et al. 2006).

Table 5.9 Antianxiety (benzodiazepines) drug–drug interactions

Drug	Interacting drug	Effect	What to do?
Diazepam (Valium), alprazolam (Xanax), midazolam (Versed), triazolam (Halcion)	Grapefruit juice	Inhibits CYP3A4 enzyme, decreasing metabolism of these drugs, thus increasing blood levels	The duration of effect of grapefruit juice – do not take juice while on these drugs
	Cimetidine (Tagamet)	Inhibits diazepam elimination Increases CNS depression	Little clinical importance
	Opioids (codeine, hydrocodone)	Increases CNS depression	Avoid taking together
	Clarithromycin	Increases benzodiazepine levels; increased sedation	Contraindicated; use alternative drugs
	HIV protease inhibitors	Increase benzodiazepine levels	Contraindicated
	HIV efavirenz/ emtricitabine/ tenofovir	Increase benzodiazepine levels	Contraindicated
	Isoniazid	Increases benzodiazepine levels	Contraindicated

Source: Data from www.drugs.com.

References

American College of Obstetricians and Gynecologists (2006). Use of hormonal contraception in women with coexisting medical conditions. *American College of Obstetricians and Gynecologists Practice Bulletin* 107: 1453–1472.

American Dental Association Council on Scientific Affairs (2002). Antibiotic interference with oral contraceptives. *Journal of the American Dental Association* 133: 880.

Bautista, L.E. and Vera, L.M. (2010). Antihypertensive effects of aspirin: what is the evidence? *Current Hypertension Reports* 12: 282–289.

Becker, D. (2011). Adverse drug interactions. *Anesthesia Progress* 28: 31–41.

Bell, W.R. (1998). Acetaminophen and warfarin. Undesirable synergy. *Journal of the American Medical Association* 279: 702–703.

Burroughs, K.E. and Chambliss, M.E. (2000). Antibiotics and oral contraceptive failure. *Archives of Family Medicine* 9: 81–82.

Cascorbi, I. (2012). Drug interactions – principles, examples and clinical consequences. *Deutsches Ärzteblatt International* 109 (33–34): 546–556.

Corrie, K. and Hardman, J.G. (2011). Mechanisms of drug interactions: pharmacodynamics and pharmacokinetics. *Anaesthesia & Intensive Care Medicine* 12 (4): 156–159.

Cupp, M.J. and Tracy, T. (1998). Cytochrome P450: new nomenclature and clinical implications. *American Family Physcian* 57: 107–116.

Dawoud, B.E.S., Roberts, A., and Yates, J.M. (2014). Drug interactions in general dental practice – considerations for the dental practitioner. *British Dental Journal* 216: 15–23.

DeRossi, S.S. and Hersh, E.V. (2002). Antibiotics and oral contraceptives. *Dental Clinics of North America* 46: 653–654.

Glasheen, J.J., Fugit, R.V., and Prochazka, A.V. (2005). The risk of overanticoagulation with antibiotic use in outpatients on stable warfarin regimens. *Journal of General Internal Medicine* 20: 653–656.

Goulet, J.P., Pérusse, R., and Turcotte, J.Y. (1992). *Contraindications to vasoconstrictors in dentistry*. Part III. *Oral Surgery Oral Medicine Oral Pathology* 74: 692–297.

Haas, D.A. (1999). Adverse drug interactions in dental practice: interactions associated with analgesics. Part III in a series. *Journal of the American Dental Association* 130: 397–407.

Hansten, P. and Horn, J. (2003). Drug–drug interaction mechanisms. www.hanstenandhorn.com/ article-d-i.html.

Henrich, W.L., Agodoa, L.E., Barrett, B. et al. (1996). Analgesics and the kidney: summary and recommendations to the Scientific Advisory Board of the National Kidney Foundation from an Ad Hoc Committee of the National Kidney Foundation. *American Journal of Kidney Disease* 27: 162–165.

Hersh, E.V. (1999). Adverse drug reactions in dental practice: interactions involving antibiotics. *Journal of the American Dental Association* 130: 236–251.

Hersh, E.V. and Giannakopoulos, H. (2010). Beta-adrenergic blocking agents and dental vascoconctrictors. *Dental Clinics of North America* 2054: 687–696.

Hersh, E.V. and Moore, P.A. (2004). Drug interactions in dentistry: the importance of knowing your CYPs. *Journal of the American Dental Association* 135: 298–311.

Hersh, E.V. and Moore, P.V. (2008). Adverse drug interactions in dentistry. *Periodontology 2000* 46: 109–142.

Hylek, E.M., Heiman, H., Skates, S.J. et al. (1998). Acetaminophen and other risk factors for excessive warfarin anticoagulation. *Journal of the American Medical Association* 279: 657–662.

Meredith, P.A. and Elliott, H.L. (1992). An additive or synergistic drug interaction: application of concentration-effect modeling. *Clinical Pharmacology & Therapeutics* 51: 708–714.

Osborne, N.G. (2002). Antibiotics and oral contraceptives: potential interactions. *Journal of Gynecologic Surgery* 18: 171–172.

Rice, P.J., Perry, R.J., Afzal, Z. et al. (2003). Antibacterial prescribing and warfarin: a review. *British Dental Journal* 194: 411–415.

Schrader, S.P., Fermo, J.D., and Dzikowski, A.L. (2004). Azithromycin and warfarin interaction. *Pharmacotherapy* 24: 945–949.

Sims, P.J. and Sims, K.M. (2007). Drug interactions important for periodontal therapy. *Periodontology 2000* 44: 15–28.

Skolnick, J.L., Stoler, B.S., Katz, D.B. et al. (1976). Rifampin, oral contraceptives, and pregnancy. *Journal of the American Medical Association* 236: 1382.

Stump, A.L., Mayo, T., and Blum, A. (2006). Management of grapefruit–drug interactions. *American Family Physician* 15 (74): 605–608.

World Health Organization (WHO) (2004). Medical Eligibility Criteria for Contraceptive Use, 3e. Geneva: Reproductive Health and Research, WHO.

Yagiela, J.A. (1999). Adverse drug interactions in dental practice: interactions associated with vasoconstrictors. Part V of a series. *Journal of the American Dental Association* 130: 701–709.

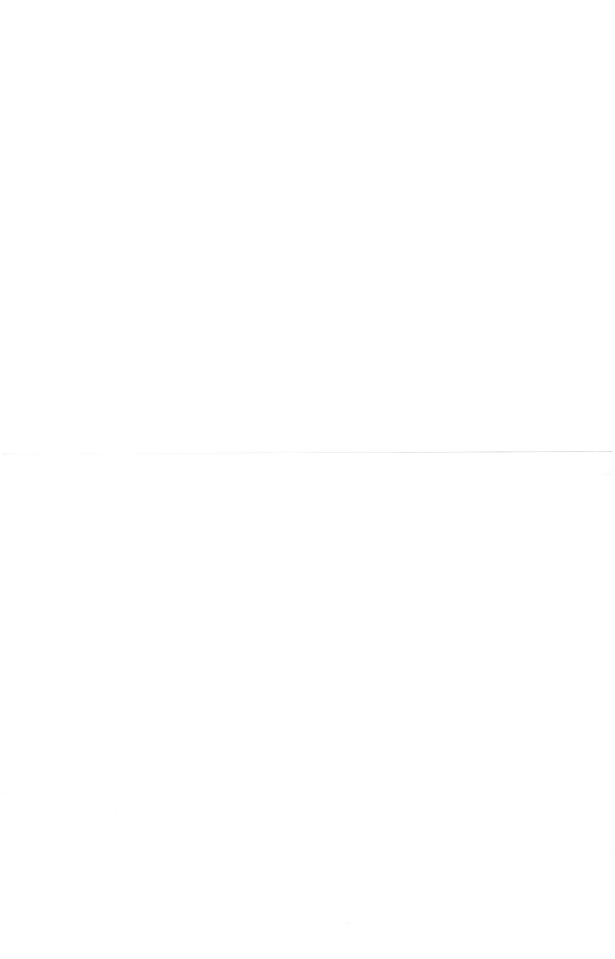

6

Evidence-Based Theory for Drug Prescribing in Dentistry

6.1 General Considerations

Q. Is it appropriate to prescribe antibiotics against postsurgical infections in implant/periodontal surgery and oral/maxillofacial surgery?

A. Yes and no. It has been reported that presurgical antibiotics and good surgical technique reduced postoperative infection to 1%. The longer the surgical procedure, the higher the incidence of postoperative infection. A single prophylactic antibiotic dose is sufficient and using antibiotics after the surgery is not indicated unless extensive surgery is performed with soft tissue manipulation, in which case it is recommended to continue antibiotics for 10 days following the surgery. The decision to use postsurgical antibiotics depends on the patient (e.g., uncontrolled diabetic patient). So, the clinical situation should be evaluated before any antibiotics are prescribed. Use of an antimicrobial rinse such as chlorhexidine gluconate can also be prescribed before and after surgery (Resnik and Misch 2008).

Q. If antibiotics are indicated before a dental surgical procedure, when should they be started?

A. To have the maximum effect, the antibiotic should be in the tissues when the bacterial contamination occurs, not after. In order for this to happen, the antibiotic needs to be administered about one hour before surgery to attain plasma levels 3–4 times the minimum inhibitory concentration (MIC) needed to kill bacteria (Peterson 1990). The antibiotic should not be given the day before or several days before the surgery (Classen et al. 1992). If antibiotic prophylaxis is required, the American Heart Association (AHA) recommends it be given between 30 and 60 minutes before a procedure.

Q. What is the usual prophylactic dose of antibiotic that should be prescribed preoperatively?

A. According to Peterson (1990), in order to achieve high levels in the plasma for the maximal therapeutic response, the dose is usually twice the regular dose; it is equivalent to administering the loading and maintenance dose. For example, if the usual dose of amoxicillin is 500 mg, prescribe 1 g, or some dentists give the same dose that the AHA recommends for prophylaxis against bacteremia, which is 2 g one hour before the dental procedure.

Q. Should there be a concern about development of bacterial resistance when prescribing short-term prophylactic antibiotics before a surgical procedure?

The Dentist's Drug and Prescription Guide, Second Edition. Mea A. Weinberg, Stuart J. Froum and Stuart L. Segelnick.
© 2020 John Wiley & Sons, Inc. Published 2020 by John Wiley & Sons, Inc.

A. No. Selective growth of resistant bacteria begins only once the host's susceptible organisms are killed, which occurs in about three days of antibiotic use. Thus, one day/time of antibiotic use does not affect the development of resistant bacteria (Peterson 1990).

Q. Does the selected antibiotic need to be effective against primarily anaerobic or aerobic bacteria?

A. Since the oral environment is usually 2 : 1 anaerobic to aerobic bacteria, it is best to choose an antibiotic effective against both periodontal pathogens (Resnik and Misch 2008). The rest of the chapter will give recommendations for using specific antibiotics with a specific bacterial infection.

Bacteria are classified as follows.

- Gram-positive facultative cocci: *Streptococcus sanguis, mitis, salvarius, Staphylococcus aureus.*
- Gram-positive facultative rods: *Actinomyces* (including *Actinomyces viscosus, A. naeslundii*).
- Gram-negative facultative rods: *Eikenella corrodens, Capnocytophaga* spp., *Aggregatibacter actinomycetemcomitans* (formerly *Actinobacillus actinomycetemcomitans*).
- Gram-positive obligate anaerobic coccus: *Peptostreptococcus* spp.
- Gram-positive obligate anaerobic rods: *Eubacterium* spp.
- Gram-negative obligate anaerobic rods: *Porphyromonus gingivalis, Prevotella intermedia, Tannerella forsynthensis* (formerly *Bacteroides forsythus*), *Fusobacterium nucleatum.*
- Gram-negative anaerobic spirochete: *Treponema* spp.
- Obligate aerobic: *Mycobacterium tuberculosis, Pseudomonas aeruginosa.*

Q. What can happen if antibiotics are used indiscriminately?

A. The indiscriminate use of systemic antibiotics could influence the emergence of bacterial strains which would be resistant to eradication by antibiotics. However, as stated in a previous question, development of resistant strains after one day of antibiotic use will most likely not happen. Allergies to drugs may also develop.

Q. What is antimicrobial stewardship and why is it important in dentistry?

A. The term "antimicrobial stewardship" refers to a program encouraging responsibility in the use of antibiotics and antimicrobials to reduce the incidence of resistance (Dyar et al. 2017). Although it is more commonly employed in hospitals, it is just as important in dentistry (Stein et al. 2018). There are numerous ways to reduce the misuse of antibiotics in dentistry, including stressing the importance of antibiotic stewardship to other dentists, setting up antibiotic stewardship in dentistry (e.g., dental societies), and changing prescribing practices (Stein et al. 2018; Tomczyk et al. 2018).

Q. Is it best to use a single antibiotic or combinations?

A. Depending upon the results of antimicrobial testing and susceptibility, combination antibiotic therapy may be necessary in mixed infections. It could be more advantageous to use combination drugs because the simultaneous use of two drugs of the same category (e.g., two bactericidal antibiotics) can achieve bactericidal synergism, allowing a reduction in dose or a shorter duration of therapy. For example, amoxicillin and metronidazole are effective against *A. actinomycetemcomitans*, where either antibiotic alone is ineffective (Jorgensen and Slots 2000). Combination drugs can also help to reduce the emergence of resistant bacterial strains. A disadvantage of using multiple antibiotics is the increased incidence of adverse effects and potential drug–drug interactions. For example, prescribing a bacteriostatic antibiotic such as tetracycline with a bactericidal drug such as amoxicillin is not advised because the bactericidal antibiotic requires active multiplying bacteria in order to destroy the bacteria.

Q. Is it appropriate to start therapy with a broad-spectrum antibiotic?

A. When prescribing antibiotics, the risk versus benefits must be considered. Broad-spectrum antibiotics increase the incidence of superinfections with *Candida* sp., enteric rods, pseudomonads, and staphylococci and increase the emergence of resistant bacterial strains.

Q. Should the prophylactic antibiotic be bactericidal or bacteriostatic?

A. Bactericidal. The antibiotic should kill the bacteria rather than inhibiting multiplication and reproduction.

Q. What is the inoculum effect?

A. The maximum concentration to have a therapeutic effect may be insufficient even with the recommended prescribed dose because of the large number of bacteria present in untreated periodontal pockets. Thus, the MIC of a certain antibiotic may actually be higher than the standard MIC for that drug.

6.2 Prescribing for Inflammatory Periodontal Diseases and Periodontal Surgical Procedures

Q. Do antibiotics have a role in the management of periodontal disease and periodontal therapy?

A. Yes. In some cases, antibiotics have been shown to be helpful in the co-management of periodontal diseases and the selective use of antibiotics will help to avoid inappropriate prescribing.

Q. If systemic antibiotics are indicated in the adjunctive management of certain periodontal diseases, when should antibiotics be started?

A. Antibiotics should never be used alone without being accompanied by mechanical debridement (scaling and root planing) and/or periodontal surgery.

Q. Why is it necessary to use antibiotics in conjunction with scaling and root planing?

A. Mechanical debridement is necessary to disrupt the bacterial biofilm (colonies). This makes it easier for the antibiotic to penetrate the bacterial cell.

Q. Has the classification for periodontal and periimplant diseases changed?

A. Yes. In 2017, the American Academy of Periodontology made changes to the 1999 classification (Caton et al. 2018). Essentially, periodontitis is no longer referred to as chronic and aggressive; however, these terms are still being used. Now, periodontitis is named according to *stages* of severity and complexity of management, *extent and distribution* and *grade* which show the risk of rapid progression and anticipated treatment response.

1) Stage I: initial periodontitis
   Stage II: moderate periodontitis
   Stage III: severe periodontitis with potential for additional tooth loss
   Stage IV: severe periodontitis with potential for loss of the dentition

2) Extent and distribution: localized, generalized, molar (first molar)-incisor distribution
   Grade A: slow rate of progression
   Grade B: moderate rate of progression
   Grade C: rapid rate of progression

6.2.1 Gingivitis, Dental Biofilm Induced

Q. What bacteria are primarily found in dental biofilm-induced gingivitis?

A. Predominant bacteria in chronic gingivitis include *Actinomyces* spp., *Capnocytophaga* spp., *Fusobacterium* spp., and *Streptococcus* spp. (*Streptococcus mitis, oralis, sanguis, gordonii, intermedius*) (Teles et al. 2007).

Q. Is antibiotic therapy used for dental biofilm-induced gingivitis?

A. Although chronic gingivitis is a bacterial infection, there is no current literature to support the use of systemic antibiotics because the infection is localized to the gingival unit with shallow probable depths which is easily treatable and reversible with mechanical debridement and optimal oral hygiene.

Q. Is there any rationale for using topical antimicrobial agents for the treatment of chronic gingivitis?

A. Topical antimicrobials including chlorhexidine gluconate may be used as an *adjunct* to scaling and root planing to help control the gingival inflammation but should never be used without mechanical debridement.

6.2.2 Periodontitis

Q. What are the bacteria found in inflammatory periodontitis?

A. Predominant bacteria in periodontitis, previously referred to as chronic periodontitis, include all of the bacteria in gingivitis in addition to obligate anaerobes: *Porphyromonas gingivalis* and *Prevotella intermedia* and facultative anaerobes: *Fusobacterium* spp., *Eikinella corrodens*, *Tannerella forsythensis* (formerly *Bacteroides forsythus*), *A. actinomycetemcomitans* (*Aa*), *A. naeslundii*, *Peptostreptococcus* spp., *A. viscosus*, *Veillonella* spp., and *Treponema denticola*.

Q. Do some bacteria invade the gingival tissues?

A. Yes. Some bacteria invade the inflamed gingival tissues rather than merely staying in the periodontal pocket. Prevalence of *Aa* in gingival tissue may be higher in localized molar-incisor periodontitis patients than in other stages of periodontitis (Thiha et al. 2007).

Q. Is systemic antibiotic therapy used in the treatment of periodontitis?

A. The use of systemic antibiotics in periodontitis is very controversial. Some studies show that the addition of antibiotics to mechanical debridement may reduce the need for further treatment, including surgery. In the 1980s, Loesche showed a benefit of using antibiotics as an adjunct (or after subgingival debridement) to conventional periodontal treatment in "reducing the need for periodontal surgery" in patients with chronic periodontitis. Actually, although defined as having chronic periodontitis, these patients could have had refractory periodontitis. In Loesche's studies, the need for surgery or extractions was determined 4–6 weeks after initial treatment which consisted of scaling and root planing and metronidazole

250 mg, three times a day for seven days. Results showed a decrease in teeth requiring surgery, pocket probing depths and subgingival bacteria (*Bacteroides* and spirochetes) and an apparent gain in periodontal attachment (Loesche et al. 1984, 1991, 1992, 1996). Metronidzole is only effective against obligate anaerobes and not *Aa*, *E. corrodens*, and *Capnocytophaga*.

Other studies using amoxicillin plus metrondizole as an adjunct to mechanical debridement have resulted in improved clinical parameters and high percentage of elimination of *Aa* and *P. gingivalis* in stage III–IV periodontitis (formerly *advanced* chronic and refractory chronic periodontitis) (van Winkelhoff et al. 1992).

Sefton et al. (1996), reported that azithromycin (500 mg once daily) consistently reduced spirochetes in chronic periodontitis patients throughout the 22 weeks of the study, but only reduced pigmented anaerobes at three and six weeks. Additional long-term studies using larger numbers of subjects need to be performed.

On the other hand, some clinical studies have documented that there are no additional treatment outcome benefits when antibiotics are used as an adjunct to scaling and root planing and periodontal pocket elimination surgery (Slots and Rams 1990). The first clinical periodontal studies using tetracycline in chronic periodontitis patients found no statistically significant differences in probing depth reduction but a slight improvement in attachment levels (Listgarten et al. 1978).

Q. What is doxycycline 20 mg?

A. Doxycycline 20 mg is a subantimicrobial dose indicated for the management of generalized Grade A, B periodontitis. The trade name was Periostat˚, but it is now available generically as doxycycline hyclate 20 mg. Usual antibiotic doses are 100–200 mg but at 20 mg doxycycline exerts anticollagenase rather than antibacterial activity. Doxycycline 20 mg inhibits the synthesis and secretion of collagenase which is an enzyme that breaks down collagen which makes up the periodontium (bone, connective tissue). This anticollagenase property does not depend on the drug's antibacterial actions. Doxycycline 20 mg is indicated for generalized periodontitis especially in cases where scaling and root planing are ineffective in halting the progression of attachment loss.

Q. Clinically, what are the outcomes of prescribing doxycycline hyclate 20 mg?

A. Gain of clinical or periodontal attachment and decreased probing depth.

Q. What does gain of clinical attachment mean?

A. After periodontal therapy (e.g., scaling and root planing), reduction of probing depths as a result of gingival recession and/or removal of inflammatory infiltrate in the gingival connective tissue with reformation of collagen fibers. Healing after conventional periodontal therapy is usually via a long junctional epithelium (repair).

Q. Do the same contraindications/precautions with doxycycline apply to doxycycline 20 mg?

A. Yes. Doxycycline 20 mg should not be used in pregnant or breastfeeding women. Inform female patients on oral contraceptives. There is possible development of resistant bacterial strains.

Q. What is the recommended dosage for doxycycline hyclate 20 mg?

A. Taken twice a day (every 12 hours) as an adjunct to scaling and root planing for up to 9 months.

Q. What are specific instructions on how to take the drug?

A. Take on an empty stomach at least one hour before or two hours after meals. Do not take concurrently with antacids, iron, zinc or multivitamins (wait two hours before or two hours after). Swallow with a full glass of water to prevent esophageal irritation. It is safe to take dairy products with doxycycline.

Q. What should be done if a dose is missed?

A. If the missed dose is close to the next dose, skip the missed dose and proceed with regular dosing regimen. Do not take two doses at once to make up the missed dose.

6.2.3 Necrotizing Periodontal Diseases

Q. What are necrotizing periodontal diseases (NPDs)?

A. NPDs, formerly known as ulcerative periodontal diseases, were renamed in the 2017 classification of periodontal diseases. Since it has been suggested that necrotizing ulcerative gingivitis (NUG) and necrotizing ulcerative periodontitis (NUP) are different stages of the same disease, they will together be referred to as NPDs. NPDs can occur in both gingivitis and periodontitis patients (Caton 2018). NPDs are bacterial infections caused specifically by *Treponema* spp., *F. nucleatum*, and *P. intermedia*.

Q. What is the treatment for NPDs?

A. It is the consensus that antibiotics are required to treat NPDs. Many different antibiotic regimens have been suggested but the first drug of choice is metronidazole (250 mg three times a day for seven days) (Malek et al. 2017; Todescan and Atout 2013). Other antibiotics that can be prescribed include tetracycline, amoxicillin and a combination of amoxicillin and metronidaloze.

Q. What can be recommended for pain control?

A. Ibuprofen 400–600 mg three times a day, if there are no contraindications or precautions including peptic ulcer disease and renal disease.

6.2.4 Refractory Periodontitis

Q. What is refractory periodontitis?

A. Refractory periodontitis was eliminated as a separate diagnostic term from the 1999 periodontal classification. In the 2017 classification, refractory periodontitis was included as a Grade C periodontitis. Antimicrobial therapy in these patients is reviewed in Table 6.1.

Table 6.1 Antibiotics that can be prescribed for Grade C periodontitis

- Clindamycin (Gram-negative) 150 mg q6h for 10 days (Gordon et al. 1990; Walker et al. 1993). Postantibiotic therapy with clindamycin results in gain of attachment and pocket depth reduction (clindamycin comes in 150 mg cap).
- Metronidazole + amoxicillin (Gram-negative obligate/facultative): 500 mg amoxicillin +500 mg metronidazole: 1 tab each q8h for seven days (van Winkelhoff and Winkel 2005).
- Amoxicillin clavulanate (Gram-positive): 250 mg tid for 10 days.
- Metronidazole (Gram-negative obligate): 250–500 mg tid for 10 days (Loesche et al. 1996; Saxén and Asikainen 1993; Winkel et al. 2001).

Q. Where are oral microbiology testing labs located in the United States?

A. The Oral Microbiology Testing Service (OMTS) Laboratory at Temple University Maurice H. Kornberg School of Dentistry (Dr Rams) in Philadelphia, Oral Microbiology Testing Laboratory at University of Southern California (Dr Slots) and Oral Microbiology Laboratory (OML) at the University of North Carolina-Chapel Hill in North Carolina.

Q. What is a DNA probe?

A. DNA probes will detect specific species and determine the antibiotic susceptibility. Molecular DNA testing uses saliva to identify and measure specific types of bacteria in periodontal diseases. Oral DNA Labs (a Quest Diagnostics Company) (www.oraldna.com/) does oral salivary DNA testing. Micro-IDent[*]plus by Hain Lifescience (www.micro-ident.de/en/products/micro-ident-and-micro-identplus) uses paper points placed in periodontal pockets to measure specific types of bacteria found in periodontal disease. They also test for GenoType IL-1 which may detect a predisposition for increased host response.

6.2.5 Molar-Incisor Periodontitis

Q. What is aggressive periodontitis?

A. The term "aggressive periodontitis" is no longer used since the new 2017 World Workshop on Classification of Periodontal Diseases. According to the 2017 World Workshop, current research does not support aggressive periodontitis as a separate disease. Instead, it is classified as periodontitis with variations in clinical presentation including *extent* and *severity* and population subsets with distinct disease (Papapanou et al. 2018). There is a genetic predisposition to aggressive periodontitis which is modified with certain risk factors such as smoking and diabetes. Localized and generalized aggressive periodontitis is currently referred to as Grade C periodontitis. In localized periodontitis, <30% of sites are involved. If >30% of periodontal sites are affected, then it is generalized periodontitis and if only the molars and incisors are effected it is called Molar/incisor pattern (MIP).

Q. Should systemic antibiotics be prescribed in patients with molar-incisor periodontitis?

A. Literature has documented the use of systemic antibiotics in molar-incisor (formerly known as aggressive) periodontitis which has high levels of *A. actinomycetemcomitans*. The use of systemic antibiotics in periodontal infections is based solely on the fact that certain bacteria invade the epithelial cells of the gingiva rather than just staying in the pocket area (Revert et al. 1990; Saglie et al. 1982). These bacteria, including *P. gingivalis* (Pg), *A. actinomycetemcomitans*, and spirochetes, invade the gingiva and avoid removal by scaling and root planing; hence, systemic antibiotics should be used. *P. gingivalis* also has the ability to invade human gingival fibroblasts. Numerous papers support the adjunctive use of systemic antibiotics in the treatment of localized and generalized aggressive periodontitis because of the invasion of these bacteria into the periodontal tissues, which cannot be eradicated by scaling and root planing or surgery alone.

Q. Which systemic antibiotics are recommended in the management of molar-incisor periodontitis?

A. Since there are many different combinations of periodontal pathogens in periodontitis, at least 10 different antibiotic regimens may be required to specifically target the various pathogen complexes (Beikler et al. 2004). Antibiotics immediately after scaling and root planing can provide more probing depth reduction and gain of attachment with healing improved up to six months (Doğan et al. 2007; Söder et al. 1989). There is no controversy regarding the use of systemic antibiotics in the adjunctive treatment of molar-incisor periodontitis. However, there may be some questions regarding the selection of antibiotic. Haffajee et al. (2003) reported a statistically significant improvement in periodontal attachment levels with tetracycline, metronidazole or metronidazole plus amoxicillin for a reduction in probing depths and clinical attachment gain (Table 6.2).

Table 6.2 Suggested antibiotic dosages used in molar-incisor periodontics

- Penicillin V (250–500 mg qid) + metronidazole (250–500 mg tid) for 8–10 days (Yek et al. 2010; Walker and Karpinia 2002)
- Azithromycin (can penetrate into both normal and diseased periodontal tissues and into polymorphonuclear leukocytes (PMNs) and has a postantibiotic effect): 500 mg qd for 4–7 days (Sefton et al. 1996)
- Clindamycin: 150–300 mg q6h for 8–10 days
- Metronidazole: 250–500 mg q8h for 8–10 days (for obligate anaerobic infections)
- Metronidazole/amoxicillin (500/500 for seven days) (McGowan et al. 2017)

Q. Can Arestin® or Atridox® be applied into the periodontal pocket in molar-incisor periodontitis patients?

A. No. Locally applied antibiotics have little or no effect on *A. actinomycetemcomitans* and do not penetrate deep into the gingival tissues.

Q. Can metronidazole be prescribed alone?

A. Metronidazole is only effective against obligate or strict or obligate anaerobes so it should be prescribed with penicillin to have better antimicrobial coverage.

6.2.6 Periodontal Therapy

6.2.6.1 Periodontal Flap Surgery: Pocket Reduction/Osseous Surgery

Q. Are systemic antibiotics necessary after pocket reduction/osseous surgery?

A. The primary rationale for using systemic antibiotics during surgical therapy is the fact that there may be an increased risk of complications including infection, pain, and delayed wound healing (Arab et al. 2006; Powell et al. 2005). Additionally, the bacterial burden of the host may be lessened with the use of systemic antibiotics (van Winkelhoff 2005). However, the prevention of infections after periodontal surgery through the routine use of antibiotics seems to be primarily based on empiricism and is very controversial and generally not recommended.

The majority of the literature does not support the use of prophylactic antibiotics in preventing postoperative infection in patients undergoing periodontal osseous surgery, including full-thickness flaps, degranulation, osteoplasty or ostectomy and sutures (Arab et al. 2006; Checchi et al. 1992; Oswal et al. 2014). Powell et al. (2005) reported that there was no statistical difference in the incidence of postoperative infections in patients undergoing periodontal surgery who did not take an antibiotic (1.81%) and those who received antibiotics pre- and/or postoperatively (2.85%). Very few studies support the use of antibiotics after periodontal osseous surgery to reduce pain swelling and improve wound healing (Peterson 1990).

Q. Why do dentists prescribe antibiotics after periodontal surgery?

A. Many dentists base their decision to use antibiotics pre- and/or postoperatively empirically. Do antibiotics reduce the incidence of infections post osseous surgery? According to Powell et al. (2005), the overall incidence of infections following different periodontal surgeries was 2.09%. Patients who received antibiotics had a 2.85% incidence of infections compared to 1.81% where antibiotics were not used. Thus, it is the opinion of the authors that there is no benefit in using antibiotics for the sole purpose of preventing postosseous surgery infections (Oswal et al. 2014).

6.2.6.2 Bone/Bone Substitutes Grafting Procedures

Q. Should antibiotics be prescribed for bone grafting procedures?

A. Yes. The difference between periodontal osseous resective surgery and periodontal/socket preservation surgery using bone grafts or bone substitute materials is that in osseous resective surgery, native bone is being either removed (ostectomy) or reshaped (osteoplasty) and the remaining bone retains its blood and lymph supply. The concern is about periodontal surgery which involves the placement of bone grafts (autogenous, bovine, freeze-dried bone) or bone substitutes (hydroxyapatite, anorganic bovine bone, bioactive glass) without an established blood supply into an infrabony defect that already has an intact blood supply. An infrabony defect is a type of intrabony vertical defect with three bony walls bordering the tooth (Weinberg and Eskow 2000). Thus, until this grafted bone material can establish a blood supply rich in inflammatory and immune cells, antibiotics may be required to aid in preventing postsurgical infections. Additionally, optimal repair and regeneration of the periodontium has been shown to be enhanced when there is suppression of the microbiota during healing (Giannopoulou et al. 2006).

During the healing phase, by 18 hours there is an accumulation of PMNs which are the first inflammatory cells to move into the wound area (Zipfel et al. 2003). After blood clot formation and inflammation, there is a two-day period of fibroblast-like mesenchymal cell chemotaxis which is driven by growth factors (Zipfel et al. 2003). By 5–9 days, blood vessel components are observed. By day 10, the first osteoblasts with new bone formation are observed (Zipfel et al. 2003). Thus, until inflammatory and immune cells are established with blood vessel formation, it may be prudent to give antibiotics one hour before and for nine days after surgery to help prevent postoperative infection. The reason for starting the antibiotic only 1–2 hours before is because most antibiotics show peak blood levels 1–2 hours after the first dose. This dose will also provide blood levels that will infiltrate the graft site. It is not necessary to start the antibiotic many days before. The duration of antibiotic therapy is for 10 days when new bone has formed.

Most of the research done on the preoperative and postoperative use of antibiotics with bone grafts/bone substitutes evaluated the clinical outcomes of the surgery, namely looking at probing depth reduction and clinical attachment gain. Some studies showed increased graft success with antibiotics while others did not support the routine administration of antibiotics (Sculean et al. 2001). In summary, antibiotics should be prescribed for bone grafting procedures (periodontal and socket preservation) until a blood supply is established.

Q. What would be the rationale for using preoperative/postoperative systemic antibiotics for bone grafting procedures?

A. To reduce postoperative infection. However, using aseptic techniques and good surgical techniques are two important factors in reducing the incidence of postoperative infections (Resnik and Misch 2008). Until blood vessel formation can be established with inflammatory and immune cells, antibiotic coverage is recommended to reduce the incidence of postoperative infection.

Some clinical trials reported that the use of systemic antibiotics in conjunction with bone material or enamel matrix proteins did not produce statistically significant pocket depth reduction and gain of clinical attachment (Sculean et al. 2001).

Q. Does research recommend the use of prophylactic antibiotics when performing surgery with enamel matrix proteins (Emdogain®)?

A. There is no standard protocol for the adjunctive use of antibiotics, before or after surgery, with Emdogain. A 2001 clinical article found that there was no advantage in prescribing systemic antibiotics as an adjunct to Emdogain infrabony surgery (Sculean et al. 2001).

Q. Should an antibiotic be mixed with the bone graft/bone substitute material for periodontal osseous defects and socket preservation?

A. There is no standardized protocol for mixing an antibiotic (e.g., opening a tetracycline or doxycycline capsule) with a bone graft or bone substitute material. Tetracycline has been very popular for many years but research has shown that tetracycline and doxycycline reduce the activity of BMP2 (bone morphogenic protein) and osteogenic protein expression and cell differentiation (Park 2011). Additionally, tetracycline may actually chelate or bond calcium and inhibit bone formation (Misch and Roknian 2016; Rupprecht et al. 2007). Misch and Roknian (2016) recommend mixing parenteral penicillin, cephalosporin or clindamycin to the graft material because they do not interfere with bone regeneration. These authors do not recommend using tablets or opening capsules as they may contain fillers and other additives.

Q. Can tetracycline be used to etch root surfaces before bone grafting periodontal defects?

A. Some clinicians compound a 5% or 10% solution of tetracycline powder with normal saline, sterile water or local anesthetic without actually knowing the exact dilution to demineralize the root surface, burnish onto the root surface to remove the smear layer and fibrin and expose the collagen matrix. This indication for topical use of tetracycline is controversial when used for periodontal regeneration. Some cases have caused root resorption and may induce an inflammatory response (Ben-Yehouda 1997; Haddad-Houri et al. 2004). The pharmacist can make up a 5% solution, which is 50 mg/mL (pH 1.6), or a 10% solution, which is 100 mg/mL. Tetracycline and doxycycline are basic compounds but after reconstitution with water the pH of doxycycline becomes 1.6–3.3. It is noted that bone forms best with an alkaline pH.

6.2.6.3 Periodontal Regenerative Surgery: Guided Tissue Regeneration

Q. Is it recommended to prescribe systemic antibiotics for guided tissue regenerative surgery?

A. It depends (Froum and Weinberg 2016). Powell et al. (1990) reported a 2.99% postoperative infection rate after guided tissue regeneration (GTR). In 1993, Mombelli et al. reported that not only was bacterial colonization of the treated sites common but there were high total bacterial counts at the time of membrane removal (using nonbioabsorbable membranes) and on exposed membranes. The numbers of *P. gingivalis*, *P. intermedia*, *Tannerella forsythensis*, and *A. actinomycetemcomitans* on retrieved expanded polytetrafluoroethylene (e-PTFE) membranes (Gore-Tex®, Gore®) were high (Ling et al. 2003).

Upon membrane retrieval, bacteria were found in the collar part of the membrane, which was partly exposed supragingivally during the healing time (DeSanctis et al. 1996). Additionally, even in cases where the barrier material had remained unexposed during the entire healing time, bacteria were found in the collar part of the membrane. DeSanctis et al. (1996) concluded that it is actually bacterial colonization rather than bacterial contamination from the surgical procedure which may alter healing following membrane exposure (Hung et al. 2002).

The type of barrier material used is critical to the incidence of bacterial contamination. Bioabsorbable polylactic acid (Guidor®) shows less bacterial colonization than e-PTFE and has the most bacterial attachment on collagen membranes (Cheng et al. 2015). Sela et al. (2009) found that cross-linked collagen membranes (e.g., Biomend Extend™, Ossix™) are primarily broken down by proteolytic enzymes of *P. gingivalis*, but they are more resistant to proteolysis than collagen membranes that were not cross-linked (e.g., Bio-Gide®). Early destruction of membranes greatly influences the success of GTR surgery. Additionally, chlorhexidine, doxycycline, and minocycline were found to inhibit the breakdown from the proteolytic enzymes and metronidazole had no effect. It was concluded that the use of antibacterial agents with cross-linked collagen membranes may significantly inhibit the breakdown of membranes. This may be good since the membrane will remain in position longer, possibly increasing its effect.

Q. Is chlorhexidine oral rinse recommended for patients after GTR surgery?

A. Chlorhexidine has been found to reduce and delay, but not prevent, early bacterial accumulation on membrane materials, especially when it becomes exposed to the oral environment which may result in surgical failure or incomplete regeneration Additionally, chlorhexidine is likely not the primary factor in reducing bacterial accumulation but rather the type of membrane material used (Chen 2003). Liu et al. (2018) reported that chlorhexidine is cytotoxic to cells including fibroblasts and osteoblasts.

Q. What are recommended antibiotics for guided tissue regenerative surgery?

A. Different antibiotic regimens have been suggested. Since it was found that *P. gingivalis* and *Aa* are the primary bacteria that colonize membranes, an antibiotic that is specific to these bacteria is recommended. Metronidazole is very effective against Gram-negative obligates (*P. gingivalis*) but not facultative anaerobes (*Aa*). Amoxicillin seems to have a good inhibitory effect on these bacteria (Cheng et al. 2015). Amoxicillin plus clavulanate potassium has been documented to be 98.8–100% effective against obligate anaerobes as well as facultative anaerobes. These bacteria have a high resistance against clindamycin (Ardila et al. 2010). It has been suggested that coverage should be for eight days. In penicillin-allergic patients, azithromycin or doxycycline 100 mg can be used.

Q. When should the antibiotic be started?

A. According to Nowzari et al. (1995), 500 mg amoxicillin/clavulanic acid (Augmentin®) was started one hour before GTR surgery, followed by 500 mg tid for eight days afterward (Nowzari et al. 1995).

Q. Can locally applied antibiotics such as Atridox or Arestin be used with GTR?

A. No. There is lack of penetration of the locally applied (into the periodontal pocket) antibiotic in the deeper parts of the tissues.

6.3 Prescribing for Dental Implant Surgery

Q. Are systemic antibiotics necessary when placing implants?

A. The use of antibiotics when performing implant surgery is controversial according to the literature. A study on the success of implants (Laskin et al. 2000) and a literature review (Ahmad and Saad 2012) demonstrated an increased success rate in patients given antibiotics. Another study (El-Kholey 2014) and literature review (Sanchez et al. 2018) concluded that a single dose of oral amoxicillin preoperatively may be sufficient to increase implant success and reduce complications. However, another review (Park et al. 2017) stated that routine doses of antibiotics in healthy patients undergoing implant therapy are not needed. Based on the most recent data (Esposito et al. 2008; Kashani et al. 2005), antibiotics are beneficial for reducing failure of dental implants in healthy patients. The regimen recommended is one dose of amoxicillin 2 g prior to surgery (or one dose prior to surgery) and one dose later in the day post surgery.

  The clinician should note that all these reviews and studies refer to healthy patients. With an increase in the number of older (≥65 years) patients living longer and having implants placed, many of these patients would not be considered "healthy" by normal standards. Many have one or more ailments (and many take medications for these). Therefore, when performing surgery on patients who do not fall into the "healthy" category, increased use of antibiotics may be prudent. When treating these patients, a consultation with their physicians would be indicated to discuss medical clearance and prophylactic antibiotic regimens. In addition, if implants are being placed in conjunction with hard or soft tissue grafting, it may be advisable to prescribe antibiotics preoperatively and postoperatively (i.e., a 7–10-day regimen to avoid infection of graft sites and other postoperative complications). This would entail prescribing 2 g amoxicillin preoperatively and 500 mg three times a day for 7–10 days postoperatively, depending on the extent of surgery and the patient's health. If the patient is allergic to amoxicillin, then azithromycin should be prescribed. Articles have been published showing that clindamycin has a 4 times more implant failures and more sinus lift failures (Salomo-Coll et al. 2018; Khoury et al. 2018).

Q. Is there concern that the use of small doses before implant surgery can increase the incidence of bacterial resistance?

A. No. Selective growth of resistant bacteria begins only once the host's susceptible organisms are killed, which occurs in about three days (48 hours) of antibiotic use. Thus, one antibiotic dose does not affect the development of resistant bacteria (Peterson 1990).

Q. What is the definition of periimplant mucositis and periimplantitis?

A. Periimplant mucositis is defined as inflammation of the mucosa surrounding the implant without loss of bone surrounding the implant (Heitz-Mayfield and Salvia 2018).

  Periimplantitis is an inflammatory process that affects the periimplant bone around a dental implant that is in function (Albrektsson and Isidor 1994; Schwarz et al. 2018).

Q. What are the definitions of the ailing, failing, and failed implant?

A. An *ailing* implant is referred to as periimplant mucositis where only the gingiva is inflamed around the implant. There is no mobility or lost bone. A *failing* implant is referred to as periimplantitis where there is bone loss (2–3 threads exposed) around the implant. A *failed* implant is mobile. The first sign of a failing implant is pain and discomfort which indicates mobility (el Askary et al. 1999).

Q. What is the pharmacological management of the ailing, failing, and failed implant?

A. Presently, there is not enough evidence to support which is the most effective therapy for peri-implantitis. However, even though there is little evidence suggesting the most effective therapy for treating periimplantitis, currently used treatments may still be effective (Esposito et al. 2006, 2010; Lindhe and Meyle 2008; Norowski and Bumgardner 2009; Pye et al. 2009). According to the Sixth European Workshop on Periodontology, there is limited evidence that the adjunctive use of systemic antibiotics could resolve many periimplantitis lesions. Also, regenerative procedures had no additional beneficial effects on treatment outcomes (Lindhe and Meyle 2008). Klinge et al. (2005) describe periimplantitis as a site-specific infection comparable to chronic periodontitis and the incidence of periimplantitis varies according to implant design and surface characteristics with the different implant systems.

Suggested treatments for periimplantitis include the following.

1) Periimplant mucositis (ailing implant) is treated with mechanical debridement, oral hygiene instruction, chlorhexidine gluconate rinse/irrigation (for about 3–4 weeks or until the inflammation has resolved) and maintenance.

2) Failing implant: -resently, there is no consistent treatment regimen for a failing implant. There are many proposed treatments including mechanical debridement, chlorhexidine rinse/irrigation, controlled locally delivered antibiotics (Arestin, Atridox), systemic antibiotics (metronidazole 250 mg tid for 10 days; amoxicillin 250 mg tid for seven days) and surgery to detoxify or deplaque the implant surface. Even though in past literature there has been much clinical improvement with regenerative procedures, a study on regenerative surgical procedures using a bone graft or enamel matrix derivative (Emdogain) covered with a collagen membrane found promising results (Froum et al. 2012). Lasers have also been used to detoxify the implant (Froum 2018).

   Which is most effective for the treatment of periimplantitis: mechanical, chemical, or laser? Froum (2018) concluded that with a variety of surface decontamination treatments and limited studies comparing different treatments, no one protocol is more effective than the other.

3) Failed implant: removal of implant (Pye et al. 2009).

6.3.1 Prescribing for Sinus Floor Elevation Surgery

Q. What is the etiology of early infection following sinus floor elevation surgery?

A. Early infection following sinus floor elevation surgery and subsequent graft and/or implant failure can occur due to many factors including:

1) contamination of the sinus by sinus or oral cavity pathogens
2) existing chronic sinusitis
3) patient smoking, resulting in delayed incision healing
4) perforation of the membrane and blockage of the maxillary ostium with graft material
5) graft becomes contaminated with saliva
6) lack of aseptic technique.

Q. Are prophylactic antibiotics recommended for sinus elevation surgery?

A. Yes. Complications during and following sinus lift surgery include bacterial contamination at the time of implant placement, perforating the Schneiderian membrane followed by sinus infection, oroantral fistula, and infection of the graft. It is important for the antibiotic to be present before the infection develops. As the sinus fills with fluid, bacteria trapped in this moist, warm environment find it an excellent place to grow. They begin to multiply and cause infection. Since it is unknown whether complications will arise, antibiotic prophylaxis is given to patients.

Q. What is the rationale for using preoperative antibiotics for sinus floor elevation surgery?

A. To have the antibiotic present at the time of bacterial contamination for the prevention of postoperative infection of the sinus and graft or soft tissue perforation. Using a loading dose (LD) at least one hour before surgery will achieve blood levels that will infiltrate the grafted site.

Q. What should be done if an infection occurs following a sinus augmentation procedure?

A. If a patient develops a complication such as infection, abscess, pus or maxillary sinusitis following the augmentation procedure, it is recommended to reopen the sinus, debride the infected graft material and take a bacterial culture. Following thorough lavage of the area and removal of granulomatous tissue, nontension closure of the flap should be performed. In a paper by Puglisi et al. (2011), aspiration from 59 patients with chronic maxillary sinusitis showed that all specimens were polymicrobial. The predominant aerobes were *S. aureus* and *Streptococcus pneumoniae*, while the more frequent anaerobes were *Peptostreptococcus* spp. and *Prevotella* spp. *Haemophilus influenzae* and *Moraxella catarrhalis* were absent in sinusitis associated with a dental origin. Overall, 22% of *S. aureus* isolates were oxacillin resistant, and 75% of *S. pneumoniae* isolates were penicillin resistant and/or erythromycin resistant; 21% of anaerobic Gram-positive bacteria were penicillin resistant and 44% of anaerobic Gram-negative bacteria were beta-lactamase positive. Vancomycin and quinopristin-dalfopristin had the highest *in vitro* activity against *S. aureus* and *Streptococcus* spp., respectively; amoxicillin-clavulanate and cefotaxime showed the highest *in vitro* activity against aerobic Gram-negative bacteria; and moxifloxacin, metronidazole, and clindamycin were the most active against anaerobic bacteria.

Therefore, if *S. aureus*, *S. pneumoniae* or *S. pyogenes* was cultured from the exudate when entering a postaugmentation sinusitis, penicillin (amoxicillin) would be the antimicrobial agent of choice.

If an isolate contained predominantly Gram-negative species, i.e. *E. coli*, *Klebsiella* spp., *H. influenzae* or *M. catarrhalis*, amoxicillin-clavulanate 1000 mg followed by 500 mg taken three times a day for 7–10 days would be the antibiotic choice.

If isolates contained anaerobic species (i.e. *Peptostreptococcus* spp., *Propionibacterium aeinis*, *Prevotella* spp., *Porphyromonas* spp., *Fusobacterium nucleatum* and *Bacteroides fragilis*) metronidazole 500 mg three times per day for 10 days would be the antibiotic of choice. In a combination aerobic/anaerobic infection, amoxicillin-clavulanate 2 g to start then 500 mg three times a day together with metronidazole 500 mg three times a day for 10 days would be the combination drugs of choice along with flap debridement of the graft and saline lavage of the sinus

Q. What antibiotic should be prescribed before sinus elevation surgery?

A. The selection of antibiotic is based on the fact that is the membrane is perforated, the maxillary sinus will be exposed and the patient will most likely develop an acute sinusitis. The antibiotic of choice should be based on current guidelines for management of acute sinusitis. The cultivable bacteria should be known. Review of sinus aspiration studies performed in adults with acute sinusitis suggests that *S. pneumoniae* is isolated in approximately 20–43%, *H. influenzae* in 22–35%, and *M. catarrhalis* in 2–10% of aspirates. Other bacterial isolates found in patients with acute sinusitis include *S. aureus* and anaerobes. Local resistance patterns vary widely, but about 15% of *S. pneumoniae* has intermediate penicillin resistance and 25% is highly resistant

(Rosenfeld et al. 2007; Sinus and Allergy Health Partnership 2004). Therefore, broad-spectrum amoxicillin would be most appropriate. If the patient has a past history of chronic or periodontic sinus infections, amoxicillin-clavulanate potassium is recommended. (Tasoulis et al. 2011). The azalides (azithromycin, clarithromycin) may also be used for patients with penicillin allergy (Rosenfeld et al. 2007; Tasoulis et al. 2011). The spectrum of activity of penicillin V is narrow and does not cover *H. influenzae* or *M. catarrhalis*. This is why amoxicillin is useful for sinus infections (Rosenfeld et al. 2007). A recent article states that clindamycin should be avoided due to development of infections and loss of grafting material (Khoury et al. 2018).

Q. What happens if the patient was previously taking an antibiotic in the past 4–6 weeks?

A. This increases the chance for bacterial resistance. Guidelines from the Sinus and Allergy Health Partnership recommend the use of high-dose amoxicillin-clavulanate (Augmentin; can write the prescription for the generic) (Rosenfeld et al. 2007; Sinus and Allergy Health Partnership 2004).

Q. What should be done if the infection does not respond to the antibiotics given?

A. Once the graft is infected and there is pus, the graft area must be irrigated and the patient placed on an antibiotic for up to three weeks. If the infection has not resolved, the graft may have to be removed. Once the infection is eliminated, the area can be regrafted (Misch 1992; Smiler 1997). A referral to an ENT practitioner may be warranted before or after sinus surgery (Cote et al. 2011; Rapsa 2017).

Q. What other medications should be given before sinus surgery?

A. Some symptoms/signs of sinusitis include infection (purulent exudates), nasal congestion and headache (Katranji et al. 2008). Patients with existing chronic sinusitis have a higher incidence of sinusitis after sinus surgery.

Prescribing nasal decongestants can help to reduce the incidence of obstruction of the ostium after surgery.

- Nasal decongestants.
  - Afrin® (oxymetazoline) nasal spray (starting a few days before surgery and continued for 10–14 days after surgery). Starts working within 10 minutes and lasts for about 12 hours. It works by causing vasoconstriction of the nasal mucosa.
- Antiinflammatory medications (to minimize postoperative swelling).
  - Ibuprofen 800 mg q8h for five days (if there are no contraindications for ibuprofen such as peptic ulcer disease, asthma [aspirin insensitivity], or patient taking warfarin).
  - Methylprednisolone dose pack (follow tapering dosage instructions on pack) *or* dexamethasone 8 mg (Decadron®) starting one hour before surgery, then 4 mg for two days.

Q. How is a prescription for methylprednisolone written (Table 6.3)?

A. If a patient is a poor candidate for corticosteroids (e.g., uncontrolled diabetes, peptic ulcer disease, osteoporosis, Cushing' syndrome, preexisting wide angle glaucoma, systemic viral disease, and psychiatric disorders), it is highly recommended that their physician be contacted. Antimicrobial rinse: chlorhexidine gluconate 0.12% rinse (Farhat et al. 2008).

Table 6.3 How a prescription for methylprednisolone is written

Rx Methylprednisolone Dosepak
Disp: 1 package
Sig: Use as directed in the instructions on the package.

6.4 Prescribing for Oral Surgery

Q. What are the most likely bacteria causing an infection after oral and maxillofacial surgery?

A. Streptococci, anaerobic Gram-positive cocci, and anaerobic Gram-negative rods.

Q. Do antibiotics routinely need to be prescribed with extractions?

A. No. A review of controlled studies for mandibular third molar surgery found little or no evidence of benefit from antibiotic prophylaxis to prevent local infection for most dentoalveolar surgery in medically healthy patients (Lawler et al. 2005). Every patient must be assessed individually. It is normal to have some inflammation with pain, swelling, redness, and trismus (limitation of jaw opening) following an extraction. This is not diagnostic of an infection (Sancho-Puchades et al. 2009).

Q. When should antibiotic prophylaxis be needed for third molar extractions?

A. There are few adequate reviews of clinical studies on antibiotic prophylaxis in oral surgery. In 2007, a Task Force of the American Association of Oral and Maxillofacial Surgeons that reviewed different aspects of third molar extractions did not even mention anything about antibiotic prophylaxis or antibiotics after extractions. Surgeons recommend that in routine nonimpacted third molar extractions, antibiotic prophylaxis is probably not necessary. Antibiotic prophylaxis using a narrow-spectrum, single, high dose of antibiotic (e.g., penicillin V) may be indicated for deep bony impactions.

Q. What is the rationale for prescribing after third molar surgical extraction?

A. Ideally, extraction procedures should be of short duration with minimal soft and hard tissue damage. Complications following surgical extraction can include inflammation and infection. The more osteotomy, tissue manipulation and longer procedures may benefit from a preoperative antibiotic prophylaxis (single dose). However, there is no literature showing this (Schwartz and Larsen 2007).

Q. What constitutes an infection following tooth extraction?

A. Hot intense swelling, presence of fluctuation, purulent discharge from the extraction site for more than 72 hours after surgery. Pain and swelling that gets worse or does not improve 48 hours after surgery (Lawler et al. 2005; Pogrel 1993).

Q. Is dry socket an infection of the socket and are oral antibiotics indicated?

A. No. Dry socket or alveolar osteitis is not considered to be an infection but rather a consequence of early wound healing with increased fibrinolytic activity. This condition usually does not require oral antibiotics; however, a 2015 article considered the use of azithromycin and chlorhexidine rinse to reduce dry socket incidence (Tarakji et al. 2015).

6.5 Prescribing for Odontogenic Infections

Q. Are odontogenic infections composed of many bacteria?

A. Yes. Odontogenic infections are polymicrobial. Studies have documented that there is an average of 4–6 different bacterial pathogens. The bacteria found in the early stages of an odontogenic infection are primarily aerobic and in the later, chronic stages (days later), it is converted from aerobic to anaerobic colonies.

Q. What is an abscess?

A. An abscess is a collection of pus or dead neutrophils (PMNs) formed by the tissue and is caused by an infection involving bacteria which are usually slow growing. The body walls off an abscess (to prevent the spread of infection) with host cells such as PMNs, which can reduce the ability of the antibiotic to penetrate the bacteria. Thus, it is important, when possible, to perform an incision and drainage (I & D) before the antibiotic is administered; it is most important to remove the reservoir of infection and reduce the bacterial load.

Q. What is the regimen for prescribing antibiotics for periodontal or endodontic abscesses?

A. There are two schools of thought concerning the optimal duration of antibiotic therapy: the duration of therapy should be either three days (high dose; short term) or 7–10 days. Of course, it depends on the severity of the infection and if there is systemic involvement.

Using antibiotics at high dose for short periods of time (e.g., three or five days versus 10 days) has been suggested because it increases patient adherence as well as targeting both sensitive and most resistant bacteria (due to the high dose), reducing both the development of resistance and the amount of antibiotic delivered to the environment. If antibiotics are prescribed over a long period (e.g., >7–10 days), there is increased incidence of bacterial resistance (Pallasch 1996) because any bacteria that survive low doses of antibiotics most likely are resistant. Medical literature favoring three-day therapy claims that prolonged exposure to antibiotics increases the risk of adverse effects, and the development of antibiotic resistant bacteria (El Moussaoui et al. 2006; Paul 2006).

Following the short-term therapy recommendations for odontogenic infections: the LD for penicillin should be 1.0 g on the first day, followed by a maintenance dose of 500 mg qid after the LD. The LD for clindamycin should be 600 mg on the first day, followed by 300 mg after the LD (American Academy of Periodontology 2004).

Some medical literature recommends that longer durations, 10 days, of treatment may be required if the initial therapy was not effective against the offending bacteria. Cunningham et al. (2009) reviewed antibiotic duration in adults hospitalized with community-acquired pneumonia. They found that there was no difference in the risk of treatment failure between the short-term versus long-term antibiotic regimens and may be it depends on the antibiotic chosen. It should be noted that these patients were hospitalized with mild to moderate community-acquired pneumonia, a potentially life-threatening condition. One of the reasons for not using short-term therapy is that after three or five days the patient may relapse.

Another clinical study comparing 4–5 days versus 10-day antibiotic therapy in patients with Group A streptococcal tonsillopharyngitis found shorter courses of penicillin were inferior to 10-day courses (Casey and Pichichero 2005).

Q. What does the term "selective pressure" of antibiotics mean?

A. Selective or selection pressure of antibiotics has led to the emergence of resistant bacteria while the susceptible bacteria die. Antibiotics can affect normal flora (bacteria not associated with the disease) which leads to the emergence of resistant bacteria inhabiting the same environment. So, antibiotics actually select for resistant strains (Albrich et al. 2004).

6.5.1 Prescribing for Endodontic Abscess

Q. How do bacteria gain access to the pulp?

A. Normally, bacteria enter the pulp through decay.

Q. Are the same bacteria in both an endodontic and periodontal abscess?

A. It is a mixed anaerobic (facultative and obligate) bacterial infection. The bacteria are similar, but every endodontic infection has a different combination of bacteria; no two infections are the same. Some bacteria types include:

- facultative Gram-positive cocci (*Streptococcus* spp.)
- anaerobic Gram-positive cocci (*Peptostreptococcus* spp.)
- Gram-negative anaerobic rods (e.g., *Prevotella* spp., *Fusobacterium necrophorum*, *Bacteroides vulgaris*) (Khemaleelakul et al. 2002).

Q. What is the healing capacity of the pulp?

A. The pulp has limited capacity to heal because it has a limited blood supply; it represents terminal circulation. When bacteria enter the pulp, an inflammatory reaction occurs, which does not heal. After the inflammatory process is initiated, it eventually leads to necrosis of the pulp.

Q. What are the different endodontic diagnoses and specific treatments?

A. Table 6.4 lists different endodontic diagnosis terminology according to the American Association of Endodontists (AAE). A complete endodontic diagnosis is made up of two parts: pulpal diagnosis and periapical diagnosis.

Table 6.4 Classification of endodontic lesions

Diagnosis	Signs and symptoms	Treatment	Antibiotics required
Pulpal diagnosis			
Normal pulp	None + cold + heat + electric pulp testing	None	None
Reversible pulpitis	++ cold (but does not linger) ++ heat (but does not linger)	Inflammation will resolve on its own and pulpal tissues return to normal	None
Irreversible pulpitis (symptomatic and asymptomatic)	Symptomatic: vital inflamed pulp. Lingering thermal (cold and heat) pain; spontaneous pain; + electric pulp testing. Asymptomatic: no clinical symptoms but inflammation due to caries or trauma	Pulpectomy or extraction	No antibiotic is required because the infection is contained within the pulpal tissue or just around the tissue. There are no signs of an infection such as fever, facial swelling or purulence
Pulp necrosis	Nonvital pulp; asymptomatic. Electric pulp testing	Root canal treatment if the tooth is restorable	None
Previously initiated therapy	Could be symptomatic	Finish endodontic therapy	None

Table 6.4 (Continued)

Diagnosis	Signs and symptoms	Treatment	Antibiotics required
Previously treated	Could be symptomatic or asymptomatic	Retreat if necessary	None
Periapical diagnosis			
Normal apical tissues	No symptoms	No treatment	None
Symptomatic apical periodontitis	Pain on percussion and biting; may or may not be associated with an apical radiolucent area	Endodontic therapy	None
Asymptomatic apical periodontitis	Apical radiolucent area; no clinical symptoms (tenderness, thermal reaction, percussion)	Endodontic therapy	None
Acute apical abscess	Spontaneous, rapid onset of pain, tenderness of tooth to pressure, pus formation and swelling	Endodontic therapy	Antibiotics are needed to prevent the spread of infection before treatment of the tooth. Medical attention may be necessary
Chronic apical abscess	Little or no discomfort to percussion with some discharge of pus through sinus tract	Endodontic therapy	None. Pus is being drained through the sinus tract.

Source: Adapted from www.aae.org/specialty/wp-content/uploads/sites/2/2017/07/endodonticdiagnosisfall2013.pdf.

Q. Is there a difference between a sinus tract and a fistula?

A. Yes, the difference depends on the lining of each tract. These two terms are often confusing to the dentist. A fistula is an internal connection between two epithelial surfaces such as a tract between the epithelial lining of the intestines and the skin epithelium. On the other hand, a sinus tract is a connection between bone (e.g., periapical lesion) and an epithelial surface (e.g., alveolar mucosa), which discharges purulent exudates (Harrison and Larson 1976). Draining sinus tracts are commonly lined with granulation tissue, not epithelium, which is chronic inflammatory tissue produced from chronic inflammation from bacterial contaminated root canals. Days after root canal therapy, microscopic analysis shows that the tract is completely gone because it is lined with chronic inflammatory granulation tissue rather than epithelium (Harrison and Larson 1976). When the source of the inflammation, the granulation tissue, is removed via endodontic procedures, the lesion will heal. On the other hand, since a fistula is lined with epithelial tissue, the lesion would probably not heal because the epithelial tissue is not a product of inflammation. Thus, in dental diagnosis, the term "fistula" is discouraged in favor of the more correct term "sinus tract" (Harrison and Larson 1976). By definition, a chronic apical abscess is a sinus tract. Because the pus is draining, sinus tracts are usually not accompanied by pain or swelling (Slutzky-Goldberg et al. 2009). On the other hand, asymptomatic apical periodontitis has an apical radiolucent area not associated with a sinus tract.

Q. How does a sinus tract develop?

A. A sinus tract develops as a result of a periapical lesion when the inflammatory process expands concentrically, and it is closer to the buccal than the lingual plate. Development of a sinus tract usually does not cause pain because it functions for drainage of the infection. If the infection is not allowed to drain through a pulpal opening (through the tooth), sinus tract or an incision, extraoral swelling and lymph node involvement will likely develop as the abscess spreads beyond the local confines of the periapical area and into the fascial planes. Sinus tracts are usually associated with chronic apical abscesses (Baumgartner 2004). Radiographically, radiolucency is usually seen apical to the abscessed tooth.

Q. What does the radiolucency around the apex indicate?

A. Periradicular bone destruction. The infected necrotic pulp is contained in the canal by either an epithelial plug or a layer of neutrophils (white blood cells) at the apical foramen which attempts to prevent the bacteria from invading the periradicular area. The invasion of bacteria past the apical foramen into the periradicular area causes the production of an abscess or cellulitis (Baumgartner 2004).

Q. How does the periapical radiolucency develop?

A. First, the radiographic periodontal ligament (PDL) widening is due to edema, resulting in accumulation of inflammatory exudates in the collagen (connective tissue) of the PDL. The PDL widening is referred to as apical periodontitis. This PDL widening can be caused by occlusal trauma (e.g., primary occlusal trauma is caused by a "high" restoration on a tooth with adequate periodontal support), orthodontic movement or tooth extrusion. Additionally, inflammatory cells present in the exudates include PMNs, which are the first inflammatory cells to arrive at the site of injury which is the pulp (e.g., due to bacterial caries involvement). The function of PMNs is to prevent the microbial invasion but unfortunately this is a "double-edged sword" because while attempting to kill the bacteria, they also cause host tissue damage during the acute phases of apical periodontitis. It is the dead PMNs within the root canal that release enzymes such as phospholipase A that induce prostaglandin E_2-mediated bone resorption. Also, proinflammatory cytokines including interleukin (IL)-1 and tumor necrosis factor (TNF)-alpha secreted by PMNs and macrophages play an additional role in periapical bone resorption and increase in collagenase production.

Q. How does an endodontic infection occur?

A. The dental pulp is sterile. The most common way bacteria enter the pulp is via dental caries. Other ways of bacterial entry into the pulp include mechanical or traumatic exposure, lateral and furcal canals or exposed noncarious dentinal tubules, cracks in the enamel–dentine junction and periodontal exposure of dentinal tubules (Baumgartner 2004). The necrosis starts from the pulp chamber and then goes through the pulpal canal to the apex.

Q. Why do some periapical lesions show radiopacity?

A. If the bone surrounding a lesion shows osteosclerosis, most likely this is caused by resistance to the pathological process resulting from osteoblastic activity.

Q. What is the difference between an acute versus a chronic apical abscess?

A. An acute lesion produces pain on biting and percussion while a chronic lesion produces little to no discomfort.

Q. What is the most current antibiotic recommendation in endodontics?

A. In 2017, the American Association of Endodontists (AAE) published *AAE Guidance on the Use of Systemic Antibiotics in Endodontics* (American Association of Endodontists 2017).

Q. When are antibiotics indicated in an endodontic infection?

A. There must be systemic signs and symptoms of infection or spread of infection: increased swelling, cellulitis, malaise, fever >37.8 °C (100 °F), lymphadenopathy, persistent infection or osteomyelitis (American Association of Endodontists 2017). According to the AAE, swellings increasing in size should be incised for drainage and adjunctive antibiotics used (American Association of Endodontists 2017). Antibiotics are indicated when the diagnosis is acute apical abscess. Also, antibiotics are recommended in immunocompromised patients.

Q. When are antibiotics not indicated?

A. Antibiotics are not indicated in endodontic therapy in the following cases (American Association of Endodontists 2017; Crumpton and McClanahan 2003).

- There is pain without signs and symptoms (e.g., swelling) of infection.
- Irreversible pulpitis with or without symptomatic apical periodontitis (older term was acute periradicular periodontitis).
- Necrotic pulp with a draining sinus tract (this acts as a pathway of drainage) (e.g., chronic apical abscess – older term was chronic periradicular abscess).
- Necrotic pulp with chronic periradicular periodontitis without swelling.

Q. Are systemic antibiotics indicated in irreversible pulpitis?

A. No. In irreversible pulpitis, antibiotics do not significantly reduce the pain, percussion perception or quantity of pain medication needed. The best way to relieve the pain is to perform a pulpotomy which will remove the inflamed pulp (Fedorowicz et al. 2005).

Q. Are antibiotics necessary in treating a combined perio/endo lesion?

A. No. Management of a combined lesion is based on basic endodontic and periodontal therapy. Remember that antibiotics are not a substitute for mechanical debridement of the root canal and root surface (Longman et al. 2000).

Q. Why are endodontic infections difficult to treat with antibiotics?

A. Infections in areas of poor blood supply (avascular), such as abscesses, necrotic areas and sinus infections, are difficult to treat because of poor distribution and concentration of the antibiotic into these regions. Additionally, the diversity of pathogens in the canal and their different sensitivities make antibiotic choice difficult.

Q. What is the antibiotic of choice for an acute apical abscess?

A. Although there are no specific guidelines suggesting an ideal antibiotic, there are some recommendations based on current evidence and microbiology. Penicillin VK is the antibiotic of choice for an acute apical abscess because most bacteria are susceptible to it and it is a narrow-spectrum antibiotic which is all that is required for the bacterial profile in an endodontic abscess. It has been recommended to prescribe a high dose for a short period of time to be effective and help reduce the development of resistance (American Association of Endodontists 2017; Baumgartner and Xia 2002; Karlowsky et al. 1993; Robertson and Smith 2005).

- The dose of penicillin V is: LD 1000 mg stat on day 1, followed by 500 mg q6h after the LD up to day 5, 7 or 10 as needed.
- If the patient is allergic to penicillin:
  - clindamycin: LD 600 mg followed by 300 mg q6h for 5–7 days, *or*
  - azithromycin: LD 500 mg on day 1, then 250 mg once a day for 2–5 days, *or*
  - clarithromycin: LD 500 mg followed by 250 mg q12h for 5–7 days.

Q. Why is clindamycin recommended for patients allergic to penicillin?

A. Clindamycin is highly effective against anaerobic bacteria and penetrates bone well (Levine 2003).

Q. What is a recommended antibiotic if the infection is not confined and is spreading?

A. Augmentin (amoxicillin-clavulanic acid) 875 mg bid. If allergic to penicillin, then prescribe Z-pack 250 mg (two tabs day 2 and then one tab days 2–5).

Q. Are any bacteria resistant to penicillin?

A. Yes. Some anaerobic bacteria from endodontic lesions are resistant to penicillin. The only way to determine this if a culture and sensitivity test was not performed is that the patient will not be getting clinically better in a few days. In these cases, it is necessary to switch to another antibiotic such as amoxicillin-clavulanic acid or clindamycin, which penetrates bone very well.

Q. For how long should antibiotics be prescribed?

A. Five to seven days, even though clinical signs and symptoms will start to decrease within 2–4 days. No longer than seven days because of potential destruction of normal oral flora.

Q. Does the severity of the abscess influence the dose of an antibiotic?

A. Yes. The larger the extent of infection, the greater the dose and concentration of the antibiotic will need to be.

Q. Why is penicillin V the best antibiotic, in nonallergic, nonimmunocompromised patients, for the management of an endodontic abscess?

A. It is ideal to choose a narrow-spectrum antibiotic. Penicillin V is well distributed into most soft tissue sites, saliva, and abscesses. It is effective against facultative bacteria including streptococci and anaerobic bacteria. Even though there are many more strains present in an infection that cannot be identified in susceptibility tests, penicillin V is effective against many of the strains in a polymicrobial infection. Also, choosing a narrow-spectrum antibiotic like penicillin allows the patient's immune response to cope with the remaining strains. This is why I & D and debriding the root canal to remove the reservoir of infection are important and reduce the bacterial load. However, if the patient is immunocompromised, then a broad-spectrum antibiotic like amoxicillin is indicated. However, a broad-spectrum antibiotic may select for resistant organisms elsewhere in the body, including the gastrointestinal (GI) and genitourinary (GU) tract. These resistant organisms may be detrimental to the patient in the future. This is why the narrower spectrum of penicillin V is recommended unless it is a life-threatening infection or the patient is immunocompromised (Baumgartner and Xia 2002).

Q. What patient instructions are important for penicillin V?

A. Take penicillin with a full glass of water one hour before or two hours after meals. Take with yogurt or acidophilus tabs.

Q. Why is amoxicillin not the drug of choice for an odontogenic infection?

A. Amoxicillin is not needed in the treatment of routine odontogenic infections because it shows slightly less activity against Gram-positive cocci but increased efficacy against aerobic Gram-negative cocci and bacilli, bacteria not commonly involved in odontogenic infections (Karlowsky et al. 1993).

Q. Are cephalosporins effective in treating periapical infections?

A. No. Cephalosporins are broad-spectrum antibiotics with limited activity in periapical infections because most periapical infections are mixed bacterial infections dominated by obligate anaerobic bacteria. Cephalosporins are not highly effective against these bacteria with less activity against many anaerobics than penicillin (Levine 2003).

6.5.2 Prescribing for Periodontal Abscess

Q. What is the treatment for a periodontal abscess?

A. The initial treatment of a periodontal abscess consists of establishing drainage, which is usually through the gingival pocket. Following effective drainage of pus, removal of the cause, which is usually subgingival calculus, is performed through scaling and root planing. The area can be irrigated with chlorhexidine or saline. Antibiotics are indicated if there is systemic involvement (e.g., fever, lymphadenopathy) or the infection has spread (e.g., cellulitis). Have the patient return to the office in about three days to evaluate. Further treatment (e.g., periodontal surgery or extraction) may be necessary.

Q. Can an antibiotic be prescribed for a periodontal abscess without scaling and root planing?

A. An antibiotic should never be prescribed without mechanical removal of the bacterial load. An antibiotic cannot penetrate the bacterial cell wall if the biofilm is not disrupted. Additionally, scaling and root planing before the start of antibiotics may minimize the microbial regrowth because microorganisms could spread and grow onto other oral surfaces. If an antibiotic is needed, a beta-lactam (e.g., penicillin V) agent is still recommended (Shweta and Prakash 2013).

References

Ahmad, N. and Saad, N. (2012). Effects of antibiotics on dental implants: a review. *Journal of Clinical Medicine Research* 4 (1): 1–6.

Albrektsson, T. and Isidor, F. (1994). Consensus Report of Session IV. In: Proceedings of the First European Workshop on Periodontology (eds. N.P. Lang and T. Karring), 365–369. London: Quintessence Publishing.

Albrich, W.C., Monnet, D.L., and Harbarth, S. (2004). Antibiotic selection pressure and resistance in *Streptococcus pneumoniae* and *Streptococcus pyogenes*. *Emerging Infectious Diseases* 10: 514–517.

American Academy of Periodontology (2004). Position paper. Systemic antibiotics in periodontics. *Journal of Periodontology* 75: 1553–1565.

American Association of Endodontists (2017). AAE Guidance on the Use of Systemic Antibiotics in Endodontics. www.aae.org/specialty/wp-content/uploads/sites/2/2017/06/aae_systemic-antibiotics.pdf.

Arab, H.R., Sargolzaie, N., Moeintaghavi, A. et al. (2006). Antibiotics to prevent complications following periodontal surgery. *International Journal of Pharmaceutics* 2: 205–208.

Ardila, C.M., López, M.A., and Guzmán, I.C. (2010). High resistance against clindamycin, metronidazole and amoxicillin in P*orphyromonas gingivalis* and *Aggregatibacter actinomycetemcomitans* isolates of periodontal disease. *Medicina Oral Patologia Oral y Cirugia Bucal* 1: e947–e951.

el Askary, A.S., Meffert, R.M., and Griffin, T. (1999). Why do dental implants fail? Part I. *Implant Dentistry* 8: 173–185.

Baumgartner, J.C. (2004). Microbial aspects of endodontic infections. *Journal of the California Dental Association* 32: 459–468.

Baumgartner, J.C. and Xia, T. (2002). Antibiotic susceptibility of bacteria associated with endodontic abscesses. *Journal of Endodontics* 29: 44–77.

Beikler, T., Prior, K., Ehmke, B. et al. (2004). Specific antibiotics in the treatment of periodontitis – a proposed strategy. *Journal of Periodontology* 75: 169–175.

Ben-Yehouda, A. (1997). Progressive cervical root resorption related to tetracycline root conditioning. *Journal of Periodontology* 68: 432–435.

Casey, R.R. and Pichichero, M.E. (2005). Metaanlysis of short course antibiotic treatment for group a streptoccal tonsillopharyngitis. *Pediatric Infectious Disease Journal* 24: 909–917.

Caton, J.B., Armitage, G., Berglundh, T. et al. (2018). A new classification scheme for periodontal and peri-implant diseases and conditions – introduction and key changes from the 1999 classification. *Journal of Periodontology* 89 (Suppl 1): S1–S8.

Checchi, L., Trombelli, L., and Nonato, M. (1992). Postoperative infections and tetracycline prophylaxis in periodontal surgery: a retrospective study. *Quintessence International* 23: 191–195.

Chen, T.Y. (2003). Attachment of periodontal ligament cells to chlorhexidine-loaded guided tissue regeneration membranes. *Journal of Periodontology* 74: 1652–1659.

Cheng, C.-F., Wu, K.-M., Chen, Y.-T., and Hung, S.-L. (2015). Bacterial adhesion to antibiotic-loaded guided tissue regeneration membranes – a scanning electron microscopy study. *Journal of the Formosan Medical Association* 114: 35–45.

Classen, D.C., Evans, R.S., Pestotnik, S.L. et al. (1992). The timing of prophylactic administration of antibiotics and the risk of surgical wound infection. *New England Journal of Medicine* 326: 281–286.

Cote, M.T., Segelnick, S.L., Rastogi, A., and Schoor, R. (2011). New York state ear, nose, and throat specialists' views on pre-sinus lift referral. *Journal of Periodontology* 82 (2): 227–233.

Crumpton, B.J. and McClanahan, S. (2003). Antibiotic resistance and antibiotics in endodontics. *Clinical Update* 25 (12). Naval Postgraduate Dental School.

Cunningham, K.E., Ellis, S., and Kripalani, S. (2009). What is the proper duration of antibiotic treatment in adults hospitalized with community-acquired pneumonia? www.the-hospitalist.org/hospitalist/article/124075/antimicrobial-resistant-infections/what-proper-duration-antibiotic.

DeSanctis, M., Xucchelli, G., and Clauser, C. (1996). Bacterial contamination of barrier material and periodontal regeneration. *Journal of Clinical Periodontology* 23: 1039–1046.

Doğan, D., Cristan, C., Dietrich, T. et al. (2007). Timing affects the clinical outcome of adjunctive systemic antibiotic therapy for generalized aggressive periodontitis. *Journal of Periodontology* 79: 1201–1208.

Dyar, O.J., Huttner, B., Schouten, J. et al. (2017). What is antimicrobial stewardship. *Clinical Microbiology and Infection* 23 (11): 793–798.

El Moussaoui, R., de Borgie, C.A.J.M., van den Broek, P. et al. (2006). Effectiveness of discontinuing antibiotic treatment after three days versus eight days in mild to moderate-severe community acquired pneumonia: randomized, double blind study. *British Medical Journal* 332: 1355–1358.

El-Kholey, K.E. (2014). Efficacy of two antibiotic regimens in the reduction of early dental implant failure: a pilot study. *International Journal of Oral and Maxillofacial Surgery* 43 (4): 487–490.

Esposito, M., Grusovin, M.G., Coulthard, P. et al. (2006). Interventions for replacing missing teeth: treatment of peri-implantitis. *Cochrane Database of Systematic Reviews* 3: CD004970.

Esposito, M., Grusovin, M.G., Talati, M. et al. (2008). Interventions for replacing missing teeth: antibiotics at dental implant placement to prevent complications. *Cochrane Database of Systematic Reviews* 3: CD004152.

Esposito, M., Grusovin, M.G., Tzanetea, E. et al. (2010). Interventions for replacing missing teeth: treatment of perimplantitis. *Cochrane Database of Systematic Reviews* 6: CD004970.

Farhat, F.F., Kinaia, B., and Gross, H.B. (2008). Sinus bone augmentation: a review of the common techniques. *Compendium of Continuing Education in Dentistry* 29 (7): 388–392.

Fedorowicz, Z., Keenan, J.V., Farman, A.G. et al. (2005). Antibiotic use for irreversible pulpitis. *Cochrane Database of Systematic Reviews* 2: CD004969.

Froum, S.J. (2018). Which is the most effective for the treatment of peri-implantitis: mechanical, chemical or laser? www.perioimplantadvisory.com/articles/2018/01/which-is-most-effective-for-the-treatment-of-peri-implantitis-mechanical-chemical-or-laser.html.

Froum, S.J. and Weinberg, M.A. (2016). Antibiotics for periodontal and implant surgery. *International Journal of Periodontics and Restorative Dentistry* 35: 418–487.

Froum, S.J., Froum, S.H., and Rosen, P.S. (2012). Successful management of peri-implantitis with a regenerative approach: a consecutive series of 51 treated implants with 3-to7.5 year follow-up. *International Journal of Periodontics and Restorative and Dentistry* 32 (1): 11–20.

Giannopoulou, C., Andersen, E., Brochut, P. et al. (2006). Enamel matrix derivative and systemic antibiotics as adjuncts to non-surgical periodontal treatment: biologic response. *Journal of Periodontology* 77: 707–713.

Gordon, J.M., Walker, C., Hovlaris, C. et al. (1990). Efficacy of clindamycin hydrochloride in refractory periodontitis: 24-month results. *Journal of Periodontology* 61: 686–691.

Haddad-Houri, Y., Karaka, L., Stabholz, A. et al. (2004). Tetracycline conditioning augments the in vivo inflammatory response induced by cementum extracts. *Journal of Periodontology* 75: 388–392.

Haffajee, A.D., Socransky, S.S., and Gunsolley, J.C. (2003). Systemic anti-infective periodontal therapy. A systematic review. *Annuals of Periodontology* 8: 115–181.

Harrison, J.W. and Larson, W.J. (1976). The epithelized oral sinus tract. *Oral Surgery Oral Medicine Oral Pathology* 42: 511–517.

Hertz-Mayfield, L.J.A. and Salvia, G.E. (2018). Peri-implant mucositis. *Journal of Periodontology* 89 (Suppl 1): 257–S266.

Hung, S.H., Lin, Y.W., Want, Y.H. et al. (2002). Permeability of *Streptococcus mutans* and *Actinobacillus actinomycetemcomitans* through guided tissue regeneration membranes and their effects on attachment of periodontal ligament cells. *Journal of Periodontology* 73: 843–851.

Jorgensen, M.G. and Slots, J. (2000). Responsible use of antimicrobials in periodontics. *Journal of the California Dental Association* 28: 185–193.

Karlowsky, J., Ferguson, J., and Zhanel, G. (1993). A review of commonly prescribed oral antibiotics in general dentistry. *Journal of the Canadian Dental Association* 59: 292–300.

Kashani, H., Dahlin, C., and Alsen, B. (2005). Influence of different prophylactic antibiotic regiments on implant survival rate: a retrospective clinical study. *Clinical Implant Dentistry and Related Research* 7 (1): 32–35.

Katranji, A., Fotek, P., and Wang, H.L. (2008). Sinus augmentation complications: etiology and treatment. *Implant Dentistry* 17 (3): 339–349.

Khemaleelakul, S., Baumgartner, J.C., and Pruksakorn, S. (2002). Identification of bacteria in acute endodontic infections and their antimicrobial susceptibility. *Oral Surgery Oral Medicine Oral Pathology Oral Radiology Endodontology* 94: 746–755.

Khoury, F., Javed, F., and Romanos, G.E. (2018). Sinus augmentation failure and postoperative infections associated with prophylactic clindamycin therapy: an observational case series. *International Journal of Oral & Maxillofacial Implants* 33 (5): 1136–1139.

Klinge, B., Hultin, M., and Berglundh, T. (2005). Peri-implantitis. *Dental Clinics of North America* 49: 661–676.

Laskin, D.M., Dent, C.D., Morris, H.F. et al. (2000). The influence of preoperative antibiotics on success of endosseous implants at 36 months. *Annuals of Periodontology* 5: 166–174.

Lawler, B., Sambrook, P.J., and Goss, A.N. (2005). Antibiotic prophylaxis for dentoalveolar surgery: is it indicated? *Australian Dental Journal* 50 (Suppl 2): S54–S59.

Levine, S.P. (2003). Endodontics. In: Dental Secrets, 3rde (ed. S.T. Sonis), 117–137. Philadelphia: Hanley & Belfus.

Lindhe, J. and Meyle, J. (2008). Peri-implant diseases: consensus report of the sixth European workshop on periodontology. *Journal of Clinical Periodontology* 35 (Suppl. 8): 282–285.

Ling, L.J., Hung, S.L., Lee, C.F. et al. (2003). The influence of membrane exposure on the outcomes of guided tissue regeneration: clinical and microbiological aspects. *Journal of Periodontal Research* 38: 57–63.

Listgarten, M.A., Lindhe, J., and Helldén, L. (1978). Effect of tetracycline and/or scaling on human periodontal disease. Clinical, microbiological, and histopathological observations. *Journal of Clinical Periodontology* 5: 246–271.

Liu, J.X., Werner, J., Kirsch, T. et al. (2018). Cytotoxicity evaluation of chlorhexidine gluconate on human fibroblasts, myoblasts, and osteoblasts. *Journal of Bone and Joint Infection* 3 (4): 165–172.

Loesche, W.J., Syed, S.A., Morrison, E.C. et al. (1984). Metronidazole in periodontitis. I. Clinical and bacteriological results after 15 to 30 weeks. *Journal of Periodontology* 55: 325–335.

Loesche, W.J., Schmidt, E., Smith, B.A. et al. (1991). Effects of metronidazole on periodontal treatment needs. *Journal of Periodontology* 62: 247–257.

Loesche, W.J., Giordano, J.R., Hujoel, P. et al. (1992). Metronidazole in periodontitis: reduced need for surgery. *Journal of Clinical Periodontology* 19: 103–112.

Loesche, W.J., Giordano, J., Soehren, S. et al. (1996). Nonsurgical treatment of patients with periodontal disease. *Oral Surgery Oral Medicine Oral Pathology Oral Radiology Endodontology* 81: 533–543.

Longman, L.P., Preston, A.J., Martin, M.V. et al. (2000). Endodontics in the adult patient: the role of antibiotics. *Journal of Dentistry* 28: 539–548.

Malek, R., Gharibi, A., Khlil, N., and Kissa, J. (2017). Necrotizing ulcerative gingivitis. *Contemporary Clinical Dentistry*. 8 (3): 496–500.

McGowan, K., McGowan, T., and Ivanovski, S. (2017). Optimal dose and duration of amoxicillin-plus-metronidazole as an adjunct to non-surgical periodontal therapy: a systematic review and meta-analysis of randomized, placebo-controlled trials. *Journal of Clinical Periodontology* 45 (1): 56–57.

Misch, C.M. (1992). The pharmacologic management of maxillary sinus elevation surgery. *Journal of Oral Implantology* 18: 15–23.

Misch, C.E. and Roknian, V.A. (2016) Keys to predictable socket grafting – part I. www.oralhealthgroup.com/features/keys-predictable-socket-grafting-part-1.

Mombelli, A., Lang, N.P., and Nyman, S. (1993). Isolation of periodontal species after guided tissue regeneration. *Journal of Periodontology* 64: 1171–1175.

Norowski, P.A. and Bumgardner, J.D. (2009). Biomaterial and antibiotic strategies for peri-implantitis. *Journal of Biomedical Materials Research Part B, Applied Biomaterials* 88: 530–543.

Nowzari, H., Matian, F., and Slots, J. (1995). Periodontal pathogens on polytetrafluoroethylene membrane for guided tissue regeneration inhibits healing. *Journal of Clinical Periodontology* 22: 469–474.

Oswal, S., Ravindra, S., Sinha, A., and Manjunath, S. (2014). Antibiotics in periodontal surgeries: a prospective randomised cross over clinical trial. *Journal of Indian Society of Periodontology* 18 (5): 570–574.

Pallasch, T.J. (1996). Pharmacokinetic principles of antimicrobial therapy. *Periodontology 2000* 10: 5–11.

Papapanou, P.N., Sanz, M., Buduneli, N. et al. (2018). Periodontitis: consensus report of workgroup 2 of the 2017 world workshop on the classification of periodontal and peri-implant diseases and conditions. *Journal of Periodontology* 89 (Supp 1): S173–S182.

Park, J.B. (2011). Effects of doxycycline, minocycline, and tetracycline on cell proliferation, differentiation, and protein expression in osteoprecursor cells. *Journal of Craniofacial Surgery* 22 (5): 1839–1842.

Park, J., Tennant, M., Walsh, L.J., and Kruger, E. (2017). Is there a consensus on antibiotic usage for dental implant placement in healthy patients? *Australian Dental Journal* 63 (1): 25–33.

Paul, J. (2006). What is the optimal duration of antibiotic therapy? *British Medical Journal* 332: 1358.

Peterson, L.J. (1990). Antibiotic prophylaxis against wound infections in oral and maxillofacial surgery. *Journal of Oral and Maxillofacial Surgery* 58: 617–620.

Pogrel, M.A. (1993). Infection management. *Oral and Maxillofacial Surgery Clinics of North America* 5: 127–135.

Powell, C.A., Mealey, B.L., Deas, D.E. et al. (2005). Post-surgical infections: prevalence associated with various periodontal surgical procedures. *Journal of Periodontology* 76: 329–333.

Puglisi, S., Privitera, S., Maiolino, L. et al. (2011). Bacteriological findings and antimicrobial resistance in odontogenic and non-odontogenic chronic maxillary sinusitis. *Journal of Medical Microbiology* 60: 1353–1359.

Pye, A.D., Lockhart, D.E.A., Dawson, M.P. et al. (2009). A review of dental implants and infection. *Journal of Hospital Infection* 72: 104–110.

Rapsa, K. (2017). Sinus lifts failure resulting in chronic sinusitis. *Journal of Otolaryngology-ENT Research* 8 (6): 00270.

Resnick, R. and Misch, C. (2008). Prophylactic antibiotic regimens in oral implantology – rationale and protocol. *Dental Implant Summaries* 17 (1): 142–150.

Revert, S.M., Wilström, G., Dahlèn, G. et al. (1990). Effect of subgingival debridement on the elimination of *Actinobacillus actinomycetemcomtans* and *Bacteriodes gingivalis* from periodontal pockets. *Journal of Clinical Periodontology* 17: 345–350.

Robertson, D. and Smith, A.J. (2005). The microbiology of the acute dental abscess. *Journal of Medical Microbiology* 58: 155–162.

Rosenfeld, R.M., Andes, D., Bhattacharyya, N. et al. (2007). Clinical practice guideline: adult sinusitis. *Otolaryngology – Head and Neck Surgery* 137: S1–S31.

Rupprecht, S., Petrovic, L., Burchhardt, B. et al. (2007). Antibiotic-containing collagen for the treatment of bone defects. *Journal of Biomedical Materials Research* 83 (2): 314–319.

Saglie, R., Newman, M.G., Carranza, F.A. Jr. et al. (1982). Bacterial invasion of gingival in advanced periodontitis in humans. *Journal of Periodontology* 53: 217–222.

Salomó-Coll, O., Lozano-Carrascal, N., Lázaro-Abdulkarim, A. et al. (2018) Do penicillin-allergic patients present a higher rate of implant failure? *International Journal of Oral & Maxillofacial Implants* 33: 1390–1395.

Sanchez, F.R., Andres, C.R., and Arteagoitia, I. (2018). Which antibiotic regiment prevents implant failure or infection after dental implant surgery? A systematic review and meta-analysis. *Journal of Cranio-Maxillo-Facial Surgery* 46: 722–736.

Sancho-Puchades, M., Herrázez-Vilas, J.M., Berini-Aytés, L. et al. (2009). Antibiotic prophylaxis to prevent local infection in oral surgery: use or abuse? *Medicina Oral Patologia Oral Cirugia Bucal* 14: E28–E33.

Saxén, L. and Asikainen, S. (1993). Metronidazole in the treatment of localized juvenile periodontitis. *Journal of Clinical Periodontology* 20: 166–171.

Schwartz, A.B. and Larsen, E.L. (2007). Antibiotic prophylaxis and postoperative complications after tooth extraction and implant placement: a review of the literature. *Journal of Dentistry* 35: 881–888.

Schwarz, F., Derks, J., Monje, A., and Wang, H.-L. (2018). Peri-implantitis. *Journal of Periodontology* 89 (Suppl 1): S267–S290.

Sculean, A., Blaes, A., Arweiler, N. et al. (2001). The effect of post-surgical antibiotics on the healing of intrabony defects following treatment with enamel matrix proteins. *Journal of Periodontology* 72: 190–195.

Sefton, A.M., Maskell, J.P., Beighton, D. et al. (1996). Azithromycin in the treatment of periodontal disease. Effect on microbial flora. *Journal of Clinical Periodontology* 23: 998–1003.

Sela, M.N., Babirtski, E., Steinberg, D. et al. (2009). Degradation of collagen-guided tissue regeneration membranes by proteolytic enzymes of *Porphyromonas gingivalis* and its inhibition by antibacterial agents. *Clinical Oral Implants Research* 20: 496–502.

Shweta, S. and Prakash, S.K. (2013). Dental abscess: a microbiological review. *Dental Research Journal* 10 (5): 585–591.

Sinus and Allergy Health Partnership (SAHP) (2004). Antimicrobial treatment guidelines for acute bacterial rhinosinusitis. *Otolaryngology – Head and Neck Surgery* 30 (Suppl): 1–45.

Slots, J. and Rams, T.E. (1990). Antibiotics in periodontal therapy: advantages and disadvantages. *Journal of Clinical Periodontology* 17: 479–493.

Slutzky-Goldberg, I., Tsesis, I., Slutzky, H. et al. (2009). Odontogenic sinus tracts: a cohort study. *Quintessence International* 40: 13–18.

Smiler, D.G. (1997). The sinus lift graft: basic technique and variations. *Practical Periodontics & Aesthetic Dentistry* 9: 885–893.

Söder, P.O., Frithiof, L., Wikner, S. et al. (1989). The effects of metronidazole in treatment of young adults with severe periodontitis. *Journal of Dental Research* 68: 710, abstr 86.

Stein, K., Singhal, S., Mara, F., and Quinonez, C. (2018). The use and misuse of antibiotics in dentistry. A scoping review. *Journal of the American Dental Association* 149 (10): 869–884.

Tarakji, B., Saleh, L.A., Umair, A. et al. (2015). Systemic review of dry socket: aetiology, treatment, and prevention. *Journal of Clinical and Diagnostic Research* 9 (4): ZE10–ZE13.

Tasoulis, G., Yao, S.G., and Fine, J.B. (2011). The maxillary sinus: challenges and treatment for implant placement. *Compendium* 32: 10–20.

Teles, R.P., Bogren, A., Patel, M. et al. (2007). A three-year prospective study of adult subjects with gingivitis II: microbiological parameters. *Journal of Clinical Periodontology* 34: 7–17.

Thiha, K., Takeuchi, Y., Umeda, M. et al. (2007). Identification of periodontopathic bacteria in gingival tissue of Japanese periodontitis patients. *Oral Microbiology and Immunology* 22: 201–207.

Todescan, S. and Atout, R.N. (2013). Managing patients with necrotizing ulcerative gingivitis. *Journal of the Canadian Dental Association* 79: D46.

Tomczyk, S., Whitten, T., Holzbauer, S.M., and Lynfield, R. (2018). Combating antibiotic resistance: a survey on the antibiotic-prescribing habits of dentists. *General Dentistry* 66 (5): 61–68.

Walker, C. and Karpinia, K. (2002). Rationale for use of antibiotics in periodontics. *Journal of Periodontology* 73: 1188–1196.

Walker, C.B., Gordon, J.M., Magnusson, I. et al. (1993). A role for antibiotics in the treatment of refractory periodontitis. *Journal of Periodontology* 64 (8 Suppl): 772–781.

Weinberg, M.A. and Eskow, R.N. (2000). Osseous defects: proper terminology revisited. *Journal of Periodontology* 71: 1928.

Winkel, E.G., van Winkelhoff, A.J., Timmerman, M.F. et al. (2001). Amoxicillin plus metronidazole in the treatment of adult periodontitis patients. A double-blind, placebo-controlled study. *Journal of Clinical Periodontology* 28: 296–305.

van Winkelhoff, A.J. (2005). Antibiotics in periodontics: are we getting somewhere? *Journal of Clinical Periodontology* 32: 1094–1095.

van Winkelhoff, A.J. and Winkel, E.G. (2005). Microbiological diagnostics in periodontics: biological significance and clinical validity. *Periodontology 2000* 39(1): 40–52.

van Winkelhoff, A.J., Tijhof, C.J., and de Graaff, J. (1992). Microbiological and clinical results of metronidazole plus amoxicillin therapy in *Actinobacillus actinomycetemcomitans*-associated periodontitis. *Journal of Periodontology* 63: 52–57.

Yek, E.C., Cintan, S., Topcuoglu, N. et al. (2010). Efficacy of amoxicillin and metronidazole combination for the management of generalized aggressive periodontitis. *Journal of Periodontology* 81: 964–974.

Zipfel, G.J., Guiot, B.H., and Fessler, R.G. (2003). Bone grafting. *Neurosurgical Focus* 14: 1–8.

7

Management of Medications Taken by Medically Complex Dental Patients

7.1 American Heart Association Guidelines for Antibiotic Prophylaxis

Q. What are the current guidelines for antibiotic prophylaxis?

A. In 2017, the American Dental Association (ADA) and the American Heart Association (AHA) published the most current guidelines for the prevention of infective endocarditis (IE). Essentially, they reinforced the 2014 recommendations. The article is: Nishimura et al. (2017).

   The Committee concluded that only a very small number of cases of IE might be prevented by antibiotic prophylaxis for dental procedures even if prophylactic therapy were 100% effective.

Q. What are the current medical conditions that require antibiotic prophylaxis?

A. See Table 7.1.

Q. Does a patient with a cardiovascular implantable electronic device (e.g., pacemaker) require antibiotic prophylaxis according to the AHA?

A. There do not seem to be any scientific studies to support the use of antibiotic prophylaxis in these patients for invasive dental procedures (Baddour et al. 2011).

Q. Are there other medical conditions that may also require antibiotic prophylaxis?

A. Yes. When in doubt, get a medical consultation from the patient's physician. Other conditions possibly requiring premedication prior to invasive dental treatment include (Lockart et al. 2007):

- renal transplants/dialysis
- hemophilia
- shunts
- immunosuppression secondary to cancer and cancer chemotherapy
- immunosuppression secondary to HIV/AIDS (ANC <500)
- systemic lupus erythematosus (SLE)
- poorly controlled insulin-dependent diabetes mellitus.

The Dentist's Drug and Prescription Guide, Second Edition. Mea A. Weinberg, Stuart J. Froum and Stuart L. Segelnick.
© 2020 John Wiley & Sons, Inc. Published 2020 by John Wiley & Sons, Inc.

Table 7.1 Conditions recommended for prophylactic antibiotics

1) Artificial heart valves or prosthetic material used for valve repair such as annuloplasty rings and chords
2) A history of IE
3) Certain specific, serious congenital (present from birth) heart conditions, including:
   a) unrepaired or incompletely repaired cyanotic congenital heart disease, including those with palliative shunts and conduits
   b) a completely repaired congenital heart defect with prosthetic material or device, whether placed by surgery or by catheter intervention, during the first six months after the procedure
   c) any repaired congenital heart defect with residual defect at the site or adjacent to the site of a prosthetic patch or a prosthetic device
4) A cardiac transplant that develops a problem in a heart valve

   According to the new guidelines, patients who have taken prophylactic antibiotics in the past but no longer need them include those with:

   mitral valve prolapse

   rheumatic heart disease

   bicuspid valve disease

   calcified aortic stenosis

   congenital heart conditions such as ventricular septal defect, atrial septal defect, and hypertrophic cardiomyopathy

---

Q. Is antibiotic prophylaxis required for patients who have been treated for heart disease (e.g., blocked arteries)?

A. No. Angioplasty can be performed to open blocked heart arteries. Stent placement is another option that can be done during angioplasty. A cardiac stent is a small mesh tube used to treat narrow or weak arteries. Balloon angioplasty involves a specially designed catheter with a small balloon tip which is guided to the point of narrowing in the artery. Once in place, the balloon is inflated to compress the fatty matter into the artery wall and stretch the artery open to increase blood flow to the heart.

Q. According to the 2017 guidelines, what dental procedures are required for patients to have antibiotic prophylaxis?

A. See Table 7.2.

Q. Is antibiotic prophylaxis required for patients taking low-dose aspirin?

A. No. Antibiotic prophylaxis is not indicated for patients taking low-dose aspirin.

Q. According to the 2017 guidelines, which is the antibiotic of choice for prophylaxis against IE?

A. The bacterium most commonly associated with endocarditis following dental and oral procedures is *Streptococcus viridans* (alpha-hemolytic streptococci). Amoxicillin remains the most recommended antibiotic for endocarditis prophylaxis. Agents such as ampicillin and penicillin VK have an equal antimicrobial effect against alpha-hemolytic streptococci, but amoxicillin is better absorbed in the gastrointestinal tract and provides higher, more sustained serum levels than the other penicillins.

Q. What are the most current AHA guidelines for antibiotic dosing for prophylaxis against IE?

A. See Table 7.3.

Table 7.2 Antibiotic prophylaxis recommendations for dental procedures

Higher incidence	Lower incidence
Dental extractions	Restorative dentistry (operative and prosthodontic)
Periodontal procedures: surgery, scaling and root planing, probing and recall maintenance	Local anesthetic injections (all except intraligamentary)
Implant placement and reimplantation of avulsed teeth	Placement of rubber dams
Root canal instrumentation when beyond apex (endodontics)	Postoperative suture removal
Subgingival placement of antibiotic fibers or strips	Placement of removable prosthodontic/orthodontic appliances
Placement of orthodontic bands (not brackets)	Taking oral impressions or radiographs
Intraligamentary local anesthesia injection	Fluoride treatment
Prophylactic cleaning of teeth and implants	

Source: Wilson, W., Taubert, K.A., Gewitz, M., et al. (2007) Prevention of infective endocarditis. Guidelines from the American Heart Association. A guideline from the American Heart Association Rheumatic Fever, Endocarditis, and Kawasaki Disease Committee, Council on cardiovascular Disease in the Young, and the Council on Clinical Cardiology, Council on Cardiovascular Surgery and Anesthesia, and the Quality of Care and Outcomes Research Interdisciplinary Working Group. Circulation, 116(15): 1736–1754 with permission from Wolters Kluwer Health.

Table 7.3 Prophylactic antibiotic regimens for oral and dental procedures

Situation	Drug	Regimen (to be taken 30–60 min before dental procedure)
Oral	Amoxicillin	Adults: 2 g Children: 50 mg/kg
Unable to take oral medications	Ampicillin or cefazolin, or ceftriaxone[a]	Adults: 2 g IM or IV Children: 50 mg/kg IM or IV Adults: 1 g IM or IV Children: 50 mg/kg
Allergic to penicillins or ampicillin – oral	Cephalexin[a] or clindamycin or azithromycin or clarithromycin	Adults: 2 g Children: 50 mg/kg Adults: 600 mg Children: 20 mg/kg Adults: 500 mg Children: 15 mg/kg
Allergic to penicillins or ampicillin and unable to take oral medications	Cefazolin or ceftriaxone[a] or clindamycin	Adults: 1 g IM or IV Children: 50 mg/kg IM or IV Adults: 600 mg IM or IV Children: 20 mg/kg IM or IV

[a] Cephalosporins should not be given to an individual with a history of anaphylaxis, angioedema, or urticaria with penicillins or ampicillin.
Source: Wilson, W., Taubert, K.A., Gewitz, M., et al. (2007) Prevention of infective endocarditis. Guidelines from the American Heart Association. A guideline from the American Heart Association Rheumatic Fever, Endocarditis, and Kawasaki Disease Committee, Council on cardiovascular Disease in the Young, and the Council on Clinical Cardiology, Council on Cardiovascular Surgery and Anesthesia, and the Quality of Care and Outcomes Research Interdisciplinary Working Group. Circulation, 116(15): 1736–1754 with permission from Wolters Kluwer Health.

Q. What happens if the patient forgot to take the antibiotic 30–60 minutes before the dental procedure?

A. If the antibiotic was not taken before the procedure, the full amount may be taken up to two hours after the dental procedure (Dajani et al. 1997; Wilson et al. 2007).

Q. What happens if a patient is already taking an antibiotic for either a medical or dental reason?

A. Patients receiving antibiotics for other reasons at the time of a routine dental visit who are considered at risk for endocarditis have specific recommendations. The antibiotic that the patient is already taking is not adequate to prevent a dentally induced bacterium. Rather than increasing the dose of the drug currently used, it is advisable to select an agent from a different class of antibiotic. Remember, if you have to choose another antibiotic, it must have the same bactericidal or bacteriostatic activity as the antibiotic taken for prophylaxis. For instance, if the patient is taking tetracycline (a bacteriostatic drug), he or she cannot take amoxicillin (a bactericidal antibiotic), but can take clindamycin, azithromycin, or clarithromycin, which are all bacteriostatic. If possible, the dental procedure is best postponed until at least 9–14 days after completion of the antibiotic. This will allow the normal oral flora to reestablish and help to reduce the incidence of bacterial resistance (Dajani et al. 1997; Wilson et al. 2007).

Q. Can I prescribe erythromycin to a patient who is allergic to penicillin?

A. Erythromycin, which was originally approved as an effective prophylactic agent for endocarditis in cases of penicillin allergy, is no longer among the recommended drugs. Erythromycin can cause severe gastrointestinal upset, and certain formulations (e.g., erythromcyin ethylsuccinate) have complicated pharmacokinetics. Instead, second-generation erythromycins, azithromycin, or clarithromycin can be prescribed because they have better absorption and produce fewer adverse effects.

Q. Is it advisable to see a patient taking antibiotic prophylaxis more than once a week or even once a week?

A. No. Since repeated use of antibiotics can lead to the emergence of antibiotic-resistant microorganisms in the oral cavity, it is recommended that there be an interval of at least seven days between dental appointments. There needs to be adequate time for the patient's normal oral flora to be reestablished and prevent the development of resistant strains.

Q. How are prescriptions written for the different antibiotics for IE prophylaxis (Wilson et al. 2007)?

A. See Table 7.4. If allergic to penicillins then prescribe as shown in Table 7.5.

Table 7.4 How the prescription is written for oral prophylactic antibiotic regimens

Rx amoxicillin 500 mg
Disp: # 4 (four) caps
Sig: Take four caps po 30 minutes to 1 hour before dental procedure

Table 7.5 How the prescription is written for oral prophylactic antibiotic regimens if allergic to penicillin

Rx clindamycin 300 mg

Disp: # 2 (two) caps

Sig: Take two caps 30 minutes to 1 hour before dental procedure

or

Rx clarithromycin 250 mg

Disp: # 2 (two) tabs

Sig: Take two tabs 30 minutes to 1 hour before dental procedure

or

Rx azithromycin

Disp: # 2 (two) caps

Sig: Take two caps 30 minutes to 1 hour before dental procedure

7.2 Antibiotic Prophylaxis for Total Joint Replacement

Q. What is the concern about antibiotic prophylaxis for dental patients with total joint replacement?

A. A problem arises in patients with total joint replacements because if an infection develops, the bacteria, usually *Staphylococcus aureus*, cannot be easily eliminated from a joint replacement implant (Paauw 2017). Bacteremias can cause hematogenous seeding of a joint implant soon after the surgery and for years afterward. However, most bacteria from dentistry are usually *Streptococcus* (Paauw 2017).

Q. What are the current guidelines for antibiotic prophylaxis for dental patients with total joint replacements?

A. Guidelines have changed over the years. In 2009, the American Academy of Orthopedic Surgery (AAOS) safety committee recommended that dentists consider antibiotic prophylaxis for all patients with total joint (e.g., knee, hip) replacement before any dental procedure whether or not that person was even at high risk for developing an infection. The AAOS stated that "given the potential adverse outcomes and cost of treating an infected joint replacement, the AAOS recommends that clinicians consider antibiotic prophylaxis of all total joint replacement patients prior to any invasive procedure that may cause bacteremia" (American Dental Association: American Academy of Orthopaedic Surgeons 2003). This recommendation followed an earlier guideline by the AAOS and the American Dental Association, who in 2003 said that antibiotic prophylaxis should only be considered *within two years post implant surgery* in high-risk patients who have high-risk dental procedures such as dental extraction, periodontal procedures, endodontic procedures, initial placement of orthodontic bands, implant placement, and oral prophylaxis with anticipated bleeding (American Dental Association: American Academy of Orthopaedic Surgeons 2003).

The most current American Dental Association guidelines as of January 2015 state that "in general, for patients with prosthetic joint implants, prophylactic antibiotics are *NOT* recommended prior to dental procedures to prevent prosthetic joint infections" (Sollecito et al. 2015).

It is emphasized that dentists must use their own clinical judgment in determining whether a patient requires antibiotic prophylaxis and if necessary, consult with the patient's orthopedist.

Q. Why is there controversy regarding the use of antibiotic prophylaxis in patients with total joint replacement?

A. Some sources say that staphylococci, the most common cause of prosthetic joint infection (PJI), are relatively uncommon commensals of the oral flora and have been rarely implicated in bacteremia occurring after dental procedures. On the other hand, viridans group streptococci make up most of the facultative oral flora and are the most common cause of transient bacteremia after dental procedures that result in trauma to the gingival or oral mucosa. However, viridans group streptococci account for only 2% of all hematogenous PJIs. Additionally, concerns about promoting antimicrobial resistance and about adverse reactions from antimicrobial use may outweigh any hypothetical benefit related to prevention of PJI (Deacon et al. 1996; Paauw 2017). Another 2011 article reported that dental procedures are not significantly associated with a risk for PJIs and the use of prophylactic antibiotics in these patients may be questioned (Skaar et al. 2011).

Q. If antibiotic prophylaxis is necessary for joint replacement, what is the suggested antibiotic prophylaxis regimen for dental patients with total joint replacement?

A. See Table 7.6.

Table 7.6 Suggested antibiotic prophylaxis regimen in dental patients with total joint replacement

Type of patient	Recommended drug	Drug dosage
Oral: patients not allergic to penicillin	Cephalexin, cephradine or amoxicillin	2 g orally (po) 1 hour prior to dental procedure
Parenteral: patients are not allergic to penicillin but cannot take or tolerate oral medications	Cefazolin or ampicillin	Cefazolin 1 g or ampicillin 2 g intramuscularly (IM) or intravenously 1 hour prior to the dental procedure
Oral: patients who are allergic to penicillin	Clindamycin	600 mg orally (po) 1 hour prior to the dental procedure
Parenteral: patients who are allergic to penicillin but cannot take or tolerate oral medications	Clindamycin	600 mg intravenously (IV) 1 hour prior to the dental procedure

Source: Adapted from American Dental Association; American Academy of Orthopedic Surgeons (2003). *Source:* Wilson, W., Taubert, K.A., Gewitz, M., et al. (2007) Prevention of infective endocarditis. Guidelines from the American Heart Association. A guideline from the American Heart Association Rheumatic Fever, Endocarditis, and Kawasaki Disease Committee, Council on cardiovascular Disease in the Young, and the Council on Clinical Cardiology, Council on Cardiovascular Surgery and Anesthesia, and the Quality of Care and Outcomes Research Interdisciplinary Working Group. Circulation, 116(15): 1736–1754 with permission from Wolters Kluwer Health.

Q. How are prescriptions written for antibiotics used as prophylaxis for dental patients with total joint replacement?

A. Oral antibiotic prophylaxis for total joint replacement.

- Standard regimen (Table 7.7).
- If allergic to penicillin (Table 7.8).

Table 7.7 How the prescriptions are written for oral antibiotic prophylaxis for total joint replacement

Rx cephalexin 500 mg
Disp: # 4 (four) caps
Sig: Take 4 caps po 30 minutes to 1 hour before dental procedure
or
Rx amoxicillin 500 mg
Disp: # 4 (four) caps
Sig: Take 4 caps po 30 minutes to 1 hour before dental procedure.

Table 7.8 How the prescriptions are written for oral antibiotic prophylaxis for total joint replacement if allergic to penicillin

Rx clindamycin 300 mg
Disp: # 2 (two) caps
Sig: Take 2 caps po 30 minutes to 1 hour before dental procedure

Q. Why is cephalexin suggested as an antibiotic?

A. Cephalexin (Keflex®) is a cephalosporin that has excellent bone-penetrating properties and is an ideal antibiotic in patients with total joint replacement. However, there is approximately a 10% cross-sensitivity between penicillins and cephalosporins, which precludes prescribing a cephalosporin to patients allergic to penicillins. In these cases, an alternative antibiotic is clindamycin (see Table 7.6).

Q. Is a patient with a titanium rod or plate in the neck required to have antibiotic prophylaxis?

A. No. According to the ADA and the AAOS, antibiotic prophylaxis is not indicated for dental patients with pins, plates, screws or rods (American Dental Association: American Academy of Orthopaedic Surgeons 2003; Rubin et al. 1976).

Q. Is antibiotic prophylaxis indicated for patients with pins, plates, or screws?

A. No. Antibiotic prophylaxis is not indicated for dental patients with pins, plates or screws in any part of the body (American Dental Association: American Academy of Orthopaedic Surgeons 2003).

Q. If the patient is allergic to penicillin, can cephalexin be prescribed?

A. No. If the patient is allergic to penicillin, cephalexin, which is a cephalosporin, should not be prescribed as there is a 10% cross-sensitivity in patients allergic to penicillin. Instead, clindamycin can be prescribed (see Table 7.8).

7.3 Cardiovascular Diseases (Marc A. Singer, MD)

7.3.1 Hypertension

Q. What is the most current classification of blood pressure for adults?

A. In 2017, the American College of Cardiology (ACC)/AHA published an updated hypertension guideline lowering the threshold for intervention and treatment (Table 7.9).

Table 7.9 Classification of high blood pressure (BP)

Blood pressure classification	Systolic BP (mmHg)	Diastolic BP (mmHg)
Normal	<120 *and*	<80
Elevated	120–129 *or*	<80
Stage 1 hypertension	130–139 *or*	80–89
Stage 2 hypertension	At least 140	At least 90
Hypertensive crisis	>180	>120

Source: Whelton et al. (2018).

Q. According to the new guidelines, how is treatment different?

A. Medications are prescribed in Stage I hypertension only if the patient had a previous cardiovascular event or is considered to be high risk for a cardiovascular event or has certain other conditions including kidney disease.

Q. What are the different classifications of medications prescribed for hypertension and what are common dental adverse effects, and how are they managed in the dental office?

A. See Table 7.10.

Table 7.10 Dental management of patients taking drugs for hypertension

Antihypertensive drug	Adverse effects	Dental management
Diuretics Thiazide diuretics: Chlorthalidone Hydrochlorothiazide (Hydrodiuril®) (HCTZ) Potassium-sparing diuretics: Amiloride (Midamore®) Triamterene (Dyrenium®) Combination diuretics: Aldactazide® (HCTZ + spironolactone) Dyazide® (HCTZ + triamterene) Maxzide® (25/50 mg (HCTZ +37.5/75 mg triamterene) Moduretic® (HCTZ + amiloride)	Xerostomia (loop diuretics cause the most xerostomia) Orthostatic hypotension Drug interaction with NSAIDs Lichenoid reactions (e.g., lichen planus-like lesions)	*Xerostomia* Xerostomia: monitor for caries, candidiasis and periodontal disease If xerostomia is severe, contact patient's physician to change to a different classification of medication For xerostomia: recommend OTC products Saliva substitutes: effects only last for a few hours. Most contain either carboxymethylcellulose or hydroxyethylcellulose (e.g., Moi-Stir® spray or oral Swabsticks®, Optimoist® spray, Salivart® aerosol, Xero-Lube® spray *or* mucopolysaccharide solutions (e.g., MouthKote® spray) *or* Saliva stimulants: Natrol® Dry Mouth Relief Saliva lubricants/moisturizers: Biotene® Dry Mouth toothpaste mouthwash, gum, moisturizing gel drink plenty of water chew sugarless gum or candy use of sodium fluoride gels or rinses

Table 7.10 (Continued)

Antihypertensive drug	Adverse effects	Dental management
		if severe, prescribe salivary stimulants (cholinergic agents) such as pilocarpine (Salgan) or cevimeline HCL (Evoxac)
		Pilocarpine is contraindicated in patients with uncontrolled asthma, narrow-angle glaucoma or iritis. Pregnancy category C. Adverse effects include excessive sweating and gastrointestinal distress. Recommended dose: Comes in 5 mg tabs: Initial dose 5 mg tid or qid; up to 3 to 6 tabs per day; not to exceed 2 Tables (10 mg) per dose. Can take up to 6 to 12 weeks to see results.
		Cevimeline (Evoxac) contraindicated in patients with uncontrolled asthma, narrow-angle glaucoma or iritis. Pregnancy category C. Adverse effects include sweating and nausea.
		Orthostatic hypotension
		After being in a supine position for dental care, slowly raise the dental chair to an upright position and have the patient sit in the upright position for a few minutes before getting out of the chair
		Assistance in helping the patient out of the chair is important
		Monitor vital signs
		NSAIDs use
		Reduce effectiveness of antihypertensive drug
		Limit use of NSAID to less than 1 week or 2. Have blood pressure monitored
		Lichenoid reactions
		Refer to patient's physician for either treatment of the reaction with topical corticosteroids or change in medication
		Use of epinephrine
		No precautions or contraindications to using epinephrine with these medications
		Monitor vital signs
		✓ Medical consultation is required if hypertension is not controlled.

(Continued)

Table 7.10 (Continued)

Antihypertensive drug	Adverse effects	Dental management
Beta-blockers Acebutolol (Sectral®) [a]Atenolol (Tenormin®) [a]Bisoprolol (Zebeta®) [b]Carvedilol (Coreg®) [b]Labetalol (Normodyne®) [a]Metoprolol (Lopressor®) Nadolol (Corgard) [a]Nebivolol (Bystolic®) Pindolol (Visken®) Propranolol (Inderal) Sotalol (Betapace®) Timolol (Blocadren)	Xerostomia, dizziness, oral lesions, orthostatic hypotension	*Xerostomia*: see above recommendations *Orthostatic hypotension*: see above recommendations *NSAIDs use* Limit use of NSAID to less than a week or two. Monitor blood pressure *Oral lesions* (Kalmar 2009) Lichen planus-like lesions, pemphigus-like lesions (especially with propranolol) *Use of epinephrine* Monitor vital signs Noncardiac selective beta-blockers: limit epinephrine to two cartridges of 1 : 100 000 because nonselective beta- blockers block both beta-1 and beta-2 receptors leaving alpha receptors for binding which causes increased blood pressure when exposed to epinephrine. Medical consultation is required if hypertension is not controlled
Adrenergic blockers Doxazosin (Cardura®) Prazosin (Minipress®) Tamsulosin (Flomax®) Terazosin (Hytrin®) *Alpha-beta blockers* Carvedilol (Coreg) Labetalol (Normodyne)	Xerostomia, dizziness, vertigo	*Xerostomia*: see above recommendations *Orthostatic hypotension*: see above recommendations *NSAIDs use*: see above recommendations *Use of epinephrine* No precautions or contraindications with the use of epinephrine with these medications
Angiotensin-converting enzyme inhibitors Benazepril (Lotensin®) Captopril (Capoten®) Enalapril (Vasotec®) Fosinopril (Monopril®) Lisinopril (Zestril®, Prinivil®) Quinapril (Accupril®) Ramipril (Altace®)	Cough (highest incidence with ramipril), orofacial angioedema (swelling of the oral cavity; tongue, soft palate and uvula) (Yagiela and Haymore 2007), less xerostomia	*Orthostatic hypotension*: see above recommendations *NSAIDs use*: see above recommendations *Orofacial angioedema*: refer to emergency medical evaluation (Rees and Gibson 1997). Orofacial angioedema is a condition with lip, facial or oral swelling. The danger of this condition is the possibility of airway obstruction (laryngeal edema). (Scully and Porter 2003) *Use of epinephrine* No precautions or contraindications with the use of epinephrine with these medications *Oral vesiculobullous lesions,* *pemphigoid-like lesions*: Captopril

Table 7.10 (Continued)

Antihypertensive drug	Adverse effects	Dental management
Calcium channel blockers Amlodipine (Norvasc) Diltiazem (Cardizem) Felodipine (Plendil®) Nisoldipine (Sular®) Nifedipine (Adalat, Procardia) Nicardipine (Cardene®) Isradipine (DynaCirc®) Verapamil (Calan®, Isoptin®)	Gingival enlargement, dizziness	*Orthostatic hypotension*: see above recommendations *Use of epinephrine* No precautions or contraindications with the use of epinephrine with these medications *Gingival enlargement* More commonly seen with nifedipine and amlodipine Strict home care (plaque control) Periodontal surgery, if necessary. If the patient continues taking the calcium channel blocker, the gingiva will return to an overgrowth state
Angiotensin receptor blockers Candesartan (Atacand®) Eprosartan (Teveten®) Irbesartan (Avapro®) Losartan (Cozaar®) Valsartan (Diovan®)	Dizziness	*Orthostatic hypotension*: see above recommendations *NSAIDs use*: see above recommendations *Use of epinephrine* No precautions or contraindications with the use of epinephrine with these medications
Central antiadrenergic Clonidine (Catapres®) Methyldopa (Aldomet®)	Rebound hypertension, orthostatic hypotension, oral lichenoid lesions, xerostomia	*Xerostomia*: see above recommendations *Orthostatic hypotension*: see above recommendations *NSAIDs use*: see above recommendations *Oral lesions*: Pemphigoid-like oral reaction *Use of epinephrine* No precautions or contraindications with the use of epinephrine with these medications

[a] Selective cardiac beta-blockers (block only beta-1 adrenergic receptors).
[b] Combined alpha/beta-blocker.

Q. If a patient is taking multiple antihypertensive medications, are the adverse effects additive?

A. Yes. This is true in the majority of cases when patients are taking more than one antihypertensive. For example, if a patient is taking more than one antihypertensive drug that causes xerostomia, the xerostomia effect will be greater (Yagiela and Haymore 2007).

Q. Are many of these antihypertensive medications also used for other heart conditions?

A. Yes. Some medications prescribed for hypertension are also prescribed for other heart conditions such as angina, arrhythmias, and heart failure.

Q. What are the effects of epinephrine on the sympathetic receptors in the body?

A. Theoretically, epinephrine binds to all sympathetic receptors (alpha-1, beta-1, beta-2) in the body. The alpha-1 receptors are located predominantly on blood vessels under the skin, mucous membranes, and gastrointestinal (GI) tract. The beta-2 receptors are located predominantly on blood vessels on certain internal organs like the lungs, liver and brain, and in blood vessels in skeletal muscle. Beta-1 receptors are primarily located on the heart. The coronary arteries have both alpha-1 and beta-2 receptors.

Epinephrine in low concentrations (up to two or three cartridges) administered systemically after anesthetic injections in dentistry is fairly selective for beta-2 receptors over alpha receptors. Epinephrine has some alpha-1 receptor effects resulting in vasoconstriction. When activated by epinephrine, the beta-2 receptors cause a decrease in peripheral vascular resistance by selectively causing vasodilation in skeletal muscle blood vessels. This opposing vasodilation limits the potential vasopressor effects of epinephrine, thus lowering peripheral resistance and therefore diastolic blood pressure which is governed by peripheral vascular resistance. At the same time, the beta-1 (and beta-2) receptors in the heart are activated, and increase cardiac output and therefore systolic blood pressure; this is influenced by peripheral vascular resistance as well, but is also heavily influenced by the cardiac output, which epinephrine increases strongly. With an increase in systolic blood pressure and a decrease in diastolic blood pressure, there is no real change in mean blood pressure; these two influences cancel each other out regarding mean blood pressure.

Higher doses of epinephrine, such as used to treat anaphylaxis, stimulate alpha-1 receptors. Since there are more of these receptors, the net effect is vasoconstriction throughout the body, and an increase in peripheral resistance. This results in an increase in both systolic and diastolic blood pressure, and a possible reflex slowing of the heart mediated by the reflux vagal stimulation of the sinoatrial (SA) node (Yagiela 1999).

Q. If more than three cartridges are needed in these patients, is it best to space the doses apart rather than injecting all at one time?

A. When epinephrine is injected and absorbed into the blood, it is rapidly converted to inactive metabolites. So injections can be administered over time (e.g., 30 minutes) to decrease the risk of side effects (Yagiela and Haymore 2007).

Q. It is a major concern of dentistry whether to use epinephrine in hypertensive patients. Does the amount of epinephrine need to be limited in the controlled hypertensive patient?

A. Knowing the mechanism of how epinephrine affects the alpha and beta receptors in the body in low and high doses should help with answering this question (see above). Remember, epinephrine is an endogenously produced neurotransmitter so that there is no real total contraindication for its use. The question that arises, then, is how much epinephrine can be injected? It also depends which antihypertensive the patient is taking.

There is no antihypertensive need to limit the amount of epinephrine used in dental local anesthesia in hypertensive patients who are controlled, so long as there are no drug interactions and no intravascular injections. However, the ADA recommends that the total dosage of epinephrine be limited to 0.04 mg (two or three cartridges) in patients with known cardiovascular disease. In uncontrolled hypertensive patients, studies have shown that even a few cartridges (up to two or three) of lidocaine with 1 : 100 000 epinephrine can be used without changing the blood pressure; however, it is recommended to delay dental treatment in uncontrolled hypertensive patients until the blood pressure is under control. Of course, extra care must be taken to aspirate and avoid intravascular injection (Budenz 2008; Yagiela and Haymore 2007).

Q. Can levonordefrin be used instead of epinephrine?

A. Levonordefrin (Neo-Cobefrin®) is half as potent a vasoconstrictor as epinephrine. However, it primarily stimulates alpha-adrenergic (sympathetic) receptors, with little to no effect on the beta adrenoceptor. Stimulation of alpha-1 receptors on tissues/organs causes vasoconstriction of blood vessels, resulting in hypertension (increased systolic and diastolic blood pressure). Epinephrine produces a greater stimulation of beta-2 than beta-1 receptors, causing vasodilation and decreasing diastolic blood pressure. Higher doses produce more vasoconstriction and increased blood pressure. Since it is less effective/potent than epinephrine, levonordefrin can be used in higher concentrations (e.g., 2% mepivacaine with 1 : 20 000 levonordefrin) and has similar adverse effects as 1 : 100 000 epinephrine. Thus, levonordefrin can be used in patients taking nonselective beta-blockers.

Q. Is there a local anesthetic that contains less of a concentration than 1 : 100 000 epinephrine as a vasoconstrictor?

A. Yes. Recommendations in cardiac patients include administering block anesthesia with mepivacaine 3% (Carbocaine®, Polocaine® plain) and then infiltrating with articaine 4% (Septocaine®) that contains 1 : 200 000 epinephrine, which is half the concentration of the standard 1 : 100 000 epinephrine.

Q. What is a safe way to administer epinephrine in a hypertensive patient?

A. It is best to inject a small amount of anesthetic solution containing epinephrine and to wait about five minutes while monitoring the patient.

Q. Can gingival retraction cord be used safely in hypertensive patients?

A. Gingival retraction cord is made of cotton with a range of options of nonimpregnated and chemically impregnated cords that have astringent (contraction–retraction; shrinkage of gingival tissues and sulcular displacement) or hemostatic (vasoconstriction; coagulation) actions. Examples of astringent/hemostatic agents include aluminum chloride, aluminum sulfate, and aluminum potassium sulfate, racemic epinephrine (equal amounts of dextrorotatory [d] and levorotatory [l] isomers) and ferric sulfate; 20–25% aluminum chloride and 15.5–20% ferric sulfate are most commonly used (Strassler and Boksman 2011). The ADA has stated that 5–10% aluminum chloride is safe and effective (American Dental Association 2002). Gingival retraction cords are also impregnated with epinephrine. About 92% of the epinephrine is systemically absorbed (Malamed 1993; Pallasch 1998). In fact, the amount of epinephrine absorbed may be equal to about 3.9 cartridges of a local anesthetic with 1 : 100 000 epinephrine. This provides a concentration of about 4% (equals 40 mg/mL) of active epinephrine which is about 40 times the concentration given for cardiac arrest or allergic anaphylaxis (Malamed 1993). Since there is controversy regarding the adverse effects of epinephrine-impregnated gingival retraction cords, it is advised to limit or avoid their use especially in cardiac patients.

Q. Can nonsteroidal antiinflammatory drugs (NSAIDs) be taken for pain by patients on cardiovascular medications?

A. Yes, but there is a limit in the number of days an NSAID can be taken with certain medications, with diuretics, angiotensin-converting enzyme inhibitors (ACEIs), beta-blockers, and angiotensin II receptor blockers (ARBs) being most susceptible in causing hypotensive effects. Calcium channel blockers do not seem to interact with these cardiovascular medications. Low dose and short courses of less than one or two weeks are recommended (Townsend 2017).

Q. What are the dental adverse effects of antihypertensives?

A. See Table 7.10. Xerostomia or dry mouth is a common adverse effect of heart medications, especially diuretics, although it may not be severe enough to interfere with oral function.

Orthostatic hypotension is common. There is no drug–drug interaction with epinephrine except for noncardiac selective beta-blockers, where the maximum amount of 1 : 100 000 epinephrine is two cartridges.

Q. If a patient is taking a nonselective beta-blocker, can epinephrine be administered?

A. Beta-blockers can be categorized as nonselective and selective. Noncardioselective beta-blockers block both beta-1 and beta-2 receptors, allowing binding to the alpha receptors, which results in vasoconstriction and possible hypertensive effects. Noncardioselective beta-blockers include propranolol (Inderal®), timolol (Blocadren®), and nadolol (Corgard®). Epinephrine should be limited to 0.04 mg or two cartridges of 1 : 100 000 epinephrine (Horn and Hansten 2009).

Cardioselective beta blockers selectively block only beta-1 receptors. Thus, there is little concern for using epinephrine in these patients.

Q. Which cardiac drugs can cause gingival enlargement?

A. Calcium channel blockers, especially nifedipine (Adalat®, Procardia®), amlodipine (Norvasc®) and, less likely, diltiazem (Cardizem®), can cause gingival enlargement.

Q. What is the mechanism of calcium channel blocker-induced gingival enlargement?

A. The exact mechanism of action is unclear. However, a proposed hypothesis involves both inflammatory factors within the gingival tissue whereby numerous inflammatory cells in the connective tissue are replaced by collagen. An alteration of the intracellular calcium level in gingival cells by nifedipine and local inflammatory factors (plaque or biofilm accumulation) are important in causing gingival enlargement (Ciancio 2004).

Q. What is the treatment of calcium channel blocker-induced gingival enlargement?

A. It is recommended to teach the patient optimum oral home care. If there is no underlying periodontal disease and adequate keratinized gingiva, a gingivectomy can be performed but it must be understood that as long as the patient is taking the medication, the gingival enlargement will return. If there is underlying periodontal disease, then periodontal flap surgery is advised. Referral to a periodontist may be necessary.

Q. Many antihypertensive drugs cause orthostatic hypotension. What precautions should the dentist follow?

A. According to the American Autonomic Society, orthostatic hypotension or postural hypotension is defined as a systolic blood pressure decrease of at least 20 mmHg or a diastolic blood pressure decrease of at least 10 mmHg within three minutes of standing (Bradley and Davis 2003). Many cases of orthostatic hypotension are due to antihypertensive medications. Most antihypertensives, except calcium channel blockers, can potentially cause orthostatic hypotension. Medications that can cause orthostatic hypotension include diuretics, beta-blockers, alpha-blockers, angiotensin-converting enzyme (ACE) inhibitors, erectile dysfunction drugs: sildenafil (Viagra®), vardenafil (Levitra®), and tadalafil (Cialis®), antidepressants (tricyclic antidepressants [TCAs]).

Q. How do beta-blockers cause orthostatic hypotension?

A. Beta-blockers block the beta adrenoceptor in the body, preventing the reflex increase in heart rate and contractility. All three of these effects impact the body's ability to appropriately respond to position changes.

Q. When can orthostatic hypotension happen in the dental patient?

A. 1) When rising from a supine position and quickly sitting up and then standing.

2) Immediately after intravenous sedation (due to vasodilation).

3) After nitroglycerin or other medication use.

Q. How can orthostatic hypotension be managed in the dental patient?

A. Make slow, careful changes in position. After being in a supine position for dental care, slowly raise the dental chair to an upright position and have the patient sit and dangle their feet a few minutes before getting out of the chair. Assistance in helping the patient out of the chair is important. Vital signs must be monitored.

Q. Is angioedema of the oral cavity dose related?

A. No. Angioedema from ACE inhibitors can occur at any time during therapy (Yagiela and Haymore 2007).

7.3.2 Angina and Other Ischemic Cardiac Conditions

Q. What is angina?

A. Angina pectoris occurs when the metabolic demands of the heart exceed the ability of the coronary arteries to supply adequate blood flow and oxygen to the heart muscle. There are different types of angina: stable angina (angina upon exercise); unstable angina (angina at rest); variant angina (Prinzmetal angina) due to a coronary vasospasm, often occurring during rest.

Q. What drugs are used to treat angina pectoris?

A. The purpose of medication prescribed for angina pectoris is to increase blood flow and oxygen to the heart, or to decrease the heart's demand. Table 7.11 reviews drugs used in the management of angina.

Table 7.11 Dental management of patients taking drugs for angina

Drug	Mechanism of action	Adverse effects and dental management
Nitrates Nitroglycerin (Nitro-Bid®, Nitrostat®, Nitro-Dur®) Isosorbide dinitrate (Isordil®)	Dilate and relax coronary blood vessels	Headache, dizziness, and/or flushing, orthostatic hypotension. Monitor blood pressure. Allow patient to sit in an upright position in dental chair for a few minutes before dismissing them. Epinephrine can be used but limit to two cartridges of 1 : 100 000 because of increased risk of developing tachycardia
Calcium channel blockers Bepridil (Vascor) Diltiazem (Cardizem) Verapamil (Calan, Isoptin)	Slow heart rate and dilate coronary arteries	Orthostatic hypotension: allow patient to sit in an upright position in dental chair for a few minutes before dismissing them. Gingival enlargement (especially with nifedipine and amlodipine). No special precautions with epinephrine and no drug interactions

(Continued)

Table 7.11 (Continued)

Drug	Mechanism of action	Adverse effects and dental management
Beta-blockers Atenolol (Tenormin) Metoprolol (Lopressor) Nadolol (Corgard) Propranolol (Inderal)	Reduce cardiac demand	NSAIDs such as naproxen sodium and ibuprofen can decrease the effectiveness of the antihypertensive, resulting in rapid elevation of blood pressure. Limit use of NSAID to one week. Orthostatic hypotension: monitor blood pressure. To avoid dizziness/fainting when a patient moves from the supine position, observe the patient seated for a few minutes before dismissing them. Vesiculobullous oral lesions (propranolol). No special concerns with epinephrine and no drug interactions

Q. Is epinephrine contraindicated in patients with angina?

A. Management of stable angina patients without a history of myocardial infarction (MI) includes the reduction of stress and anxiety, so that the concentration of epinephrine should be limited to two cartridges of 1 : 100 000. Profound anesthesia is necessary to prevent stressful situations whereby large amounts of endogenous epinephrine are synthesized and released from the adrenal medulla in response to pain. A local anesthetic with 1 : 200 000 epinephrine can also be used (e.g., articaine 4% or prilocaine 4%). In a 1.7 mL cartridge, 1 : 200 000 dilution concentration contains 0.0085 mg of epinephrine versus 0.017 mg in 1 : 100 000 concentration. Short appointments are recommended. Mild or moderate (conscious) sedation may be indicated.

Epinephrine should be avoided and no elective dental treatment in patients with unstable angina or in cases of stable angina with MI within six months of recent coronary artery bypass surgery. Consultation with the patient's physician is recommended.

Q. What local anesthetic should be administered if emergency dental treatment is necessary in the unstable angina patient or one who had a MI within the last six months?

A. Stress and anxiety reduction is important, as mentioned above, so it is safe to limit the amount of local anesthetic to one or two cartridges.

Q. If patients are taking nitroglycerin, should they have it with them at every dental visit?

A. Yes. It should be out on the table in case it is needed quickly. However, the nitroglycerin in the emergency medical kit in the dental office may have "fresher" nitroglycerin than the pills the patient is taking.

7.3.3 Heart Failure

Q. What is heart failure?

A. Systolic heart failure is defined as the heart's inability to meet the body's demands. Decreases in cardiac output activate reflex responses in the sympathetic nervous system, which attempt to compensate for the reduced cardiac output.

Q. What is the dental management of patients taking medications for heart failure?

A. See Table 7.12.

Table 7.12 Dental management of patients taking medications for heart failure

Drug	Dental management and adverse effects
Diuretics Thiazides: hydrochlorothiazide (Hydrodiuril) Loop diuretics: furosemide (Lasix®)	NSAIDs such as naproxen sodium (Aleve®) and ibuprofen can decrease the effectiveness of the antihypertensive action of the thiazide diuretic, resulting in rapid elevation of blood pressure. Only use NSAIDs for one week. Monitor blood pressure. Orthostatic hypotension: monitor blood pressure. To avoid dizziness/fainting when a patient moves from the supine position, have the patient sit in an upright position for a few minutes before dismissing them. Monitor blood pressure. Xerostomia: monitor for dental caries, periodontal disease and candidiasis; monitor salivary consistency. No drug interactions with the use of epinephrine
Cardiac glycosides Digoxin (Lanoxin®)	No interactions with NSAIDs. No xerostomia. Limit amount of local anesthetic to two cartridges of 1 : 100 000 epinephrine because epinephrine may cause arrhythmias in patients taking digoxin. Avoid concurrent use with clarithromycin (Biaxin®) and tetracyclines. Use penicillin, clindamycin or azithromycin
Vasodilators Hydralazine (Apresoline®)	NSAIDs such as naproxen sodium (Aleve) and ibuprofen can decrease the effectiveness of the antihypertensive action of the ACE inhibitor, resulting in rapid elevation of blood pressure. Only use for one week. Monitor blood pressure. Orthostatic hypotension: monitor blood pressure. To avoid dizziness/fainting when a patient moves from the supine position, have the patient sit in an upright position for a few minutes before dismissing them. Monitor blood pressure. Xerostomia: monitor for dental caries, periodontal disease and candidiasis; monitor salivary consistency. No special precautions or interactions with the use of epinephrine
ACE inhibitors Captopril (Capoten) Enalapril (Vasotec) Lisinopril (Prinivil, Zestril) Quinapril (Accupril) Fosinopril (Monopril) *Angiotensin receptor blockers* Candesartan (Atacand) Eprosartan (Teveten) Irbesartan (Avapro) Losartan (Cozaar) Valsartan (Diovan)	NSAIDs such as naproxen sodium (Aleve) and ibuprofen can decrease the effectiveness of the antihypertensive action of the ACE inhibitor, resulting in rapid elevation of blood pressure. Limit use to one week. Monitor blood pressure. Orthostatic hypotension: monitor blood pressure. To avoid dizziness/fainting when a patient moves from the supine position, have the patient sit in an upright position for a few minutes before dismissing them. Monitor blood pressure. Xerostomia: monitor for dental caries, periodontal disease and candidiasis; monitor salivary consistency. Lichen planus-like oral lesions: captopril – develop oral lesions that mimic or resemble idiopathic lichen planus (Kalmer 2009). No special precautions or interactions with the use of epinephrine
Calcium channel blockers Diltiazem (Cardizem) Verapamil (Calan, Isoptin) Amlodipine (Norvasc) Felodipine (Plendil) Isradipine (DynaCirc) Nicardipine (Cardene) Nifedipine (Adalat, Procardia) Nisoldipine (Sular)	OK to recommend or prescribe NSAIDs. Orthostatic hypotension: Monitor blood pressure. To avoid dizziness/fainting when a patient moves from the supine position, have the patient sit in an upright position for a few minutes before dismissing them. Monitor blood pressure. Monitor for gingival enlargement especially with nifedipine and amlodipine. Xerostomia: monitor for dental caries, periodontal disease and candidiasis; monitor salivary consistency. No special precautions or interactions with the use of epinephrine

Q. Can epinephrine be used safely in a patient with heart failure?

A. It is advised to limit the amount of epinephrine to two cartridges of 1 : 100 000 epinephrine, especially if taking digoxin.

Q. Is lidocaine contraindicated in patients with heart failure?

A. Yes. Lidocaine is contraindicated in patients allergic to lidocaine, heart failure, cardiogenic shock, second- or third-degree heart block (if no artificial pacemaker), Wolff–Parkinson–White syndrome (this may be controversial), and Stokes–Adams syndrome.

7.3.4 Patient on Low-Dose Aspirin and Other Antiplatelet Drugs

Q. Should the term "baby aspirin" be used?

A. No. All products containing 81 mg are called "low-dose aspirin" and not "baby aspirin" because the term "baby" was ambiguous, and many people would give the "baby" aspirin to babies. All labeling is now "low-dose" aspirin. Low-dose aspirin products contain 81 mg of aspirin.

Q. Is aspirin an antiplatelet or anticoagulant drug?

A. Aspirin is an antiplatelet drug with a totally different mechanism of action from warfarin and heparin, which are anticoagulant drugs. Aspirin is also used as an antithrombotic agent because of its action of inhibiting platelet aggregation.

Q. What are the different antiplatelet drugs?

A. Irreversible platelet inhibitors

- Aspirin (acetylsalicylic acid or ASA)
- Clopidogrel (Plavix®)
- Ticagrelor (Brilinta®)
- Prasugrel (Effient®)
- Aspirin-dipyridamole (Aggrenox®).

Reversible platelet inhibitors

- Dipyridamole (Persantine®)

Q. Which is the newest antiplatelet drug?

A. Prasugrel (Effient) is an antiplatelet (aggregation inhibitor) indicated to reduce the rate of thrombotic cardiovascular events such as stent thrombosis in patients with unstable angina, non-ST segment elevation MI, or ST elevation MI (STEMI) managed with percutaneous coronary intervention (stent placement). There is a **Black Box Warning** that prasugrel may cause significant or fatal bleeding. Consult with the patient's physician before dental procedures. There is no evidence for discontinuing prasugrel prior to dental surgery. Discontinuing prasugrel as well as any antiplatelet drug may lead to increased risk of cardiovascular events. However, consultation with the patient's physician is important.

Q. What is dipyridamole (Persantine)?

A. Dipyridamole is sometimes used with aspirin to reduce the risk of death after a heart attack and to prevent another heart attack. Dipyridamole is used with other drugs to reduce the risk of blood clots after heart valve replacement. It works by preventing excessive blood clotting.

Q. What is clopidogrel?

A. Clopidogrel (Plavix) is a reversible platelet inhibitor. The combination of aspirin and clopidogrel is usually standard treatment for one month after stent placement and long-term use can significantly reduce the risk of major cardiovascular events after percutaneous coronary intervention (Patrono et al. 2004). Clopidogrel works differently from aspirin by inhibiting the binding of fibrinogen to platelets, which is an important step for platelets to clot or aggregate (Awtry and Loscalzo 2000). Clopidogrel is frequently used by patients who cannot tolerate the adverse gastrointestinal effects of aspirin or are allergic or intolerant to aspirin (American Dental Hygiene Association 2011).

Q. What is the difference between irreversible and reversible platelet inhibitors?

A. Irreversible inhibitors of platelet aggregation require new platelets (about 5–10 days) to be produced to reverse their effect and get normal bleeding times. When reversible inhibitors of platelet aggregation are stopped, the affected platelets regain aggregation function more quickly, usually within about two days (American Dental Association 2011).

Q. What is the mechanism of aspirin's antiplatelet action and does it differ from regular antiinflammatory/analgesic dose aspirin?

A. Basically, the beneficial antiplatelet effects of aspirin for secondary or primary prevention of cardiovascular disease result from irreversible acetylation of the active site of cyclooxygenase (COX) in platelets which prevents the formation of thromboxane A_2 (TXA_2), resulting in inhibition of platelet aggregation or clotting (www.uptodate.com/contents/benefits-and-risks-of-aspirin-in-secondary-and-primary-prevention-of-cardiovascular-disease?source=see_link). (See "Benefits and risks of aspirin in secondary and primary prevention of cardiovascular disease.")

How does this happen? Aspirin permanently inactivates the COX-1 and COX-2 activity in platelets, preventing the formation of TXA_2, and in endothelial cells, preventing the formation of prostacyclin (PGI_2). COX-1 is considered to be the "protective" enzyme and is normally found in the gastrointestinal tract, kidneys, uterus, and platelets. Under the influence of COX-1, prostaglandins maintain and protect the gastric mucosa, maintain normal platelet function and regulate renal blood flow. COX-2 is produced only during inflammation and is found in low amounts in the tissues. Antiinflammatory drugs work to reduce the inflammation and pain caused by COX-2. TXA_2, found in platelets, strongly induces platelet aggregation and vasoconstriction (prevents bleeding), while prostacyclin, formed in endothelial cells (lining of blood vessels), has the opposite effect, inhibits platelet aggregation and induces coronary artery vasodilation. Thus, prostacyclin has beneficial and desirable effects by protecting cells from platelet deposition and causing coronary artery vasodilation.

The antiplatelet effect occurs when aspirin or acetylsalicylic acid is broken down or metabolized to acetic acid and salicylic acid (salicylate). It is the acetic acid that *irreversibly/permanently* binds covalently to the COX enzyme in the platelet. However, in anucleated (without a nucleus) platelets, new COX is formed about every 10–14 days, which is the life span of platelets; the antiplatelet effect will persist for about five days which is when 50% of platelet function returns to normal. On the other hand, in endothelial cells which have a nucleus, more COX is formed immediately. This allows the endothelial cell to continue to produce prostacyclin (Page 2005). Thus, since aspirin is very effective at low doses (75–325 mg/day) to COX-1 rather than to COX-2 and TXA_2 is derived from COX-1 in platelets, it can be concluded that aspirin in low doses and longer dosing intervals has a lasting antiplatelet effect by inhibiting platelet aggregation via inhibition of TXA_2 formation (Page 2005).

In contrast, at daily regular analgesic/antiinflammatory dosages of greater than 1000 mg (this is considered to be an antiinflammatory dose, not an antithrombotic dose), aspirin inhibits both TXA_2 and prostacyclin, which negates the entire antiplatelet effect, while lower doses (antithrombotic) of 75–325 mg/day preferentially inhibit TXA_2, resulting in the antiplatelet phenomenon (Page 2005). The reason why higher doses and shorter dosing interval are required for an antiinflammatory/analgesic effect is that COX-2, which is responsible for pain and inflammation, is much less sensitive to the actions of aspirin (Page 2005). Therefore, regular antiinflammatory doses most likely will not result in bleeding, while low-dose aspirin could result in bleeding.

Q. How soon after taking aspirin is an antiplatelet effect noticed?

A. Aspirin is absorbed in the upper gastrointestinal tract and exhibits its effect within 60 minutes, which is associated with a prolonged bleeding time (Awtry and Loscalzo 2000; Patrono et al. 1998).

Q. Does low-dose aspirin inhibit both COX-1 and COX-2?

A. Yes. Low-dose aspirin inhibits both COX-1 and COX-2 but is a more potent inhibitor of COX-1, thereby suppressing TXA_2 production and irreversibly inhibiting platelet aggregation for the life of the platelet, which is about 10–14 days.

Q. What happens to the antiplatelet effect when NSAIDs are given with aspirin?

A. The effect of oral ibuprofen on *in vitro* platelet aggregation was evaluated in a study in which healthy volunteers were treated with aspirin two hours before or two hours after ibuprofen. When ibuprofen was given before aspirin, TXA_2 production by activated platelets was approximately twofold higher and inhibition of platelet aggregation was negligible at 24 hours. Ibuprofen had no effect on the action of aspirin when given two hours after aspirin and neither acetaminophen nor diclofenac affected the activity of aspirin.

Q. Does aspirin cause gastrointestinal tract toxicity (e.g., GI tract bleeding)?

A. Yes. However, aspirin-induced gastrointestinal toxicity is dose dependent, so even at lower doses aspirin can cause serious GI bleeding, especially in patients with preexisting gastric ulcers (Patrono et al. 2004).

Q. What is the dosage of low-dose aspirin?

A. The accepted dosage of low-dose aspirin is controversial because aspirin is antithrombotic in a wide range of doses (Patrono et al. 2004). Low dose can be considered to be between 81 and 325 mg/day or even twice weekly. This dosage is adequate because approximately 10% of the platelets are replenished daily so that once-a-day dosing can completely inhibit the formation of TXA_2 (Patrono et al. 2004).

Q. Should I ask every patient if they are taking aspirin?

A. Yes. Sometimes patients may take the aspirin on their own without physician input. It is important to ask every patient if the aspirin or other antiinflammatory was prescribed by a physician.

Q. Does low-dose aspirin interfere with bleeding time? Are patients who take prophylactic low-dose aspirin more prone to bleeding during invasive dental procedures?

A. It has been published that low-dose aspirin may not significantly alter bleeding time (Ardekian et al. 2000; AAP 1996). Only about 20–25% of patients taking aspirin have an abnormal bleeding time (Randall 2007). The increase in bleeding time lasts for the lifetime of the platelet or until new platelets are formed, which is about 10–14 days. About 50% of platelet function returns to normal within five days after aspirin is stopped. Consultation with the patient's physician is recommended.

Q. Should aspirin be discontinued before dental surgery (e.g., periodontal/implant/oral surgery) because of the risk of excessive bleeding?

A. It is the consensus that if an antiplatelet drug is used as monotherapy (only one drug), it does not need to be discontinued or altered in dose. The frequency of oral bleeding complications after invasive dental procedures is low to negligible for patients taking antiplatelet drugs. Bleeding will still occur but the risks of altering or discontinuing use of antiplatelet medications outweigh the low risk of postoperative oral bleeding complications resulting from dental procedures that can be usually controlled with local measures (Ardekian et al. 2000; Brennan et al. 2008; Madan et al. 2005; Napeñas et al. 2009). However, if more than one antiplatelet drug is being taken then the patient's physician or cardiologist must be contacted because outpatient procedures would be excessively risky.

A clinical study reported that the only significant relationship found between bleeding and all antiplatelet drugs, not just aspirin, was between bleeding and the number of teeth extracted. It was concluded by this research group that no more than three teeth should be extracted at one dental sitting and that ideally the teeth should be adjacent to each other (Cardona-Tortajada et al. 2009).

Q. Do clopidogrel (Plavix) or other antiplatelet agents other than aspirin increase bleeding?

A. Yes. Antithrombotic/antiplatelet agents may increase the risk of bleeding during invasive dental procedures (Little et al. 2002). In fact, clopidogrel is considered to be a more potent antiplatelet agent and can prolong the bleeding time by 1.5–3 times the normal value (Randall 2007). Also, sensitivity to antiplatelet agents varies in different people (Randall 2007). Some clinical reports have recommended continuing monotherapy (either aspirin or clopidogrel) or dual therapy for invasive dental procedures (Napeñas et al. 2009). Consultation with the patient's physician is recommended.

Q. Is there an increased risk of bleeding if a patient is taking two antiplatelet agents?

A. Yes. There is an increased bleeding tendency if two antiplatelet agents are used together. This must be taken into consideration before performing invasive dental procedures. Consultation with the patient's physician is recommended.

7.3.5 Oral Anticoagulants

Q. Which patients will be taking anticoagulation drugs?

A. Patients with prosthetic valves, cardiac stents, thromboembolic conditions (pulmonary embolus, deep vein thrombosis), stroke, atrial fibrillation.

Q. Are there different types of anticoagulants?

A. Currently, there are three classifications of oral anticoagulants: oral direct thrombin inhibitors (e.g., dabigatran [Pradaxa®]), oral direct factor Xa inhibitors (e.g., rivaroxaban [Xarelto®], apixaban [Eliquis®], edoxaban [Savatsa®]) which are often referred to as novel oral anticoagulants (NOACs), and warfarin (Coumadin).

Q. What is warfarin (Coumadin)?

A. Warfarin, a synthetic anticoagulant, exhibits its anticoagulant effects as a vitamin K antagonist. It is prescribed to decrease the tendency for thrombosis (clot) or as secondary prophylaxis in individuals who have had a previous thrombotic effect. Warfarin extends the time for blood to clot. Indications for using warfarin include atrial fibrillation or hypercoagulable state, artificial heart valves, deep venous thrombosis, and pulmonary embolism.

Q. What is the mechanism of action of warfarin?

A. Warfarin inhibits vitamin K epoxide reductase, an enzyme that recycles oxidized vitamin K to its reduced form; it is sometimes referred to as a vitamin K antagonist. Onset of action takes a few days until clotting factors in the liver have adequate time to be depleted once metabolized. Warfarin inhibits the formation of blood clots within blood vessels by inhibiting the synthesis of liver clotting factors II, VII, IX, and X (extrinsic clotting pathway). A single dose of warfarin has a duration of action of about three days with a range of 2–5 days. The half-life of factor II is about three days which is the longest half-life of all the factors involved (VII, IX, and X).

Q. What is INR?

A. INR stands for international normalized ratio and is a reproducible number that represents the degree of anticoagulation by warfarin. Prothrombin time (PT) standards vary between laboratories so INR was developed to allow a standardized measurement of anticoagulation. The INR should be measured prior to dental procedures to gauge bleeding risk.

Q. How do patients measure their INR?

A. Usually patients can get their INR levels at the cardiologist's office or other medical facility (e.g., lab). Also, there are numerous testing devices such as INRatio PT Monitoring System (www.hemosense.com) and Philips PT/INR self-testing (Philips Healthcare) that can be used at home or the dentist's office.

Q. When should the INR be taken?

A. It is recommended to measure the INR within 24 hours (the same day) of the dental procedure, but not more than 72 hours (Kassab et al. 2011). This is the time that the earliest changes in INR are seen after warfarin administration (Kuruvilla and Gurk-Turner 2001). The INR is applicable only for patients who have been on a stable warfarin regimen.

Q. What is the recommended INR level for dental procedures?

A. It depends on the procedure but usually it should be 2.0–3.0 in patients with pulmonary embolus, deep vein thrombosis, and atrial fibrillation and in a range 2.5–3.5 in patients with mechanical heart valves and recurrence of embolism while on warfarin. Individuals not taking warfarin have an INR of 0.8–1.2 (Kassab et al. 2011). Anticoagulation drug alteration is required if INR >4 and invasive surgical procedures are contraindicated until anticoagulant therapy is stable.

Q. What causes elevated INR?

A. An INR can be elevated when a patient is taking warfarin and if the liver is so severely damaged that vitamin K-dependent coagulation factors cannot be synthesized. Certain medications interfere with warfarin metabolism, such as antibiotics (metronidazole, azithromycin, and ciprofloxacin), which can elevate INR. Dietary factors, such as green leafy vegetables, can lower INR.

Q. For which dental procedures should a patient get an INR?

A. Nonsurgical dental procedures have a significantly lower risk for bleeding than invasive surgical procedures (Kassab et al. 2011).

- Low risk for bleeding: radiographs, impressions.
- Low–moderate risk for bleeding (INR >3: do not perform dental procedures): simple restorative procedures, scaling and root planing, endodontic procedures, oral prophylaxis.
- High risk for bleeding (INR >3.5: do not perform dental procedures): simple extractions for not more than three teeth, periodontal surgery, crown and bridge.

However, Jeske and Suchko (2003) reported that dental procedures can be performed safely on patients with an INR ≤4, independent of the type of medical condition and the reason warfarin was prescribed.

Q. Is it necessary to check a patient's INR when performing periodontal probing?

A. A recent article found that anticoagulated patients did not bleed more than nonanticoagulated patients when periodontal probing was performed (Almiñana-Pastor et al. 2017). However, it is prudent to have the INR levels.

Q. Does warfarin have a narrow therapeutic index or window?

A. Yes. A narrow therapeutic index or window is defined as a very close margin between the therapeutic dose in the blood and the lethal/toxic dose of a drug. Drugs that have a narrow therapeutic index include warfarin, lithium, digoxin, phenytoin, clozapine, cyclosporine, metaproterenol, and levothyroxine. The goal of warfarin therapy is to administer the lowest effective dose to maintain the target INR (Kuruvilla and Gurk-Turner 2001). Initiation of warfarin therapy is difficult and often patients given a loading dose reach a supratherapeutic INR level, resulting in prolonged bleeding (Kuruvilla and Gurk-Turner 2001).

Q. Should warfarin be held before a dental procedure?

A. The major risk for thromboembolic events in a patient with atrial fibrillation can occur if warfarin is stopped for three days before a dental procedure. Remember that warfarin has a duration of action of about three days (range 2–5 days) so that if a physician decides to stop warfarin, it must be stopped for at least three days prior to the procedure because of this prolonged effect. The major reason for discontinuing warfarin is to prevent excessive bleeding. Most of the bleeding can be easily treated with local measures. Always get a medical consult from the patient's physician (Jeske and Suchko 2003).

Q. If warfarin is not stopped, is there a higher incidence of postoperative bleeding?

A. Yes. Continuing warfarin during dental surgery will increase the incidence of postoperative bleeding but discontinuing warfarin does not really guarantee that there will not be excessive bleeding. (Surgical management of the primary care dental patient on warfarin. UK Medicines Information. www.dundee.ac.uk/tuith/Static/info/warfarin.pdf.)

Q. How should patients taking NOACs be handled during invasive dental procedures?

A. The problem is that when a patient is taking warfarin, the dose can be adjusted according to the INR; NOACs have fixed doses and cannot be adjusted. For multiple and extensive extractions, it is best to refer to an oral surgeon. For other invasive procedures, consultation with the patient's physician is necessary. Sometimes, a less invasive procedure can be done, such as endodontics instead of extraction. Any invasive dental procedures should be postponed until the patient has been off the NOAC for 48 hours. For instance, the decision to stop apixaban (Eliquis) before dental procedures is based on the risk of hemorrhaging and the renal status of the patient and this is up to the patient's physician (Daly 2016). For some dental procedures that have a low risk for bleeding, apixaban may not need to be stopped. In this case, the dental procedure can be performed 12 hours after the last dose (Daly 2016).

Q. Why is an INR not required for NOACs (e.g., Eliquis)?

A. Because NOACs do not have a narrow therapeutic range, as does warfarin, so small changes in the medication dose do not have an effect on clotting.

Q. What is hypercoagulation?

A. Stopping warfarin may lead to a "rebound" hypercoagulable state where there is an increase in clotting factors and thrombin activity after discontinuing the warfarin. Warfarin inhibits the synthesis of "new" clotting factors II, VII, IX, and X but does not interfere with already synthesized and circulating factors in the blood. These factors are still able to function until their half-lives are over so that until the remaining coagulation factors are degraded, there will always be a risk of abnormal coagulation. This results in a transient hypercoagulation. The half-life of factor II is 60 hours; factor VII is 4–6 hours; factor IX is 24 hours; and factor X is about three days (http://emedicine.medscape.com/article/821038-overview#a0104).

Q. Besides clotting factors II, VII, IX, and X, are there any proteins involved in clotting?

A. Yes. Warfarin also inhibits anticoagulant proteins C and S. It takes about two days for these proteins to disappear; half-life of protein C is eight hours and protein S is 30 hours. Thus, a transient hypercoagulation state can also occur due to inhibition of protein C and S soon after treatment with warfarin. Once protein C disappears (shortest half-life), there is a temporary procoagulation until warfarin has time to decrease the production of the clotting factors.

Q. Do aspirin and warfarin have the same mechanism of action?

A. No. Aspirin (an antiplatelet) can cause bleeding, but it is definitely an inferior anticoagulant.

Q. Why are there so many drug interactions with warfarin?

A. There are several mechanisms of warfarin's drug–drug interactions. Warfarin is metabolized by the liver cytochrome P450 enzymes (CYP1A2) and it is highly protein bound (about 98%) to albumin in the blood, which allows other highly protein-bound drugs to displace warfarin.

Q. How do antibiotics interfere with warfarin?

A. Certain antibiotics, especially broad-spectrum antibiotics such as amoxicillin, metronidazole, erythromycin, clarithromycin, and azithromycin, inhibit bacterial production of vitamin K activity because they reduce the normal bacterial flora in the gastrointestinal tract or decrease the metabolism of warfarin via cytochrome P450 enzymes in the liver. It is advisable to check the antibiotic you are prescribing to see if there are interactions with warfarin.

Q. What happens if a patient on warfarin needs to have antibiotic prophylaxis?

A. A single 2 g dose of amoxicillin does not cause any interaction. If the patient is allergic to penicillin, a single dose of 600 mg clindamycin will not cause any interaction. Since there is a major interaction between warfarin and clarithromycin and azithromycin, these two antibiotics should be avoided due to increased bleeding (www.drugs.com).

Q. What analgesics can be prescribed or recommended to a patient taking warfarin?

A. There is an undesirable synergistic effect when acetaminophen is taken with warfarin, resulting in dangerously elevated INRs (Bell 1998). Care must be taken not to prescribe a narcotic–acetaminophen combination drug such as Vicodin®. NSAIDs such as ibuprofen or naproxen should be avoided due to increased risk of bleeding.

Q. If a patient is also taking warfarin, can an NSAID or acetaminophen also be taken?

A. No. when a NSAID or acetaminophen is taken with warfarin, the interaction is synergistic, resulting in the possibility of increased bleeding. It has been demonstrated that administering acetaminophen to a patient who is stable on warfarin may increase the INR within 18–48 hours. Thus, careful monitoring of patients taking warfarin and acetaminophen is necessary. Currently, there are no specific clinical guidelines to follow when recommending acetaminophen to patients taking warfarin. If a patient requires acetaminophen for mild pain, the dose should be the lowest possible with the shortest duration of acetaminophen therapy (Hylek et al. 1998). It has been recommended that if acetaminophen is necessary at doses >2 g a day for more than one day, an extra INR measurement may be necessary (Hughes et al. 2011).

7.3.6 Low Molecular Weight Heparins

Q. What are low molecular weight heparins (LMWHs)?

A. LMWHs are heparin salts used as an anticoagulant. If patients are taking warfarin and are at high risk for developing a thromboembolism, they can be given prophylactic LMWHs while the warfarin is stopped. In the past, these high-risk patients needed to be hospitalized. Now with the development of LMWHs which are self-administered by injection, the patient does not need to be hospitalized. Also, since LMWHs have about a 95% bioavailability, constant INR testing is not needed. The most common LMWH is enoxaparin (Lovenox®). The patient's physician must be consulted before any dental procedures because a decision must be made to place the patient on LMWH. Usually dental surgery should be performed 18–24 hours after the last dose of LMWH (Ganda 2008).

Q. What is the best analgesic for a patient taking warfarin?

A. Aspirin and NSAIDs such as ibuprofen or naproxen sodium are contraindicated in patients taking warfarin because of an increased risk for bleeding. Any morphine analogs, including hydrocodone (Vicodin), can be used but only for a few days. Extra-strength Tylenol® taken with warfarin may cause a substantial increase in INR. So, the recommended analgesic is regular-strength Tylenol.

7.3.7 Myocardial Infarction

Q. How soon after a patient has had a MI can dental treatment be started?

A. As a general rule, treatment should not be started for six months post MI and three months post coronary artery bypass graft surgery (CABG) (Lifshey 2004).

Q. What are common post-MI medications?

A. In order to reduce the chance of another MI, a patient may be taking:

- a low-dose aspirin for its antiplatelet actions
- a beta-blocker to reduce the workload of the heart by blocking the beta-1 receptors on heart muscle cells: the beta-blocker binds to the beta receptors on the heart muscle cell and prevents them from being stimulated) (see earlier discussion)
- an ACE inhibitor: blocks angiotensin in the blood, allowing for vasodilation and lowering blood pressure. It also has a direct action on the heart which has a protective effect
- a cholesterol-lowering drug such as a "statin": mechanism of action is to reduce the amount of cholesterol made in the liver.

Q. What should be done if you suspect a patient is having a MI in the dental office?

A. The emergency medical system (EMS) should be activated. Have the patient lie down on the floor and assess the airway, breathing, circulation (ABCs) and monitor vital signs (American Academy of Periodontology 1996).

7.3.8 Cardiac Arrhythmias

Q. What is a cardiac arrhythmia?

A. An arrhythmia or abnormal heart rhythm occurs when either the impulse rhythm does not start in the sinoatrial node or the rate of heartbeats is abnormal (normally the heart beats about 70–80 times per minute). Classification of arrhythmias is based on the anatomical site where the abnormal rhythm originates: atrial (atrium), ventricular (ventricle), or supraventricular (atrium or above the ventricles). When the heart is beating too slowly but at a regular rate, it is called sinus bradycardiIf the heart is beating too fast, it is called sinus tachycardiSigns and symptoms of arrhythmia include skipped beats, palpitations, chest pain or shortness of breath.

Q. What drugs are used in the management of cardiac arrhythmias?

A. Many drugs used in the treatment of hypertension and angina are also used in the treatment of arrhythmias. See Table 7.13.

Table 7.13 Medications used for cardiac arrhythmias

Common drugs	Common oral adverse effects
Class I: Sodium channel blockers	
Class I-A	
Quinidine (Quinidine®)	Lupus erythematosus-like oral lesions
Procainamide (Pronestyl®)	Lupus erythematosus-like oral lesions
Disopyramide (Norpace®)	Severe xerostomia
Class I-B	
Lidocaine (Xylocaine®)	When given intravenously, nothing related to dentistry
Phenytoin (Dilatin®)	Gingival enlargement
Mexiletine (Mexitil®)	Blood disorders: gingival bleeding
Class I-C	
Flecainide (Tambocor®)	Dizziness, fainting (care taken when arising from dental chair)
Propafenone (Rythmol®)	Dizziness, metallic taste

Table 7.13   (Continued)

Common drugs	Common oral adverse effects
Class II: Beta-adrenergic blockers	
Metoprolol (Lopressor)	Nonselective cardiac beta-blocker; limit epinephrine use
	Caution use with antihypertensives (limit to five days)
Propranolol (Inderal)	Nonselective cardiac beta-blocker; limit epinephrine use
	Caution use with antihypertensives (limit to five days)
	Pemphigus and lichen planus-like oral lesions
Class III: Potassium channel blockers	
Amiodarone (Cordarone®)	Oral ulcers, neuralgic pain
Dofetilide (Tikosyn®)	
Sotalol (Betapace®)	Also, a beta-blocker, xerostomia
Amiodarone (Cardarone®)	No oral adverse side effects
Class IV: Calcium channel blockers	
Diltiazem (Cardizem)	Gingival enlargement (less likely than nifedipine)
Nifedipine (Adalat, Procardia)	Gingival enlargement
Verapamil (Calan)	Gingival enlargement (less likely than the other two)

Q. It seems that there are some antiarrhythmic drugs that can cause vesiculobullous lesions that mimic or resemble the real autoimmune disease.

A. Yes. Clinically, lesions can develop in patients taking certain drugs. This condition is called drug-related lichenoid reactions. See Table A2.1 (Kalmer 2009; Scully and Bagan-Sebastian 2004).

Q. Is epinephrine contraindicated in patients with cardiac arrhythmias?

A. Treatment modification is needed to avoid triggering an arrhythmiThe amount of epinephrine should be limited to two cartridges of 1 : 100 000 epinephrine to prevent an epinephrine-induced tachycardia.

Q. For patients with arrhythmias, is it necessary to get a medical consultation before dental treatment?

A. Yes. If a pacemaker or defibrillator has recently been implanted (within six months), antibiotic prophylaxis may be needed, although there is a low risk for the development of IE and the AHA does not recommend antibiotic prophylaxis. With newer pacemakers that are well insulated (shielded), there is most likely no problem with impairing function when an electric dental device is used; however, due to the scarcity of human studies and medico-legal reasons, ultrasonic scalers should be avoided.

7.3.9   Valvular Heart Disease

Q. What is valvular heart disease?

A. Valvular heart disease includes conditions associated with valvular stenosis and regurgitation. Essentially, it can involve the mitral, aortic, pulmonary or tricuspid heart valves. Valvular heart disease can occur from other pathological medical conditions such as rheumatic fever, congenital heart defects, mitral valve prolapse, Kawasaki disease, and SLE. With mitral valve prolapse, it is important to determine whether there is regurgitation and the degree.

Q. Is antibiotic prophylaxis required for mitral valve prolapse or heart murmur?

A. According to the 2007 Guidelines on IE from the AHA, mitral valve prolapse even with heart murmur does not require antibiotic prophylaxis before invasive dental procedures causing bleeding. If necessary, obtain a medical consult from the patient's physician (Wilson et al. 2007).

Q. How is valvular disease treated?

A. Either with medications or valve replacement.

Q. Is antibiotic prophylaxis required for patients with heart valve replacement?

A. There is a 2017 update for management of patients with valvular heart disease (Nishimura et al. 2017). This update made no changes from the 2007 guidelines. Antibiotic prophylaxis is required for patients with heart valve replacement and palliative shunts, but *not* for cardiac stents. In a baby with congenital heart disease, a shunt diverts blood from one area of the heart to another to allow blood to flow to the lungs to receive oxygen.

Q. What medications are taken by patients with valvular disease?

A. Warfarin, aspirin, clopidogrel (Plavix), aspirin-dipyridamole (Aggrenox). Bleeding is to be monitored. Obtain a consult from the patient's physician. INR is required for warfarin.

Q. What other medical conditions are patients with valvular heart disease more prone to develop?

A. Heart failure, arrhythmia, and IE (American Academy of Periodontology 1996).

7.4 Pregnant and Nursing Patient

Q. When is the safest time to treat a pregnant patient?

A. Preventive dental care should be provided to the pregnant patient as early as possible. The first trimester is from week 1 to 12; second trimester week 13–28 and; third trimester week 29–40 or delivery.

Elective dental care is contraindicated in the first 10 weeks of pregnancy because at this time teratogenic risks are greatest. Routine care (e.g., scaling and root planing, restorative procedures) should be performed between 14 and 27 weeks, but it is best early in the second trimester. Emergency care (e.g., active infection or abscess) during the first trimester may outweigh the risks if treatment was not done. Radiographs can also be taken as needed following all precautions. If there are any reservations concerning treatment of the pregnant patient, consult with the patient's physician (American Academy of Periodontology 2004a,b).

Q. Is epinephrine containing local anesthetics safe to administer to the pregnant patient?

A. Yes. As mentioned earlier, epinephrine is a natural hormone produced in the body. Epinephrine acting as a vasoconstrictor actually reduces the toxicity of the local anesthetic. Intravascular injection should be avoided. According to Michalowicz et al. (2008), essential dental treatment (e.g., scaling and root planing, temporary or permanent restorations, endodontic therapy or extraction) with the administration of topical anesthetics and local anesthetics containing 1 : 100 000 epinephrine is safe and did not significantly increase the risk of any adverse events in pregnant women at week 13–21 of gestation. In this clinical study, different anesthetics were used including topical 5% lidocaine and 1% dyclonine and injected local anesthetics such as 2% lidocaine with 1 : 100 000 epinephrine, 4% prilocaine with epinephrine and prilocaine without a vasoconstrictor. The authors conclude that data from larger clinical studies are needed to confirm the safety of dental care in pregnant women.

Q. Is lidocaine the safest local anesthetic to administer to the pregnant patient?

A. Yes. Lidocaine, an amide, is associated with the least medical/dental complications.

Q. Are topical anesthetics safe in pregnant women at 13–21 weeks?

A. Caution should be used with ester topical anesthetics since allergic reactions are possible. However, an article in the *Journal of the American Dental Association* reports the use of topical and local anesthetics is safe in pregnant women at 13–21 weeks' gestation (Michalowicz et al. 2008).

Q. So, epinephrine is safe to administer during pregnancy?

A. Yes. Lidocaine with 1 : 100 000 epinephrine (0.017 mg of epinephrine in a 1.7 mL cartridge of lidocaine) is safe to administer during pregnancy (Lee and Shin 2017). The concern about epinephrine is its effect on uterine muscle but there are no studies to confirm this effect in pregnant women (New York State Department of Health 2006). Additionally, the concerns with epinephrine are most likely from higher doses and not 1 : 100 000 used in dentistry. Doses should also be kept to a maximum of two cartridges. Lidocaine can also be administered without epinephrine.

Q. What other precautions should be followed when treating a pregnant patient?

A. During the second and third trimester, the patient should be positioned in the dental chair on her left side to avoid or relieve supine hypotensive syndrome. Blood pressure should be monitored.

Q. Can nitrous oxide be administered safely to a pregnant patient?

A. It is recommended to consult with the patient's prenatal care provider regarding use of nitrous oxide.

Q. What antibiotics should not be prescribed to a pregnant patient?

A. Tetracycline, doxycycline, and minocycline, especially in the second and third trimesters during tooth development

7.5 Corticosteroids and Thyroid Medication

Q. What is cortisol?

A. The adrenal cortex normally produces and secretes cortisol, an endogenous hormone. When exogenous steroids (e.g., prednisone, methylprednisolone) are taken, the adrenal gland shuts off. In the normal, nonstressed person, about 8–10 mg of cortisol is produced per day which is equivalent to about 5–7 mg of prednisone. Cortisol is released in a highly irregular manner, with peak secretion in the early morning, which then tapers out in the late afternoon and evening. When a person is stressed, cortisol production is increased to about 50–300 mg a day. Cortisol functions to regulate energy by selecting the right type and amount of substrate (carbohydrate, fat or protein) that is needed by the body to meet the physiological demands placed upon it. Cortisol mobilizes energy by moving the body's fat stores (in the form of triglycerides) from one area to another or delivering it to hungry tissues such as working muscle. During stressful times, higher levels of cortisol are released, which have been associated with several medical conditions including suppressed thyroid function and hyperglycemiHowever, when taking exogenous steroids, there may not be enough endogenous cortisol to handle the body's stressful demands so that patients on long-term systemic steroids have been advised to take supplemental glucocorticoids.

Q. When are systemic glucocorticoid steroids indicated?

A. Chronic persistent asthma, Addison disease, rheumatoid arthritis, pemphigus, pemphigoid, psoriasis, SLE, and gastrointestinal diseases such as Crohn disease and ulcerative colitis.

Q. Does a patient taking systemic long-term glucocorticoid steroids such as prednisone or prednisolone need any specific adjustments in dosage during stressful dental procedures?

A. An "older" theory concerning the need for steroid supplementation in patients taking steroids was the "rule of twos" which stated that if the patient was currently on 20 mg of cortisone (equivalent to 5 mg prednisone) daily for two weeks or longer within the past two years then it was necessary to give supplemental steroids to prevent an adrenal crisis.

Addison or adrenal crisis is associated with a stressful event that is caused by the failure of cortisol levels to meet the body's increased requirements for cortisol and is primarily a mineralocorticoid steroid deficiency, not a glucocorticoid deficiency. Mineralocorticoids (e.g., aldosterone) maintain the level of sodium and potassium in the body. Adrenal crisis is a medical emergency characterized by abdominal pain, weakness, hypotension, dehydration, nausea and vomiting. Actually, adrenal crisis is primarily due to an insufficiency of mineralocorticoids.

It has been concluded in clinical studies that patients on long-term steroid drugs do not require supplemental "steroid coverage" for routine dentistry, including minor surgical procedures under profound local anesthesia with adequate postoperative pain control. The low incidence of significant adrenal insufficiency precludes the addition of supplemental steroids (Gibson and Ferguson 2004). For major oral/periodontal surgery under general anesthesia, supplemental steroids may be required depending upon the dose of steroid and duration of treatment. It is important to obtain a medical consultation from the patient's physician.

Schedule the patient in the morning and make sure the patient took the steroid within two hours of the dental procedure.

Q. Can epinephrine be used safely in patients taking a systemic steroid such as prednisone?

A. Yes. Epinephrine is synthesized and secreted by the adrenal medulla.

Q. What is the appropriate corticosteroid supplementation for a patient taking steroids and undergoing dental treatment?

A. The conclusion is that adrenal crisis is a rare event in dentistry, especially for patients with secondary adrenal insufficiency who develop this condition from taking steroids for common medical conditions. Most routine dental procedures, including nonsurgical periodontal therapy (scaling and root planing) and restorative procedures, can be performed without glucocorticoid supplementation. See Table 7.14.

Table 7.14 Dental guidelines for corticosteroid supplementation: preoperative considerations

Risk category and dental procedure	Supplemental steroids
Minimal risk: e.g., nonsurgical dental procedures	Not needed – regular steroid dose
Possible risk: e.g., *minor* periodontal and oral surgery with local anesthetic	Adrenal insufficiency is prevented when circulating levels of glucocorticoids are about 25 mg of hydrocortisone equivalent/day which is equivalent to a dose of about 5–6 mg of prednisone (prednisone is supplied as 1, 2.5, 5,10, 20, 50 mg tabs). This should be taken 1–2 hours before treatment
Moderate to major risk: e.g., major dental surgery (multiple extractions, quadrant periodontal surgery, multiple implants under general anesthesia longer than 1 hour [usually in the hospital])	Need glucocorticoid levels of 50–100 mg per day of hydrocortisone equivalent on the day of surgery and for at least one day after surgery. Intramuscular injection of 100 mg hydrocortisone one hour prior to surgery. Prescribe 25 mg hydrocortisone for 24 hours, then return to normal dose

Source: Data from Little et al. (2008).
See also Gibson and Ferguson (2004).

Q. Are there any precautions or contraindications for thyroid patients?

A. In most cases, hypothyroid patients receiving thyroid medication who have normal blood levels are treated without any special requirements and no antibiotic prophylaxis is needed. If the hypothyroid patient is untreated, it is best to obtain a medical consult and postpone dental treatment until the condition is under control.

In patients who are hyperthyroid and untreated, it is advised to avoid any surgical procedures as well as epinephrine because this could cause hyperthyroid crisis (thyroid storm, thyrotoxicosis) which may result in high blood pressure and/or cardiac arrhythmias. Since there is sympathetic overactivity in the hyperthyroid patient, epinephrine's effects will be additive. Epinephrine should *not* be used if the patient is currently being treated for hyperthyroidism with propylthiouracil (PTU) or methimazole (Tapazole®). Once the patient with hyperthyroidism is treated and is euthyroid (normal thyroid) then proceed as normal with no special requirements; epinephrine can be used but limited to two cartridges of 1 : 100 000.

7.6 Asthma Medications

Q. What is asthma?

A. A chronic respiratory disease associated with:

- reversible airflow obstruction
- bronchial hyperresponsiveness
- airway inflammation.

Q. Are there any dental materials that can exacerbate an asthmatic attack?

A. Yes. Fissure sealants, methyl methacrylate, dentifrices.

Q. What medications are taken in the management of asthma?

A. The patient will be taking a rescue bronchodilator, usually a short-acting beta-2 adrenergic receptor agonist. Some patients with persistent symptoms will require one or more controller medications. These usually consist of leukotriene modifiers, immunomodulators, inhaled corticosteroids, and long-acting beta-2 agonists. See Table 7.15.

Table 7.15 Medications for short-term and long-term control of asthma

Rescue inhalers (bronchodilators) for bronchospasm (intermittent asthma)
Adrenergic (short-acting)
Albuterol (Proventil®, Ventolin®)
Pirbuterol (Maxair®)
Terbutaline (Brethine,® Brethaire®)
Metaproterenol (Alupent®)
Levalbuterol (Xopenex®)
Anticholinergics
Ipratropium bromide HFA (Atrovent®)
Ipratropium bromide and albuterol sulfate (Combivent®)
Tiotropium bromide (Spiriva®)
Long-term control of asthma
Corticosteroids (antiinflammatory)
Beclomethasone dipropionate (Beclovent®, Vanceril®)
Budesonide (Pulmicort®)
Flunisolide (AeroBid®)
Fluticasone (Flovent®, Advair®)
Mometasone (Asmanex®)
Triamcinolone (Azmacort®)
Selective beta-2 agonists (long-acting) (bronchodilator)
Salmeterol (Serevent®)
Formoterol (Foradil®)
Methylxanthines (bronchodilator)
Theophylline (Slo-Phyllin®, Theo-Dur®, Theo-24®)
Mast cell stabilizers (antiinflammatory)
Cromolyn sodium (Inta®l)
Nedocromil (Tilade®)
Leukotriene modifiers (antiinflammatory)
Zafirlukast (Accolate®)
Montelukast (Singulair®)
Zileuton (Zyflo®)
Immunomodulators (antiinflammatory)
Omalizumab (Xolair®)

Q. How is an asthma patient managed in the dental chair?

A. If the patient is using an inhaler for acute bronchospasm, it should be on the treatment table in easy reach in case an attack occurs. Ask the patient when the last attack was and what triggered it. Be prepared if the patient has an asthmatic attack in the dental chair. The dental provider should be prepared to manage an acute bronchospasm if the rescue inhaler does not relieve symptoms. Dental care is performed only on well-controlled asthmatics.

Q. What should be done if the patient is taking corticosteroids for long-term use?

A. See section on adrenal insufficiency. Additionally, an adverse effect of corticosteroids that could affect dental treatment is the development of diabetes. In this case, a medical consultation from the patient's physician is advised to determine if the patient needs cortisone supplementation.

Q. Is epinephrine contraindicated in asthma patients?

A. This is very controversial. Epinephrine 1 : 100 000 is safe to use in a well-controlled asthmatic patient. Actually, there are some OTC products for asthma (e.g., Primatine Mist®) that contain epinephrine. Epinephrine is also used for the treatment of acute exacerbations refractory to bronchodilator inhalers.

   Some articles have reported not to use vasoconstrictors in asthmatic patients because of sodium metabisulfite, a sulfite preservative/antioxidant for the vasoconstrictor to stop it being degraded by light; however, epinephrine has been used safely in these patients. Methylparaben is only added to multiple-dose vials (Steinbacher and Glick 2001).

Q. Can a patient be allergic to epinephrine?

A. No, because epinephrine is an endogenous hormone produced by the adrenal medulla in the body.

Q. What is Samter's triad?

A. Samter's triad is a medical condition characterized by the presence of asthma + aspirin (and NSAID) sensitivity + nasal polyps. This condition can occur in asthmatic patients who experience worsening of asthma after taking aspirin or NSAIDs. Patients who have Samter's triad also have nasal polyps. Before recommending or prescribing an analgesic to an asthmatic, it is important to confirm that the patient does not have nasal polyps and if there has been no problem taking NSAIDs before. Acetaminophen is the preferred analgesic for asthmatic patients.

Q. What antibiotics should not be prescribed to an asthmatic?

A. If the patient is taking theophylline for asthma, ***erythromycin and clarithromycin (Biaxin) are contraindicated***. This is a severe drug–drug interaction that can result in death (Rieder and Spino 1988).

7.7 Diabetes Medication

Q. What is the classification of diabetes?

A. Type 1 and type 2. The underlying cause of type 1 diabetes is autoimmune destruction of the beta cells in the pancreas. Since the beta cells do not produce any insulin, exogenous insulin must be used. Insulin is needed in the body because it helps the blood glucose get into the tissue cells which use it for energy. When this does not happen, glucose stays in the blood, resulting in hyperglycemiAfter a meal, excess glucose not taken up by the tissue cells is stored in the liver in the form of glycogen and can be used later when energy is required. Type 1 diabetics are prone to diabetic ketoacidosis where fat is broken down to glycerol and fatty acids due to energy needs. The fatty acids are converted to elevated ketone levels which are excreted in the urine. Type 1 diabetics require insulin.

Risk factors for type 2 diabetes include genetics, obesity, and increasing age. Insulin is being produced but there is insulin resistance where insulin is not recognized by the tissue cells, resulting in hyperglycemia, which can cause the pancreas to produce more insulin, resulting in hyperinsulinemia. Type 2 diabetics do not always need exogenous insulin since it is being produced but require oral forms of medications that act differently so that an individual may be on more than one oral medication. See Table 7.16.

Table 7.16 Oral medications for diabetes

Sulfonylureas
First-generation agents: stimulate release of insulin from beta cells
Chlorpropamide (Diabinese®)
Tolazamide (Tolinase®)
Tolbutamide (Orinase®)
Second-generation agents: stimulate release of insulin from beta cells
Glipizide (Glucotrol®)
Glyburide (DiaBeta, Micronase®)
Glyburide, micronized (Glynase®)
Glimepiride (Amaryl®)
Biguanides: shut off the liver's excess glucose production
Metformin (Glucophage®)
Combination drugs
Glyburide/metformin (Glucovance®)
Metformin/glipizide (Metaglip®)
Metformin/rosiglitazone (Avandamet®)
Thiazolidinediones: target insulin sensitivity; mechanism unclear
Pioglitazone (Actos®)
Rosiglitazone (Avandia®)
Alpha-glucosidase inhibitors: slow postprandial (after meals) carbohydrate absorption in the blood. Used when diet alone is not enough
Acarbose (Precose®)
Miglitol (Glyset®)
Meglitinides: increase insulin secretion from beta cells, which reduces glucose levels
Repaglinide (Prandin®)
Nateglinide (Starlix®)

Q. What are some important diabetic complications associated with dentistry?

A. Diabetics are at increased risk for macrovascular (arteries) complications, including coronary artery disease, and microvascular (the terminal ends of blood vessels of capillaries and arterioles) complications of the eye (retinopathy), gingiva (periodontal disease), kidneys, nerves (neuropathy), and extremities (e.g., foot ulcers). This occurs because of excessive accumulation of glycated proteins (referred to as AGEs or advanced glycation endproducts) in the walls of large blood vessels. This causes impaired collagen turnover due to accumulation of AGE-modified collagen, resulting in increased levels of low-density lipoproteins and narrowing of the blood vessels.

Q. What must be known about a diabetic patient before rendering dental treatment?

A. How well controlled is the patient? Results from two different tests must be known before dental treatment is started: fasting glucose and glycosylated hemoglobin (HbA1c). Hemoglobin A1c provides an average of blood glucose control over 2–3 months and is used in conjunction with home blood glucose monitoring. HbA1c levels represent blood glucose that combines with hemoglobin and becomes glycated. Therefore, the average amount of glucose in the blood is determined by measuring HbA1c level. A consult with the patient's physician is necessary to know the patient's control and HbA1c levels.

    The fasting blood glucose is just as important as HbA1c because the risk of infection may be directly related to fasting blood glucose. Fasting glucose levels are done by the patient (from the fingertip) in the morning before eating. When levels are <206 mg/dL there is no risk for developing infection. With blood glucose levels >230 mg/dL, there is an increased risk for developing an infection.

    HbA1c levels (Mealey and Oates 2006) are as follows.

- Normal level: treatment can precede 5.0–6.0%
- Treatment goal: treatment can precede <7.0%
- Alternative diabetic management required >8.0%; increased risk for complications such as delayed wound healing)

Q. What dental conditions are diabetics prone to develop?

A. Periodontal diseases, xerostomia, fungal infections (e.g., psuedomembranous candidiasis – dental sore mouth), taste disturbances, burning mouth syndrome, dental caries, glossodynia.

Q. Should diabetic patients have antibiotic coverage to decrease the incidence of infection and increase wound healing?

A. In patients who are poorly controlled dental treatment should be delayed until control is established. If dental treatment cannot wait, antibiotic prophylaxis may help prevent impaired and delayed wound healing. If the patient is wellcontrolled antibiotic coverage is not necessary (www.health.am/db/diabetes-mellitus-and-oral health/#1).

Q. What medical condition in diabetics taking insulin is commonly seen in dental offices?

A. Hypoglycemia usually occurs with insulin treatment but can occur with oral hypoglycemics. It happens due either to too much insulin being injected or improper timing of the injections with meals. Symptoms of hypoglycemia may not be apparent until blood glucose levels fall <60 mg/dL but can occur at any blood glucose level. Hypoglycemia is characterized by nervousness, anxiety, sweating, headache, hunger, pallor, coldness, palpitations, and tachycardiTreating hypoglycemia is targeted to getting blood glucose to normal by eating 10–20 g (3–4 oz) of carbohydrate in the form of sugar such as orange juice or pure sugar. Also, vital signs must be monitored. If the patient becomes unconscious, call 911. Glucagon 1 mg SC or IM or 20 mL of 50% dextrose IV is administered along with oxygen and monitoring vital signs (Lamster et al. 2008; Ship 2003).

Q. Is epinephrine safe to administer to diabetics?

A. Many factors may increase the body's insulin requirements which could worsen the diabetic state. Epinephrine, which is released during stressful times, causes gluconeogenesis which is the production of glucose. Also, epinephrine inhibits the release of insulin from the pancreas, resulting in less glucose uptake into the cells which is used for energy. The risk of metabolic complications after the administration of small doses of epinephrine used in dentistry is much less than when used in larger doses in medicine. Additionally, there is a higher risk of complications in patients taking insulin than being controlled with diet alone or hypoglycemic oral drugs (Pérusse et al. 1992).

7.8 Psychiatric and Neurological Medications

Q. Why should oral health practitioners care about psychiatric medications?

A. Mental illness is a ubiquitous set of behavioral and cognitive pathologies that all healthcare providers encounter on a regular basis and dental professionals are no exception. There is evidence that people with mental illness may have a disproportionate amount of dental pathology. In order to ensure that these patients receive dental treatment that integrates into their allopathic care, there are many notable medication interactions and risks associated with prescribing other medications that the clinician should be aware of.

People with mental illness are at increased risk of poor oral health because of behavioral tendencies related to their underlying disease and side effects of commonly prescribed psychiatric medications. Some of these risk factors include the following (Kisely 2016).

- Poor nutritional habits like consuming sugary beverages due to low education level, lack of insight or other related substance use.
- Malnutrition due to disorganized and disordered thinking or eating disorders like anorexia nervosa.
- Poor hygiene in general and oral hygiene in particular.
- Extremely high rates of tobacco use (as high as 80% in people with schizophrenia) and alcohol use.
- Barriers to accessing care, whether no access to care or being unable to make it to scheduled dental visits.
- Xerostomia, a side effect of many psychotropic medications, especially those with anticholinergic effect and a common finding in anorexia nervosa.
- Erosive fluids in mouth; a well-known finding in patient with bulimia nervosa is erosion of lingual surfaces of maxillary incisors.

These risk factors exacerbate common dental diseases including dental erosion, caries, and periodontal diseases. These pathologies can ultimately result in edentulism, which can worsen these already vulnerable people's nutritional status, level of functioning, and thus quality of life. These patients are also high risk for oral cancer, given poor oral hygiene and high-risk substance use. Because they have such difficulty accessing care, cancerous lesions are less likely to be identified early and this can ultimately be life threatening. An additional concern may be a higher risk of endocarditis that results from seeding with oral bacteria (this is not established but a theoretically increased risk) (Kisely 2016).

Q. How common is mental illness?

A. Mental illness and substance use disorders are pervasive, which means dentists have a high likelihood of regular contact with patients who have these disorders. According to the National Alliance on Mental Illness (NAMI), in 2016 44.7 million US adults experienced mental illness and this number appears to be growing. One in five American adults experiences mental illness. Broken down by disease: 2.4 million adults live with schizophrenia (1 out of every 100), 6.1 million live with bipolar disorder (2.6% of the population), 16 million live with major depression (6.9%), and 42 million live with anxiety disorders (18.1%). About 10.2 million adults have co-occurring addiction and mental health disorders. Depression is the leading cause of disability worldwide. A 2010 survey of dental patients by Giglio and Laskin (2010) found that one in five had a history of being diagnosed with a psychiatric condition.

According to a report by the Substance Abuse and Mental Health Service Administration (SAMHSA), in 2016, about 20.1 million people aged 12 or older had a substance use disorder, with alcohol use disorder accounting for about 15.1 million and illicit drug use disorders accounting for 7.4 million. The most common illicit drug use disorder was for marijuana (4 million people). An estimated 2.1 million people had an opioid use disorder, which includes 1.8 million with a prescription pain reliever use disorder and 0.6 million people with a heroin use disorder (Substance Abuse and Mental Health Services Administration 2017).

Q. How do I know what qualifies as a psychiatric medication and why does it matter?

A. Psychiatric medications include many classes of drugs, broken down into categories based on the pathology they are most commonly prescribed for. For example, antidepressants are used most often for depression, mood stabilizers for bipolar disorder, antipsychotics for psychotic disorders, stimulants for ADHD, cognitive enhancers for dementia, wakefulness-promoting drugs for narcolepsy, and anxiolytics and sedative/hypnotics for anxiety disorders. Within each of these classes there are subclasses; for example, within antidepressants, there are selective serotonin reuptake inhibitors (SSRIs), monoamine oxidase inhibitors (MAOIs), TCAs, and serotonin-norepinephrine reuptake inhibitors (SNRIs), among others. These categories are not rigid; many drugs have FDA approved and nonapproved indications besides their primary use. For example, atypical antipsychotics are frequently prescribed as adjunctive treatment for depression. Because of the diversity of their mechanisms of action, these drugs have an immense number of drug–drug interactions and side effects, that at best are a nuisance and at worst fatal. This amalgamation of heterogeneous drugs with varying mechanisms and side effect profiles can, understandably, be difficult for practitioners to keep track of.

Q. What are the classes of psychiatric medications and which medications are in each class (Stahl 2008)?

A.

Antidepressants

Generic name	Common brand names	Type
Imipramine	Tofranil®	TCA
Amitriptyline	Elavil®	TCA
Clomipramine	Anafranil®	TCA
Doxepin	Sinequan®, Adapin®	TCA
Desipramine	Norpramin®	TCA
Nortriptyline	Aventyl®, Pamelor®	TCA
Phenelzine	Nardil®	MAOI
Tranylcypromine	Parnate®	MAOI
Selegeline	Emsam®	MAOI
Fluoxetine	Prozac®	SSRI
Paroxetine	Paxil®	SSRI
Sertraline	Zoloft®	SSRI
Fluvoxamine	Luvox®	SSRI
Citalopram	Celexa®	SSRI
Escitalopram	Lexapro®	SSRI
Venlafaxine	Effexor®	SNRI
Duloxetine	Cymbalta®	SNRI
Bupropion	Wellbutrin®, ForFivo®, Zyban®	[a]
Mirtazapine	Remeron®	[a]
Trazodone	Desyrel®, Oleptro®	[a]
Desvenlafaxine	Pristiq®, Khedezla®	SNRI
Vilazodone	Viibryd®	[a]
Isocarboxazid	Marplan®	MAOI
Levomilnacipran	Fetzima®	SNRI
Vortioxetine	Brintellix®	[a]

[a] Other mechanism of action.

MAOI, monoamine oxidase inhibitor; SNRI, serotonin-norepinephrine reuptake inhibitor; SSRI, selective serotonin reuptake inhibitor; TCA, tricyclic antidepressant.

Anxiolytics

Generic name	Common brand names	Type
Clonazepam	Klonipin®	Benzodiazepine
Diazepam	Valium®, Diastat®	Benzodiazepine
Chlordiazepoxide	Librium®	Benzodiazepine
Oxazepam	Serax®	Benzodiazepine
Lorazepam	Ativan®	Benzodiazepine

Generic name	Common brand names	Type
Alprazolam	Xanax®	Benzodiazepine
Buspirone	Buspar®	5HT1A partial agonist
Propranolol	Inderal®, Innopran®	Beta-blocker
Clonidine	Catapres®	Alpha-2 agonist
Prazosin	Minipress®	Alpha-1 antagonist
Hydroxyzine	Atarax®, Vistaril®	Antihistamine – H1 antagonist
Zolpidem	Ambien®	Hypnotic
Zaleplon	Sonata®	Hypnotic
Eszopiclone	Lunesta®	Hypnotic
Ramelteon	Rozerem®	Melatonin receptor agonist

Antipsychotics

Generic name	Common brand names	Type
Chlorprimazine	Thorazine®	FGA
Thioridazine	Mellaril®	FGA
Perphenazine	Trilafon®	FGA
Pimozide	Orap®	FGA
Fluphenazine	Prolixin®	FGA
Haloperidol	Haldol®	FGA
Risperidone	Risperdal®	SGA
Olanzapine	Zyprexa®, Zyprexa Zydis®	SGA
Quetiapine	Seroquel®	SGA
Ziprasidone	Geodon®	SGA
Aripiprazole	Abilify®	SGA
Clozapine	Clozaril®, FazaClo®	SGA
Paliperidone	Invega®, Invega Sustenna®	SGA
Iloperidone	Fanapt®	SGA
Asenapine	Saphris®	SGA
Lurasidone	Latuda®	SGA

FGA, first-generation antipsychotic; SGA, second-generation antipsychotic.

Mood stabilizers

Generic name	Common brand names
Lithium carbonate	Lithobid®, Eskalith®
Divalproex sodium, valproic acid, valproate	Depakote®, Depakene®
Carbamezapine	Tegretol®, Carbatrol®, Equetro®
Lamotrigine	Lamictal®

Cognitive enhancers

Generic name	Common brand names	Type
Methylphenidate	Ritalin®, Concerta®, Daytrana®, Metadate®, Methylin®, Quiillivant®	Stimulant
Dexmethylphenidate	Focalin®	Stimulant
Amphetamine salts	Adderall®	Stimulant
Dextroamphetamine	Dexedrine®, DextroStat®, Procentra®	Stimulant
Lisdexamfetamine dimesylate	Vyvanse®	Stimulant
Atomoxetine	Strattera®	SNRI
Clonidine extended release	Kapvay®	Alpha-2 agonist
Guanfacine ER	Intuniv®	Alpha-2a agonist
Donepezil	Aricept®, Memac®	Cholinesterase inhibitor
Memantine	Namenda®	NMDA/glutamate antagonist
Modafinil/Armodafinil	Provigil®/Nuvigil®	Dopamine reuptake inhibitor

NMDA, N-methyl-D-aspartate; SNRI, selective norepinephrine reuptake inhibitor.

Substance use disorder treatments

Generic name	Common brand names	Type
Methadone	Dolophine®, Methadose®	Opioid agonist and analgesic
Buprenorphine	Subutex®	Opioid agonist
Buprenorphine/naloxone	Suboxone®	Partial opioid agonist with opioid antagonist
Acamprosate	Campral®	GABA analog
Disulfiram	Antabuse®	Aldehyde dehydrogenase inhibitor
Naltrexone	ReVita®, Vivitrol®	Opioid antagonist
Varenicline	Chantix®	Nicotine acetylcholine receptor agonist
Nicotine	Nicoderm patch, Commit® lozenges, Nicorette® gum, Nicotrol® inhaler and nasal spray	Nicotine replacement therapy

GABA, gamma-aminobutyric acid.

Q. Which psychiatric medications are my patients most likely to be on?

A. It is hard to say what psychiatric medications patients presenting for dental care will most likely be on. There are data based on the Medical Expenditure Panel Survey (MEPS), estimating the number of times medications are prescribed annually (www.meps.ahrq.gov/mepsweb). A list of the 200 most prescribed medications based on MEPS can be found at http://clincalc.com/DrugStats. Utilizing this information, we can get a sense of what psychiatric medications are most common in society, thus increasing the odds of these medications being found on dental patients' medication lists. Of the 25 most prescribed medications in the US by number of times that medication has been filled in 2018, it is estimated that five are medications with

FDA indications for psychiatric pathology. For example, sertraline hydrochloride is the 14th most often filled medication overall, with about 38 877 836 prescriptions for this medication in 2015. For comparison, the number 1 drug on this list is simvastatin, with about 112 923 790 fills. Although this is not a precise measure of how many patients are actively on this medication at a given time, it does indicate that a lot of patients are on sertraline overall, increasing the odds that someone on this medication will present for dental care.

Other medications on this list are fluoxetine (#20, 28 311 454 prescriptions); citalopram (#21, 28 069 030 prescriptions); trazodone (#22, 27 564 196 prescriptions); alprazolam (#23, 27 051 071 prescriptions); bupropion (#25, 26 198 463); escitalopram (#31, 24 068 904 prescriptions); clonazepam (#38, 21 817 867 prescriptions); zolpidem (#46, 19 185 054 prescriptions); duloxetine (#48, 17 890 815 prescriptions); venlafaxine (#50, 17 109 915 prescriptions); lorazepam (#55, 15 698 434 prescriptions); paroxetine (#57, 14 808 496 prescriptions); methylphenidate (#58, 14 521 828 prescriptions); propanolol (#63, 13 854 897 prescriptions); lamotrigine (#70, 12 096 327 prescriptions); clonidine (#76, 10 896 072 prescriptions); topiramate (#77, 10 752 428 prescriptions); amitriptyline (#83, 9 664 825 prescriptions); quetiapine (#87, 9 195 115 prescriptions); diazepam (#91, 8 899 752 prescriptions); hydroxyzine (#95, 8 297 684 prescriptions); divalproex (#120, 6 112 173 prescriptions); risperidone (#130, 5 575 236 prescriptions); aripiprazole (#133, 5 410 931 prescriptions); lithium (#173, 3 787 926 prescriptions).

Q. QT prolongation: what is it, why does it matter, and which medications prescribed by dentists can interact with psychiatric medications, potentially worsen QT interval?

A. One risk that dentists should keep in mind when prescribing medications for a patient is that of torsades de pointes (TdP), a polymorphic ventricular tachyarrhythmia that can lead to death even if treated properly. One way to avoid this potentially life-threatening condition is to obtain a thorough cardiac history from all patients or have access to their medical records. QT interval is often referred to as "QTc." QTc, or "corrected" QT interval, takes into account the heart rate of the individual during the EKG reading and is thought demonstrate a more accurate risk assessment for TdP.

Prolongation of the electrocardiographic QT interval is an established risk factor for TdP, though the relationship between prolonged QT and TdP is complex (Malik and Camm 2001). Some patients may have long QT syndrome (LQTC), a genetically inherited condition caused by hundreds of mutations in 10 identified genes (Roden 2008). Medications are another common cause of QT prolongation, with up to 3% of medications believed to prolong QTc, including antidepressants, antipsychotics, and nonpsychiatric medications such as antiarrhythmics, antibiotics, antifungals, and antimalarials (Beach et al. 2013). It is important to point out that not all medications that have been shown to increase the QT interval have been linked to TdP. Alcohol and illicit drugs such as cocaine and stimulants have also been shown to prolong the QTc interval (Zemrak and Kenna 2008). It is also known that the QTc can vary throughout the day up to 75–100 ms, with sleep being a risk factor for prolonged QTc interval (Yap and Camm 2003).

Drug interactions can lead to TdP either via a pharmacodynamic or pharmacokinetic interaction. In the former, the cumulative effect of two QTc-prolonging agents places the patient at risk. In the latter, co-prescribing medications in which one inhibits cytochrome P450 isoenzymes causing an increased concentration of a second QT-prolonging medication results in increased risk of TdP. Agents that are known to contribute to QTc prolongation via pharmacokinetic interactions include macrolide antibiotics, antifungal agents, the antiretroviral agent ritonavir, and grapefruit juice (Alvarez and Pahissa 2010). Decreased liver function may also lead to higher serum drug levels and elevate the risk for TdP and it is therefore helpful to have a recent liver panel (e.g., liver transaminases, alkaline phosphatase, and bilirubin) when prescribing medications that may prolong the QTc interval (Beach et al. 2013).

Q. Is there a risk of causing bleeding when prescribing NSAIDs to patient on SSRIs?

A. Blood clot formation relies on the release of serotonin from platelets, which combines with other prothrombotic factors (Napenas et al. 2011). Clotting may be prolonged (and therefore bleeding time increased) in some patients who are unable to store serotonin in their platelets. This risk is increased in patients on SSRIs, antiplatelet agents (e.g., aspirin, clopidogrel) and anticoagulant warfarin (Sadock et al. 2017). Clinicians should perform a risk assessment when considering prescribing NSAIDs to at-risk patients taking SSRIs, as the combination of these two drug classes increases the risk of GI bleeding events compared with either drug alone (Pinto et al. 2009).

Q. Cytochrome (CYP) P450 enzyme drug interactions: what are they, why do they matter, and how to avoid them?

A. Certain medications prescribed by dentists can affect the metabolism of some psychiatric medications, leading to subtherapeutic or elevated, sometimes even toxic blood levels. For example, the macrolide antibiotics erythromycin and clarithromycin influence the hepatic metabolism of a large number of medicines by inhibiting cytochrome isoenzymes CYP 3A4 and CYP 1A2. Patients on TCAs or SSRIs who are prescribed a course of erythromycin or ciprofloxacin can suffer from anticholinergic and alpha-1-blocking activity because of CYP inhibition from the antibiotics. This can cause xerostomia, constipation, increased intraocular pressure, tachycardia, dysrhythmias, confusion, and orthostatic hypotension. It is reasonable to replace erythromycin or clarithromycin with azithromycin because these antibiotics do not influence the hepatic metabolism of other drugs by inhibition of the CYP isoenzymes.

Prescribing tetracyclines or metronidazole to patients taking lithium for mood stabilization should also be done with caution to avoid possible lithium toxicity. Lithium toxicity is characterized by confusion, ataxia, and kidney damage. The reduction in lithium clearance by tetracyclines and metronidazole can increase lithium serum levels beyond the toxic threshold and is a possible mechanism for these adverse effects. However, only metronidazole has been shown (albeit in several case reports) to invoke this drug interaction.

Other drug interactions to consider include increased photosensitivity with tetracycline and St John's wort (a dietary supplement often used for depression) and co-administration and accelerated metabolism of doxycycline by carbamazepine (an antiepileptic also used as a mood stabilizer), reducing the efficacy of the antibiotic.

The above interaction with St John's wort highlights the importance of taking a full medical history from patients, including any possible substance use, herbal or homeopathic remedies, prescription drugs and OTC medicines to avoid drug–drug interactions and related side effects.

Unfortunately, there is a lack of studies exploring drug interactions in the area of dental and antidepressant medications. A good rule of thumb, however, is that the more specific the action of the antidepressant (e.g., on a specific receptor), the safer it is for co-administration with other drugs. That is, older antidepressants such as MAOIs and TCAs are much more likely to have drug interactions than newer generation antidepressants such as the SSRIs (Lambrecht et al. 2013).

Opiates are metabolized via phase I metabolism by the CYP pathway, phase II metabolism by glucuronidation or both. Phase I metabolism involves the CYP3A4 and CYP2D6 enzymes, the former metabolizing 50% of all drugs. Due to its key role in metabolism, opiates metabolized by CYP3A4 have an increased risk for drug–drug interactions. Drugs metabolized by CYP2D6 have an intermediate risk of drug–drug interactions due to it metabolizing fewer drugs.

Fentanyl and oxycodone are primarily metabolized by CYP3A4 enzyme, although a small portion of oxycodone is metabolized to oxymorphone by CYP2D6. Tramadol is metabolized by both CYP3A4 and CYP2D6. Methadone involves quite significant interaction potential as it is metabolized by six different CYP enzymes (primarily CYP3A4 and CYP2B6 but also by CYP2C8, CYP2C19, CYP2D6, and CYP2C9).

CYP3A4 substrates or inhibitors can increase opioid concentrations, potentially increasing their duration and adverse effects such as sedation and respiratory depression. In contrast, CYP3A4 inducers can reduce the pain-killing abilities of opiates. Besides medications, commonly consumed food products such as bergamottin (a strong CYP3A4 inhibitor found in grapefruit juice) and cafestol (a CYP3A4 inducer found in coffee) should be considered when prescribing opiates for analgesia.

When using medications that induce CYP3A4 enzymes, particular care should be taken when prescribing tramadol, which has been associated with seizures, even when using acceptable doses. Seizure risk increases when using tramadol with CYP3A4 inducers such as carbamazepine, or with SSRIs, TCAs or other serotonergic medications.

Hydrocodone, codeine, and dihydrocodeine are entirely metabolized by the CYP2D6 enzyme with subsequent processing of their respective metabolites by phase II glucuronidation. These opioids (and to a lesser extent oxycodone, tramadol, and methadone) may interact with SSRIs, TCAs, beta-blockers, and antiarrhythmics; other drugs are substrates, inducers, or inhibitors of the CYP2D6 enzyme.

Clearance of medications via CYP enzyme induction is also dependent on the patient's genome. For example, it is thought that approximately 5–10% of Caucasians possess allelic variants of the *CYP2D6* gene that are associated with decreased clearance of drugs metabolized by this isoenzyme, and between 1% and 7% of Caucasians carry CYP2D6 allelic variants associated with rapid metabolism. The prevalence of poor metabolizers is lower among Asian populations (≤1%) and is highly variable in African populations (0–34%). The prevalence of rapid metabolizers of opioids has not been reported in Asian populations while estimates in African populations are high but variable (9–30%).

This variance in the clearance of medications based on a person's genetic make-up can be seen when treating pain with codeine. Poor opioid metabolizers do not fully benefit from codeine treatment because they are not able to efficiently metabolize it into morphine, codeine's active molecule. Conversely, rapid opioid metabolizers might feel greater pain relief (or increased side effects) with a normal dose of codeine due to rapid metabolism generating greater concentration of morphine.

Morphine, oxymorphone, and hydromorphone are all metabolized by phase II glucuronidation and there is therefore much reduced potential for metabolically based drug interactions. For example, oxymorphone has no known pharmacokinetic drug–drug interactions, and morphine has few. Pharmacodynamic drug–drug interactions are possible with all opioids, however, and additive interactions with benzodiazepines, antihistamines, or alcohol and antagonistic interactions with naltrexone or naloxone should all be considered.

One should still consider, however, that the enzymes responsible for glucuronidation reactions may also be subject to a variety of factors that may alter opioid metabolism, the most important of which is the enzyme UGT2B7. This discussion is beyond the scope of this text (Smith 2009).

Q. How do I manage dental pain in patients on opioid replacement therapy?

A. Prescribing opiates to patients on opiate agonist therapy (OAT) for acute pain can be a challenge to clinicians for many reasons. It is helpful to have some general knowledge about the different opiate agonists used for opiate use disorder (OUD). Methadone and buprenorphine (often combined with naloxone to reduce its abuse potential) are the two OATs available in the US to treat OUD. Both of these medications have analgesic properties for 4–8 hours while their opioid withdrawal suppression properties last as long as 24–48 hours.

A dentist may hesitate to prescribe opioids to patients already on OAT due to fear of inducing an overdose (e.g., death by respiratory suppression). One should remember, however, that tolerance to the respiratory and CNS depressant effects of opioids occurs rapidly and reliably, so one need not worry more about overdose in the OAT population than the general population. Also, of reassurance, some evidence suggests that acute pain serves as a natural antagonist to opioid-associated respiratory and CNS depression.

In fact, patients being treated for OUD with methadone or buprenorphine may require increased and more frequent doses of opioids to achieve acute pain control. This may be because cross-tolerance develops between opioids used for OAT and those used for acute pain. Also, there may be a component of latent hyperalgesia due to long-term exposure to opioids. This complicates the treatment of acute pain in the patient already tolerant to opioids due to being on OAT, but these patients of course should still be treated.

Another reservation a dentist may have about prescribing opioids to a patient on OAT is not wanting to cause the patient to relapse to opioids. However, no evidence exists that exposure to opioid analgesics in the presence of acute pain increases relapse rates in patients on OAT. In fact, relapse prevention theories would suggest that the stress associated with unrelieved pain is more likely to trigger relapse than adequate pain treatment (Alford et al. 2006).

Q. Is it safe to prescribe medications metabolized by the liver, like Tylenol, to patients with alcohol use disorder or cirrhosis?

A. Alcohol abuse is extremely prevalent in the general population. When asking patients about their alcohol use, underreporting is quite prevalent due to the patients' fear of judgment, stigmatization and other personal and societal factors. Consequences of long-term heavy alcohol use include hepatitis (also can be occur with short-term use), fibrosis or even cirrhosis of the liver (Kaplan and Sadock 2017). Tylenol, or acetaminophen, is a common non-NSAID analgesic used for mild to moderate pain after many dental procedures. Tylenol is also often combined with several more powerful analgesics, such as the opioids hydrocodone (e.g., Vicodin) or oxycodone (e.g., Percocet), when more severe acute pain management is needed. Since Tylenol is metabolized by the liver, and acute Tylenol toxicity from an overdose (either intentional or iatrogenic) can be fatal, a cautious dentist may hesitate to prescribe Tylenol to a patient who either admits to or is suspected to drink heavily (Budnitz et al. 2011). Luckily, this concern does not seem to be supported in the literature. On the contrary, in well-nourished patients and in those without cirrhosis, doses of Tylenol up to 3–4 g daily for short periods of time is reasonable. In patients with decompensated alcoholic liver disease (ALD), there are not good data to strongly support a particular treatment regimen. For patients with alcoholic cirrhosis, 3–4 g daily may be reasonable for acute pain in the short term, but 2–3 g daily may be safer if analgesia is required for longer than 14 days (Hayward et al. 2016).

Q. What is tardive dyskinesia (TD) and how do I tell it apart from edentulous orofacial dyskinesia?

A. TD is a hyperkinetic movement disorder, induced by treatment with dopamine-blocking agents. TD is a characterized by a wide variety of involuntary movements that typically start while the patient is taking the offending agent and can continue after it is withdrawn, sometimes lifelong. The most common offending agents are neuroleptics (first-generation antipsychotics) and antiemetics metoclopramide and prochlorperazine. The most common manifestations of TD are the oro-bucco-lingual and facial dyskinesias, but there are also forms with limb, trunk, and respiratory manifestations. Tongue movements range from subtle sliding back and forth to full-on twisting and protrusions. Lip movements include puckering and smacking. Cheek movements include bulging and retraction of corners of the mouth. Jaw movements are typically characterized by chewing movements. At its worst, TD can interfere with chewing, swallowing, speech, and breathing.

TD can be confused with edentulous orofacial dyskinesia, a rare movement disorder of the jaw associated with edentulism, treated with denture fabrication and placement. The rhythmic, jaw swinging nature of this disorder can look a lot like TD. The best way to differentiate the two is based on the patient's history. You can ask whether the patient has been on (or is currently on) neuroleptics or other dopamine-blocking agents, or if these movements started organically, originating when the patient lost most or all of their teeth.

As the first line of oral healthcare, there is a good chance you might be the only person to inspect your patient's tongue and mouth closely on a regular basis. This gives you the unique ability to observe subtle hyperkinetic movements that may be early signs of TD. Making the patient and psychiatrist aware of these findings has the potential to prevent the patient from suffering from a very unpleasant, potentially lifelong, disorder of movement (Singh et al. 2015).

Q. I've heard lithium can be toxic – can I prescribe medications to my dental patients and not cause lithium toxicity?

A. Lithium is an element from the periodic table that is typically used to treat bipolar disorder, and sometimes depression and aggressive behavior as well. It is one of the most senior psychoactive medications, with knowledge of its effect first written up in the literature in the late 1940s, and due to its effectiveness, will continue to be a commonly prescribed medication for the foreseeable future. Lithium is ubiquitous in the body, is involved in many processes and it has therefore been difficult to ascertain the mechanism of action that drives lithium's efficacy in treating the above conditions. Lithium is notable for reducing the risk of suicide attempts in patients with bipolar disorder by up to 80% (this population has a suicide rate as high as 15%) (Cipriani et al. 2013).

Lithium's importance in treating bipolar disorder cannot be overstated; at the same time, it is important not to lose sight of the risks associated with it. Lithium undergoes renal excretion and has a very narrow therapeutic range. In other words, any medication that alters renal function in any way may alter plasma concentration of lithium. Plasma concentration for treatment is typically between 0.4–1.2 mmol/L, depending on clinical setting and patient's presenting illness, while toxicity occurs at levels greater than 1.5 mmol/L. Symptoms of lithium toxicity with plasma concentration between 1.5–2 mmol/L include weakness, drowsiness, confusion, ataxia, tremor, twitching, nausea, diarrhea, and poor appetite. Levels of above 2 mmol/L can lead to worsening confusion, seizures, and even death (Cipriani et al. 2013).

NSAIDS are frequently prescribed by oral health professionals and carry the risk of altering lithium levels. They decrease renal blood flow, thus increasing reuptake of lithium, subsequently increasing lithium plasma concentration. The effect of NSAIDs on lithium plasma level is unpredictable, with documented increases of 10% to greater than 400% in concentration. This can easily be the difference between therapeutic and toxic levels. This effect can happen within days of initiating NSAID treatment in some patients and months into treatment in others. It is important to bear in mind that when prescribing NSAIDs to patients on lithium, it is essential for them to remain hydrated, so their kidneys continue to clear lithium, preventing toxic build-up in the plasma. It is also recommended that if it is necessary to treat a patient on lithium with NSAIDs, NSAID dosing be regular and not prn, and that lithium levels be monitored more frequently than they otherwise would be (Teicher et al. 1987).

NSAIDs can be given to patients on lithium – just make sure to be in contact with the prescribing physician or psychiatrist to coordinate care in order to minimize the development of toxicity.

Q. Are there other medications I should be wary of prescribing when a patient is on lithium?

A. Antibiotics such as metronidazole and tetracycline have been noted to increase renal absorption of lithium and thus increase plasma concentration. Teicher et al. (1987) presented case reports of metronidazole and tetracycline increasing serum lithium levels in several patients, even to the point of producing symptoms of lithium toxicity. It is best to avoid these medications if your patient is on lithium, but if they require one of these drugs or it has already been started, it is important to be in touch with their psychiatrist about monitoring lithium serum concentration and serum creatinine in order to avoid toxicity (Stahl 2008; Teicher et al. 1987).

Q. MAOI/TCA/SSRI and epinephrine – is there a risk of hypertensive crisis?

A. Vasoconstrictors (adrenaline, noradrenaline, isoprenaline and phenylephrine) are often added to local anesthetics in order to increase localized efficacy of these numbing agents. Although the anesthetic effects may be localized, small amounts of both anesthetic and vasoconstrictor likely enter systemic circulation. Some antidepressants – specifically TCAs and possibly MAOIs – may prevent reuptake or metabolism, respectively, of the vasoconstrictors, resulting in a systemic vasoconstriction effect that could be dangerous.

In their survey of the literature, Lambrecht et al. (2013) found conflicting information regarding TCAs. There are studies showing increased sensitivity to epinephrine in healthy patients on recently initiated TCAs, no case reports of this interaction in the literature and articles suggesting that long-term use of TCAs actually results in a paradoxical effect, where postsynaptic desensitization results in systemic vasodilation (Saraghi et al. 2018). In terms of MAOIs, whether an interaction with vasoconstrictors/catecholamines exists at all is controversial. Many authors theorize that since catecholamines are primarily metabolized by cathechol-O-methyltransferase (COMT) and MAO, there should be no systemic effect in patients on MAOIs.

Given the controversy over TCA and epinephrine interaction due to lack of current dental case studies, it is advised to reduce the amount of epinephrine given or give it over a prolonged period of time, as slow administration may reduce systemic absorption (Lambrecht et al. 2013). Additionally, systemic effect is likely dose dependent and when patients are on small doses of TCAs for pain, nocturnal bruxism or insomnia, there may not be a clinically significant interaction (Saraghi et al. 2018).

The mechanism of action of SSRIs is quite different from the older TCAs and does not have the same concerns as TCAs and thus there is no direct interaction with epinephrine.

Q. Why is there a limit on the amount of epinephrine in patients taking a TCA?

A. The current theory of depression is that there are low amounts of norepinephrine and serotonin. The "older" TCAs work by blocking the reuptake of norepinephrine by inhibiting the noradrenergic reuptake pump. This allows more norepinephrine to accumulate in the synapse, increasing the levels of norepinephrine. Epinephrine functions in a similar manner. Epinephrine is partially inactivated by the noradrenergic pump. So, if TCAs inhibit the noradrenergic reuptake pump, this allows the accumulation of epinephrine in the synapse which can increase epinephrine levels in addition to norepinephrine, substantially resulting in a hypertensive crisis. Therefore, the amount of epinephrine should be limited to two cartridges of 1 : 100 000. Levonordefrin (in 2% mepivacaine) should not be used (Pérusse et al. 1992; Yagiela 1999). Since SSRIs only affect serotonin and not norepinephrine, there are no precautions regarding the use of epinephrine.

Q. Is there an interaction between epinephrine and antipsychotics?

A. There is some literature showing an interaction with antipsychotics especially if there is systemic absorption of epinephrine. This interaction clinically will worsen the hypotensive side effect of the antipsychotic (Higuchi et al. 2014).

Q. Do psychiatric medications bind to different receptors?

A. Yes. Adverse effects of TCAs and antipsychotics are caused by the different receptors they block (acting like an antagonist): muscarinic (cholinergic) receptors cause xerostomia; alpha-1 adrenergic receptors result in orthostatic hypotension, reflex tachycardia, and myocardial depression; histamine receptors result in sedation and weight gain (Weinberg 2002). It should be noted that different drugs have different affinities to the different receptors so that one drug may not have as many adverse effects as another. The SSRIs have a low affinity for adrenergic, histaminic, and muscarinic receptors resulting in fewer adverse effects than the "older" TCAs. In fact, "newer" formulations of "older" medications were developed to be more specific to the targeted receptor, resulting in fewer adverse effects.

Q. Are there any precautions to follow for patients with Parkinson's disease?

A. See Table 7.17.

Q. Are there any precautions to follow for patients on antiseizure medications?

A. See Table 7.17.

Q. Are there any precautions to follow for patients with attention deficit hyperactivity disorder (ADHD)?

A. See Table 7.17.

Table 7.17 Dental management of patients taking neurological and psychiatric drugs

Classification	Drug	Dental care
Antipsychotics (for schizophrenia and other psychiatric disorders including bipolar disorder)	Atypical antipsychotics: Clozapine (Clozaril®)	A medical consultation is required if dental surgery (e.g., extractions, periodontal/implant surgery). Clozapine has a **Black Box Warning** because of a significant risk of agranulocytosis, which is a condition involving dangerous leukopenia or lowered white blood cell (WBC) count; infection and delayed healing can occur. It is highly recommended to obtain a physician's consult regarding the WBC count. Patients usually have blood tests taken every week to determine WBC count and absolute neutrophil count. After 1 year on clozapine blood monitoring can be done once a month. Thrombocytopenia: low blood platelet count; increased bleeding problems. Reported only in a few case reports. Postpone dental care until WBC have returned to normal Xerostomia: monitor caries, periodontal diseases and oral candidiasis Orthostatic hypotension can occur. Raise the dental chair slowly from the supine position and have patient remain in upright position a few minutes before getting up from the chair. Extrapyramidal side effects can impair the patient's ability to perform oral home care. Use vasoconstrictors cautiously; Use low dose epinephrine (two cartridges of 1 : 100 000)
	Other atypical antipsychotics: risperidone (Risperdal) quetiapine (Seroquel), olanzapine (Zyprexa) ziprasidone (Geodon)	Do not have the same risk of lowering WBC or platelets as does clozapine. Use low-dose epinephrine (two cartridges of 1 : 100 000). Xerostomia: monitor caries, periodontal diseases and oral candidiasis. Orthostatic hypotension can occur. Raise the dental chair slowly from the supine position and have patient remain in upright position a few minutes before getting up from the chair. Extrapyramidal side effects can impair the patient's ability to perform oral home care
Antidepressants	Tricyclic antidepressants (TCAs): amitriptyline (Elavil) imipramine (Tofranil) nortriptyline (Aventyl) doxepin (Sinequan)	TCAs inhibit the reuptake of norepinephrine so limit the amount of epinephrine to two cartridges of 1 : 100 000 to avoid hypertensive crisis; monitor heart rate and blood pressure; epinephrine uses the same noradrenergic reuptake pump as norepinephrine

Table 7.17 (Continued)

Classification	Drug	Dental care
	Selective serotonin reuptake inhibitors (SSRIs): paroxetine (Paxil) fluoxetine (Prozac) sertraline (Zoloft) citalopram (Celexa)	SSRIs do not involve norepinephrine and epinephrine; selectively inhibit the reuptake of serotonin; epinephrine can be used
	Monoamine oxidase inhibitors (MAOIs): phenelzine (Nardil) isocarboxazid (Marplan) tranylcypromine (Parnate)	MAOIs act by inhibiting the activity of monoamine oxidase (MAO; MAO-A and MAO-B), an enzyme that breaks down monoamine neurotransmitters (epinephrine, norepinephrine, serotonin, melatonin). Although the risk of an interaction with epinephrine is low, it is best to limit use to two cartridges of 1 : 100 000 epinephrine to avoid hypertensive crisis; monitor heart rate and blood pressure
Bipolar disorder	Lithium Carbamazepine (Tegretol) Valproic acid (Depakote) Atypical antipsychotics are also used (see above notes)	Lithium has a narrow therapeutic index which requires frequent blood tests to avoid overdosing and adverse effects including fine hand tremors and polydipsia (excessive thirst). Modest rise in lithium levels. Avoid metronidazole with lithium. Lithium: limit to two cartridges of 1 : 100 000 epinephrine. Epinephrine can be used with carbamazepine and valproic acid. Valproic acid inhibits platelet aggregation which can cause altered bleeding times; monitor platelet counts and it is recommended to obtain a physician consult for invasive dental procedures
Acetylcholinesterase inhibitors (Alzheimer disease)	Donepezil (Aricept®) Galantamine (Reminyl®) Rivastigmine (Exelon®) Memantine (Namenda®) Tacrine (Cognex®)	Alzheimer's drugs act by increasing the levels of acetylcholine in the brain. Epinephrine can be used safely
Attention deficit hyperactivity disorder (ADHD)	Atomoxetine (Strattera) Amphetamine or amphetamine-like stimulants: amphetamine (Adderall), methylphenidate (Concerta, Ritalin), dexmethylphenidate (Focalin XR)	Similar actions as tricyclic antidepressants (inhibiting the reuptake of norepinephrine and dopamine and increasing their release from the presynaptic neuron into the synaptic space resulting in an increased level of both catecholamines); limit dosage of epinephrine to two cartridges of 1 : 100 000 epinephrine

(Continued)

Table 7.17 (Continued)

Classification	Drug	Dental care
Parkinson disease drugs	*Dopamine precursors*: Levodopa/carbidopa Anticholinergics: trihexyphenidyl (Artane®) Benztropine (Cogentin®) *Dopamine antagonists*: Bromocriptine (Parlodel®) Pramipexole (Mirapex®) Ropinirole (Requip®) *Catechol-O-methyl-transferase inhibitors*: Entacapone (Comtan®) Tolcapone (Tasmar®) *Antiviral*: Amantadine	Epinephrine can be used but use minimum amount (two cartridges) of 1:100 000 epinephrine with COMT inhibitors. Avoid clarithromycin, tetracycline, doxycycline with dopamine antagonists
Antiepileptic drugs	Phenytoin (Dilantin®) Carbamazepine (Tegreto®l) Phenobarbital Clonazepam (Klonopin®) Oxcarbazepine (Trileptal®) Lorazepam (Ativan®) Ethosuximide (Zarontin®) Valproic acid (Depakene®) Divalproex (Depakote®) Levetiracetam (Keppra®) Tiagabine (Gabitril®) Lamotrigine (Lamictal®) Gabapentin (Neurontin®) Pregabalin (Lyrica®) Felbamate (Felbatol®) Topiramate (Topamax) Zonisamide (Zonegran)	Epinephrine can be used. Phenytoin: monitor for gingival enlargement; optimal oral hygiene and if necessary, refer to periodontist. As long as the patient is taking phenytoin, even if the gingival overgrowth is surgically removed, the gingival enlargement will continue to occur

7.9   Organ Transplantation (Antirejection) Medications

Q. Is a medical consultation with the patient's nephrologist necessary before dental care is started?

A. Yes. Several factors are involved in preparing a patient before dental care is given. Antibiotic prophylaxis may be required to prevent systemic infection. If an antibiotic is needed as prophylaxis against infection or if the patient has an active infection (e.g., abscess), the choice of antibiotic should be confirmed with the patient's physician (Segelnick and Weinberg 2009). Many renal transplant patients have comorbidities (e.g., hypertension, diabetes) and are taking numerous medications that the dentist should be aware of (Georgakopoulou et al. 2011).

Q. Are organ transplant patients more prone to developing bacterial infections?

A. Yes. Bacterial infections occur in 33–68% of liver transplant recipients, 54% of lung transplant recipients, 47% of kidney transplant recipients, 35% of pancreas transplant recipients, and

21–30% of heart transplant recipients, usually within two months after transplantation. The risk of infection after transplantation is primarily determined by the transplant recipient's epidemiological exposures and the degree of immunosuppression. Some sources of infection in the transplant recipient include the environment and the recipient's endogenous flora (Patel and Paya 1997; Rubin et al. 1994; Soave 2001).

Q. Should a patient going for a major organ transplant be seen by the dentist before the operation?

A. Yes. It is important to remove any forms of inflammation and infection before the transplantation to reduce the incidence of transplant failure or rejection (Segelnick and Weinberg 2009). Treatment of dental caries, abscesses, necessary extractions, and periodontal diseases is important before transplantation since postoperative immunosuppression reduces a patient's ability to fight off systemic infection.

Q. Is it important to see the patient after transplantation?

A. Yes. It is very important to have the posttransplantation patient return to the dental office for regular maintenance. Usually, the patient should not have any dental care for six months post transplantation because this is the period of highest risk of organ rejection and the high dosage of immunosuppressant agents taken during this time puts the patient at risk for systemic infections (Georgakopoulou et al. 2011). At six months, the patient should only have emergency and preventive treatment done. At every appointment a thorough medical history update is done and the patient should bring in a current list of medications.

Q. Should the postorgan transplant patient receive antibiotic prophylaxis?

A. Yes. Preoperative antibacterial prophylaxis aimed at preventing wound infections (Georgakopoulou et al. 2011).

Q. What local anesthetics can be used in patients who are going to have a liver transplant?

A. These patients are treated as patients with liver failure. All injectable local anesthetics used in dentistry are amides and are metabolized in the liver. The patient's physician will have blood values for the liver enzymes. Any local anesthetic can be used but with a maximum of two cartridges at each dental visit.

Q. Can bleeding be a problem in organ transplant candidates?

A. Yes. Also, excessive bleeding can occur in organ transplant patients due to organ dysfunction or medications the patient is taking. Many patients may be taking an anticoagulant and have decreased platelet counts. For example, patients with end-stage liver disease may have excessive bleeding because the liver is not making enough clotting factors. A medical consultation with the physician is necessary (National Institute of Dental and Craniofacial Research. Dental Management of the Organ Transplant Patient. www.nidcr.nih.gov).

Q. What drugs are organ transplant patients taking?

A. Patients who had a major organ transplant are taking an immunosuppressant drug such as azathioprine (Imuran®), cyclosporine (Sandimmune®), tacrolimus, sirolimus, Prograf/FK506, or prednisone.

Q. Are there any concerns or potential adverse effects of azathioprine related to dental care?

A. Azathioprine is an antimetabolite indicated as an adjunct for the prevention of rejection in renal transplantation. It reduces inflammation and interferes with the growth of rapidly dividing cells.

There is a warning about chronic immunosuppression being associated with an increased risk of malignancy. It functions to prevent organ rejection by inhibiting the production of blood cells in the bone marrow. Serious infections are a constant concern for patients receiving azathioprine and any other immunosuppressive drug. The medical consultation with the patient's physician should address the potential for severe infections while the patient is taking azathioprine. The dentist should have the most recent results of the complete blood count (CBC) before dental treatment is started. There is an increased risk of bleeding, oral sores or swelling of the face, lips, tongue or throat. There are no drug interactions that would be of concern in dentistry.

Q. Are there any concerns or potential adverse effects of tacrolimus related to dental care?

A. Tacrolimus is an immunosuppressive drug (decreases the immune system's response to a transplanted organ) used to prevent rejection of liver and kidney organ transplant. There is a warning about *increased susceptibility to infection* and the possible development of lymphomThe medical consultation from the patient's physician should address the potential for severe infections while the patient is taking tacrolimus. Since hypertension is a common adverse effect, patients may be taking a calcium channel blocker which could cause gingival enlargement. There is a drug interaction with clarithromycin and erythromycin so these two antibiotics should not be taken with tacrolimus. Also, do not take with antifungal drugs such as clotrimazole, fluconazole, and ketoconazole as this may result in toxic plasma levels of tacrolimus.

Q. What are some adverse effects of cyclosporine?

A. Cyclosporine is a potent immunosuppressive agent that prolongs survival of many transplants such as kidney, liver, and heart. Patients taking cyclosporine usually have hypertension and are taking a calcium channel blocker such as amlodipine or nifedipine, which may cause gingival enlargement. So, gingival enlargement is a known side effect of both cyclosporine and nifedipine. Meticulous oral home care is important with these patients and maintenance/recare appointments should be scheduled every three months.

Because it is an immunosuppressant, cyclosporine may increase the susceptibility to infection. The medical consultation from the patient's physician should address the potential for severe infections that may occur while the patient is taking cyclosporine.

Cyclosporine can cause nephrotoxicity (including structural kidney damage) and hepatotoxicity. Ciprofloxacin (Cipro) and naproxen may potentiate renal dysfunction if taken with cyclosporine. Cyclosporine is a substrate and inhibitor of CYP3A4. If cyclosporine is taken with azithromycin (Zithromax), clarithromycin (Biaxin), erythromycin, fluconazole (Diflucan), or ketoconazole (Nizoral), increased concentrations of cyclosporine may occur.

Q. If the patient is taking cyclosporine and requires antibiotic prophylaxis and is allergic to penicillin, what antibiotic can be prescribed?

A. Do not prescribe clarithromycin because there is a drug–drug interaction. If the patient is allergic to penicillin it is recommended to prescribe clindamycin.

Q. What precautions should be followed if the patient is taking a corticosteroid?

A. Usually the posttransplant patient will be taking many drugs so that the corticosteroid (e.g., prednisolone) will probably be taken in a lower dose because by itself it is not adequate to prevent organ transplant rejection (Georgakopoulou et al. 2011). Corticosteroids mask inflammation, which may occur less since the dose is lower than the usual one.

Q. Are there any concerns or potential adverse effects of sirolimus related to dental care?

A. Sirolimus (Rapamune®) is an immunosuppressant only indicated for kidney transplantation. There is an increased susceptibility to infection with the development of lymphoma or other malignancies. The only dental adverse effect is oral ulcerations. Other adverse effects include hypertension, coughing up blood (hemoptysis), high cholesterol, peripheral edema (swelling of extremities), abnormal healing, bleeding, and low white blood count.

　　Sirolimus is a substrate for cytochrome P450 3A4 (CYP3A4). Inducers of CYP3A4 decrease sirolimus concentrations and inhibitors of CYP3A4 may increase sirolimus levels. Some dental drug inducers are carbamazepine (Tegretol; for trigeminal neuralgia). Some strong dental drug inhibitors are ketoconazole, clotrimazole (antifungal agent), erythromycin, and clarithromycin; avoid prescribing them to patients taking sirolimus.

7.10　Recreational and Illicit Drugs

Q. Can epinephrine be used in a patient who uses cocaine?

A. Cocaine is the most powerful vasoconstrictor. It works in two ways: as a topical anesthetic and as a recreational drug. As a topical anesthetic, cocaine acts by reversibly binding to and inactivating the sodium channels on the nerve, resulting in inhibition of a nerve impulse. As a recreational drug, cocaine works similarly to TCAs by blocking the reuptake of norepinephrine via the norepinephrine reuptake pump back into the nerve. This will result in excessive cocaine remaining in the synapse which could cause tachycardia, hypertension, diaphoresis, mydriasis, and tremors. Also, cocaine binds to dopamine reuptake transporters on the presynaptic membranes of dopaminergic neurons. This binding inhibits the removal of dopamine from the synaptic synapse and its subsequent degradation by monoamine oxidase in the nerve terminal. Dopamine remains in the synapse and binds to postsynaptic receptors which then activate the dopaminergic reward pathway leading to the feelings of euphoria and the "high" associated with cocaine use. Deaths have been caused by induction of heart stimulation, increased blood pressure and arrhythmias. If a local anesthetic containing epinephrine is injected in a patient who has just used cocaine, the concentration of norepinephrine plus epinephrine can put the patient into cardiac arrest. Epinephrine should not be used within 48 hours after the last dose of cocaine (Weinberg 2002).

Q. Why is it important to know about patients taking cannabis?

A. Cannabis, also known as marijuana, comes from the dried flowers, leaves, and stem of the *Cannabis* plant. Cannabis in the forms of hashish and hash oil is more potent than marijuan-Cannabis is known to contain up to 400 chemicals, but the primary psychoactive chemical is tetrahydrocannabinol (THC), which changes the person's perception and mood. Cannabis affects almost every system of the body, particularly the cardiovascular, respiratory, and immune systems. Cannabis's vasoactive effects include dose-related tachycardia and increased heart rate which can result in a cardiac ischemia in some individuals. Even in acute doses, marijuana causes tachycardia and peripheral vasodilation (Horowitz and Nersasian 1978; Nahas and Latour 1992). There is a mild vasodilation that causes the eyes to be "red" in marijuana users. There is a high incidence of xerostomia, which needs to be addressed – improve oral health, monitor for caries and periodontal diseases, avoid alcohol-containing mouth rinses such as chlorhexidine. Recommend GUM® chlorhexidine gluconate rinse (this is a nonalcoholic chlorhexidine rinse; OTC).

Smoke from cannabis acts as a carcinogen, which is related to dysplastic changes and premalignant lesions in the oral cavity, Because of its immunosuppressive actions, users may be more prone to oral infections (Cho et al. 2005).

Marijuana users may experience an acute anxiety attack in the dental office due to a parasympathetic response. The dentist must be prepared to handle these situations.

Q. Can epinephrine be used in a patient who uses cannabis?

A. Ask the patient at every dental visit update if they use marijuana and when it was last used. Marijuana and epinephrine could have a synergistic effect; marijuana's vasoactive effects in acute doses cause tachycardia and a decrease in blood pressure due to peripheral vasodilation (widening of the blood vessels, which causes a decrease in peripheral resistance to blood flow with a lowering of blood pressure) and the possibility of the patient having an acute anxiety response. Thus, epinephrine may cause an increase in these responses which could be life-threatening.

It is unclear exactly how long marijuana stays in the body. However, it has been documented that inhaled marijuana is rapidly absorbed from the bloodstream and metabolized in the body. This is why blood testing is not used for the detection of marijuana although some metabolites have been detected up to 13 days after use (http://alcoholism.about.com/od/pot/a/marijuana_test.htm).

Horowitz and Nersasian (1978) recommended that patients stay off marijuana for at least one week before epinephrine is used in dental treatment. It is probably safest to use a local anesthetic without a vasoconstrictor.

Q. Is marijuana legal to use?

A. As of May 2011, medical marijuana is legal to use in 17 states (Alaska, Arizona, California, Colorado, DC, Delaware, Hawaii, Maine, Michigan, Montana, Nevada, New Jersey, New Mexico, Oregon, Rhode Island, Vermont, and Washington) as an antiemetic in cancer patients, and an analgesic in chronic pain.

Q. Can nitrous oxide be administered safely in marijuana users?

A. Nitrous oxide is also used for illicit/recreational uses. One study reported that marijuana use could enhance some of the subjective effects induced by nitrous oxide inhalation (Yajnik et al. 1994).

Q. Are there any dental considerations for a patient abusing methamphetamine?

A. Methamphetamine is an addictive substance that is closely related chemically to its parent compound, amphetamine, but with more central nervous system effects. The chemical name of methamphetamine or, as it sometimes called, methylamphetamine is *n*-methyl-1-phenyl-propan-2-amine. Methamphetamine or "meth" is synthesized illegally in laboratories. Inhaled by smoking, methamphetamine releases high levels of dopamine, which stimulates brain cells, enhancing mood and body movement but also is toxic to brain cells containing dopamine and serotonin. It is referred to as "ice" or "crystal" when inhaled by smoking. With long-term use, there seems to be a depletion of dopamine, resulting in Parkinson-like symptoms. Methamphetamine is also taken orally, inhaled through the nose or injected.

Amphetamine analogs are prescription drugs (e.g., Adderall, Ritalin) indicated for the management of attention deficient hyperactivity disorder (ADHD) (http://chemistry.about.com/od/medicalhealth/a/crystalmeth.htm).

Methamphetamine is a stimulant that binds to alpha receptors throughout the body, resulting in a sympathetic "fight or flight" response, similar to amphetamine. Methamphetamine causes cardiovascular problems including increased heart rate, increased blood pressure, and cardiac arrhythmias. Other long-term effects include respiratory conditions, stroke, dilated pupils, excessive sweating, violent behavior, agitation, panic, hallucination, mood swings, confusion, permanent brain damage, and death. Oral signs of specific methamphetamine abuse include tooth attrition due to bruxism/clenching (due to excessive neuromuscular activity), xerostomia (by binding to alpha-2 receptors in the salivary glands), and dental caries. The term "meth mouth" was coined to designate rampant, untreated dental caries found specifically on the buccal and smooth surfaces of posterior teeth and interproximal surfaces of anterior teeth. Meth mouth is due to many factors including decreased salivary flow, poor oral hygiene, and consumption of carbonated sugar-containing drinks. The etiology of the rampant caries is the possible presence of phosphoric, sulfuric or muriatic acid in the methamphetamine (Muzzin and O'Brien 2010). There is also a high incidence of poor oral hygiene in these patients.

Q. Can epinephrine and nitrous oxide be used in a patient who uses methamphetamine?

A. If the patient is a methamphetamine abuser, a medical consultation is recommended. The adrenergic–sympathetic response in the body caused by methamphetamine can stimulate the synthesis and release of epinephrine and norepinephrine from the adrenal medulla which contributes to the increased heart rate and blood pressure. Care should be taken if the patient recently used meth. The use of epinephrine as a vasoconstrictor in local anesthetics synergistically can create a potentially life-threatening cardiac situation. It is recommended to use a local anesthetic that does not contain a vasoconstrictor for at least 24 hours after the patient's last dose of methamphetamine. This is because the duration of action of methamphetamine is anywhere from eight to 24 hours, depending on how much the patient used. It has been documented that the cardiovascular effects are stopped before the drug is completely eliminated from the body (Newton et al. 2005). The patient's vital signs (heart rate, blood pressure) should be monitored during each visit. Tolerance to the local anesthetic can occur which requires more of the anesthetic solution. A neutral sodium fluoride mouth rinse, toothpaste, or gel should be included in the patients' daily home care regimen. Fluoride varnish should be applied to areas of decalcification. Regular maintenance/recare appointments should be planned at three-month intervals (Donaldson and Goodchild 2006; Goodchild and Donaldson 2007; Klasser and Epstein 2006). Consultation with the physician may be necessary if postoperative analgesics are required due to respiratory depression of the opioids (Goodchild and Donaldson 2007).

Nitrous oxide should be used cautiously with patients taking methamphetamine.

Q. Are there any precautions to take with a patient who uses heroin?

A. Heroin is a semisynthetic opioid synthesized from morphine by acetylation. When injected intravenously, it produces euphoria or a "rush" within 10 seconds and the effects last for up to four hours. Systemic adverse effects of heroin include constipation, addiction, physical dependence, "pinpoint pupils," bacteremia, xerostomia, tongue discoloration, low blood pressure, bluish-colored lips and fingernails, disorientation, drowsiness, and infectious diseases. Death is usually due to respiratory depression. An overdose of heroin is managed similarly to an overdose with any narcotic. Naloxone (Narcan®), a narcotic antagonist, is injected intramuscularly. Get a medical consultation if you suspect the patient is a current heroin addict.

7.11 Antiresorptive Agents

Q. What are antiresorptive and anabolic drugs?

A. Antiresorptive medications slow the breakdown of bone. Examples of antiresorptive drugs include:

1) bisphosphonates (Table 7.18)
2) estrogen therapy or hormone therapy
3) selective estrogen receptor modulators (SERMs); raloxifene (Evista®)
4) monoclonial antibodies: denosumab (Prolial®)
5) calcitonin.

Q. Are anabolic drugs used for osteoporosis?

A. Yes. Anabolic drugs make new bone and increase bone density. Teriparatide (Forteo®) is an anabolic drug (Eastell and Walsh 2017).

Q. What are bisphosphonates and their indications for use?

A. Bisphosphonates are antiresorptive drugs that were introduced in the mid-1990s and prescribed as alternatives to hormone replacement therapies (HRTs) for osteoporosis and osteopenia to prevent spine and hip fractures and to treat osteolytic tumors and possibly slow tumor development. Bisphosphonates are powerful inhibitors of bone resorption by decreasing the action of osteoclasts, which are cells that break down bone. Also, bisphosphonates inhibit the increased osteoclastic activity and skeletal calcium release into the bloodstream induced by various stimulatory factors released by tumors.

Q. How are bisphosphonates used in cancer therapy?

A. Generally, hypercalcemia with malignancy occurs in patients who have breast cancer, squamous cell tumors of the head and neck or lung, renal cell carcinoma, and some blood malignancies such as multiple myelomExcessive release of calcium into the blood occurs as bone is resorbed, resulting in pain. In patients with hypercalcemia of malignancy (HCM), intravenous bisphosphonates decreased serum calcium and phosphorus and increased urinary calcium and phosphorus excretion.

Q. What oral adverse effects of bisphosphonates are seen in dentistry?

A. There have been major dental concerns regarding the development of antiresorptive agent-related osteonecrosis of the jaw (ARONJ). The mechanism of this adverse reaction is not clear. One proposed mechanism is that bone turnover is depressed; bisphosphonates inhibit bone removal or resorption of "old or diseased" bone by osteoclasts (remember bisphosphonates inhibit osteoclastic activity), thereby interfering with bone repair and bone turnover. The bisphosphonates irreversibly alter the metabolism of the osteoclasts which results in no or poor bone resorption even if the blood supply is adequate. This causes osteoblasts to build new bone around the diseased bone. However, one proposed mechanism is that if the necrotic bone cannot be resorbed by the osteoclasts (remember bisphosphonates inhibit osteoclastic activity) during healing, then the necrotic bone will inhibit healing and affect blood supply to the area.

Q. What are the risk factors for developing ARONJ?

A. Risk factors for the development of ARONJ include:

- currently taking or history of taking bisphosphonates (especially IV formulations but also oral for more than two years)

Table 7.18 Bisphosphonates

Generic name	Brand name	Generation 1st: nonnitrogen 2nd: nitrogen	Route of administration	Elimination half-life	Indication	Potency factor
Alendronate	Fosamax; Fosamax plus D	2nd	Oral	10 years	Osteoporosis	
Clodronate	Bonefos®	1st	Oral	157 hours	Hypercalcemia (bone metastases); osteoporosis	
Etidronate disodium	Didronel®	1st	Oral	1–6 hours	Paget disease	1
Risedronate	Actonel®	2nd	Oral	1.5–480 hours	Osteoporosis	10
Tiludronate	Skelid®	1st	Oral	150 hours	Paget disease	10
Ibandronate	Boniva	2nd	Oral/IV	37–157 hours	Osteoporosis	500
Pamidronate	Aredia®	2nd	IV	21–35 hours	Hypercalcemia, with or without bone metastases	2000
Zoledronate	Zometa®	2nd	IV	0.24–1.87 hours; terminal 146 hours	Bone metastases	1000
Pamidronate	Aredia	2nd	IV	21–35 hours	Bone metastases	100
Zoledronate	Zometa	2nd	IV	0.24–1.87 hours; terminal 146 hours	Bone metastases	10000

- individuals older than 65 years
- history of cancer (breast, lung, prostate, multiple myeloma or metastatic disease to the bone), osteoporosis, Paget disease, chronic renal disease on dialysis.

The following are local dental risk factors for ARONJ in patients taking intravenous or oral (less likely than IV but still can occur) bisphosphonates:

- periodontal surgery
- extractions (highest incidence)
- dental implant surgery
- ill-fitting dentures that is irritating to the tissues
- less likely with endodontic therapy, orthodontics, scaling and root planing
- bisphosphonate-related osteonecrosis of the jaw (BRONJ) can also occur spontaneously without any prior dental procedure.

Q. Are there any other medical/dental comorbidities related to the development of ARONJ?

A. Yes. Possible comorbidities include diabetes, patients with dentures, smoking, and periodontitis. Corticosteroid use is no longer considered a risk factor (Barasch et al. 2011).

Q. What are the clinical signs and symptoms of ARONJ?

A. Osteonecrosis is necrosis or death of bone and can cause severe, extensive, and irreversible damage to the jawbone (occurs more frequently in the mandible than maxilla). Oral lesions appear similar to those of radiation-induced osteonecrosis. Patients with BRONJ do not have a history of radiation to the jaws. There usually is delayed or completely absent healing of the periodontium after dental extraction or surgery for more than six weeks or it can occur spontaneously.
The following are signs and symptoms of ARONJ.

- Irregular mucosal ulcer with exposed bone in the maxillofacial area
- Pain or swelling in the area
- Infection
- Pain
- Mobility of teeth
- Numbness or heavy sensation
- Bone sequestrum

Q. Do patients taking oral bisphosphonates have the same incidence of developing BRONJ as patients taking IV bisphosphonates?

A. In 2007, the American Association of Oral and Maxillofacial Surgeons published a position paper on BRONJ. It concluded that patients being treated with oral bisphosphonates are at a considerably lower risk for osteonecrosis than those taking IV bisphosphonates. The concern is that once bone is exposed, it will most likely become necrotic and infected. Once the bone is exposed, it is difficult to treat. Patients who have been taking bisphosphonates for more than six months are at highest risk for developing ARONJ (Grewal and Fayans 2008; Ruggiero et al. 2004).

Q. What is the most recent information regarding the incidence of developing BRONJ in patients taking oral bisphosphonates?

A. In 2011, Jeffocoat et al. reported that oral bisphosphonates do not increase the risk for osteonecrosis of the jaw but found a sixfold increased risk in patients taking intravenous bisphosphonates (Jeffcoat et al. 2011).

Q. When could BRONJ occur while a patient is taking a bisphosphonate?

A. A survey conducted in 2005 concluded that the mean time of onset of BRONJ is about 18–22 months after the initiation of bisphosphonate therapy, although most cases have occurred after prolonged therapy, up to 3–5 years after the start of oral bisphosphonates. According to the American Dental Association on Scientific Affairs, antiresorptive drugs for low bone mass put the patient at a lower risk of developing BRONJ but it still can occur. Additionally, the risk of developing ARONJ is less for patients not being treated for cancer.

Q. Does the amount of accumulated bisphosphonate in the bone affect the poor healing response seen during dental treatment?

A. Yes. It was found that the total accumulated concentration of bisphosphonates in bone can predict toxic levels which could possibly result in poor healing of dental wounds (Jones et al. 2011; Landesberg et al. 2008). Additionally, there may be a higher incidence in the development of ARONJ based on the size of the person's skeleton or the total quantity of bone mineral into which bisphosphonates concentrate (Jones et al. 2011). Basically, individuals with higher total bone mineral content (larger skeletal frames versus smaller frames) took longer to reach toxic concentrations of the bisphosphonate (Jones et al. 2011).

Q. Why is the mandible especially prone to ARONJ?

A. The jawbone is more prone to developing ARONJ because it has a higher turnover rate than long bones.

Q. Why is there a higher incidence of developing ARONJ in patients taking IV bisphosphonates rather than oral?

A. Because an IV dose of bisphosphonate is incorporated into the bone while with an oral dose, very little is absorbed via the gastrointestinal tract into the bloodstream.

Q. How about implant surgery and the risk of ARONJ in patients taking oral or IV bisphosphonates?

A. Implant or any type of dental surgery, including extractions, is contraindicated in patients taking IV bisphosphonates for the past six months. Marx and colleagues (2007) suggested that there is an increased risk for implant failure or ARONJ around the implants once the oral bisphosphonate has been taken for more than three years. If a patient has been taking the drug for less than three years, then most likely they can be treated normally. However, these patients should be informed of the small risk of ARONJ for every person taking bisphosphonates and that the risk increases after three years of drug use. It has been suggested that being on oral bisphosphonates for more than two years increases the risk of developing ARONJ. So, not only is there about a 2.69 times higher risk for implant failure in middle-aged (>40 years) women taking oral bisphosphonates but there is also a risk, although low (<1%), for implant failure when oral bisphosphonates are started after successful implant placement (Goss et al. 2010; Yip et al. 2012).

Q. What is the half-life of oral bisphosphonates?

A. See Table 7.18. Oral bisphosphonates accumulate slowly in bone because very little is absorbed by the gastrointestinal tract into the bloodstream and slowly gets released from the bone when the drug is stopped. The half-life is the amount of time it takes the body to clear half of the medication. For example, the elimination half-life of Boniva® is up to 157 hours, which is about 6.5 days. However, once the first 50% is gone at 6.5 days, it will take the body up to another 6.5 days to clear 50% of the remaining medication. Usually it takes about five half-lives to clear 99%

of the medication. In the case of Boniva, it is about 32 days. Fosamax® has the longest half-life so it takes many years (>10 years) for the drug to be totally eliminated from the body. Discontinuing an oral bisphosphonate may result in gradual improvement but may not reduce or eliminate the chance of developing ARONJ. The AAOMS states that discontinuation of oral bisphosphonates for 6–12 months may result in either spontaneous sequestration or resolution following debridement surgery (AAOMS 2009).

Q. What are specific recommendations from the 2011 American Dental Association Council on Scientific Affairs for patients taking bisphosphonates for prevention and treatment of osteoporosis?

A. Currently, there is no established standard of care or protocol regarding dental treatment of patients on bisphosphonates. The American Dental Association Council on Scientific Affairs recommends the following regarding dental treatment in patients *without cancer* receiving antiresorptive therapy.

1) Inform patients about the risks of developing ARONJ while taking antiresorptive drugs.
2) Dentists do not need to alter routine dental procedures.
3) Antiresorptive drug therapy for low bone mass puts the patient at low risk but does not eliminate the chance of developing ARONJ.
4) A dental health program consisting of optimal oral hygiene care and regular dental appointments will help to minimize the risk of developing BRONJ (Nicolatou-Galitis et al. 2011).
5) The dentist has to make the decision to treat or not treat the patient.
6) It is not advisable not to treat active dental disease (including caries, abscesses or inflammatory periodontal diseases). Leaving dental disease untreated may exacerbate osteonecrosis and be a risk factor for ARONJ.
7) Best to prevent ARONJ by limiting extensive dental involvement.

Q. What are recommendations for patients without cancer concerning periodontal therapy?

A. It is recommended to treat periodontal diseases with nonsurgical therapy followed by a revaluation 4–8 weeks later (Segelnick and Weinberg 2006). The Council says that periodontal surgery is not contraindicated but patients should be monitored regularly.

Q. What are the 2011 recommendations concerning implant placement?

A. Reports have documented that although there are cases of ARONJ at implant sites, the incidence is small. Additionally, there is a small incidence of implant failure in patients taking bisphosphonates (Fugazzotto et al. 2007). Fugazotto et al. (2007) found that a history of oral bisphosphonate use for a mean time of 3.3 years was not a contributing factor to the development of ARONJ.

Q. What are the 2011 recommendations concerning extractions?

A. According to the Council, extractions are a major risk factor for developing ARONJ, but are not contraindicated. It is recommended, if necessary, to perform endodontics followed by removal of the clinical crown. This would allow the root to exfoliate instead of doing an extraction.

Q. What are the current thoughts about restorative and prosthetic procedures in patients taking bisphosphonates?

A. According to the American Dental Association Council on Scientific Affairs (2011), all routine restorative procedures should be performed. Any irritating or rough area on a dental prosthesis should be removed and smoothed. Additionally, malocclusion, occlusal trauma or masticatory forces do not increase the risk of developing ARONJ.

Q. What are the current thoughts about orthodontic procedures in patients taking bisphosphonates?

A. According to the American Dental Association Council on Scientific Affairs (2011), there are not enough studies concerning orthodontics increasing the risk of developing ARONJ. However, there are reports of inhibited tooth movement during orthodontic therapy, but orthodontic therapy is not contraindicated (Rinchuse et al. 2007).

Q. How do we manage these patients?

A. There is no consensus on the management of these patients. Take a thorough medical history and written consent. Get a consultation from the patient's physician. The patient should be counseled on the practicality of developing ONJ. In 2006, the American Dental Association Council on Scientific Affairs published its expert panel's recommendations on how to manage patients on antiresorptive drugs.

Q. What are the recommendations for treating patients taking oral bisphosphonates and what is a three-month drug holiday?

A. The three-month holiday is as follows: if on an oral bisphosphonate for <3 years, treat as usual. If the patient is on an oral bisphosphonate for >3 years, then discontinue for three months before a dental procedure. Serum CTX is not a valid preoperative test to accurately determine the risk of a patient developing ARONJ (Lee and Suzuki 2010). The 2011 ADA recommendations for managing the dental care of patients taking antiresorptive drugs for the prevention and treatment of osteoporosis state that "discontinuing bisphosphonate therapy may not eliminate the risk of developing ARONJ." It is advised to have patients rinse for one minute with 0.2% chlorhexidine rinse before dental treatment and to continue twice a day for one week after treatment.

Q. Is there a higher risk for implant failure in postmenopausal women?

A. A 2010 article reported that dental implant survival in postmenopausal women is the same regardless of their history of bisphosphonate use. Postmenopausal women taking bisphosphonates who have dental implant surgery are at low risk for ARONJ and a "drug holiday" would not be indicated in these patients (Koka et al. 2010).

Q. If the patient develops ARONJ, what is its management?

A. It is very difficult to treat ARONJ and it is not reversible. If ARONJ is diagnosed, it could last from as few as eight weeks to a lifetime. First, the bisphosphonate should be stopped.

The AAOMS has published risk category stages of ARONJ with the appropriate management (AAOMS 2009) (Table 7.19).

Oral hygiene and conservative systemic antibiotic therapy are pivotal in healing an elimination of pain in these patients (Nicolatou-Galitis et al. 2011). Systemic antibiotics (e.g., amoxicillin or levofloxacin [Levaquin®] 500 mg every day and metronidazole 500 mg bid) to prevent secondary infection. Chlorhexidine gluconate 0.12% mouth rinse and irrigation with hydrogen peroxide and surgical debridement are also done. Hyperbaric oxygen is used to counteract the necrosis by promoting periosteal blood supply to the bone. Any movable segments of bony sequestrum should be removed without exposing uninvolved bone (AAOMS 2009).

Table 7.19 Risk category stages of ARONJ with the appropriate management

At-risk category: patients taking oral or IV bisphosphonates with no apparent signs or symptoms of BRONJ. No treatment is indicated besides oral hygiene instruction

Stage 0: no clinical evidence of necrotic bone, but there are nonspecific clinical findings and symptoms. Management consists of pain medications and antibiotics

Stage 1: bone is exposed and/or necrotic, but patient is asymptomatic, and no infection is seen. Management consists of use of antibacterial oral rinse such as chlorhexidine, patient education, and a follow-up four times a year

Stage 2: exposed and necrotic bone associated with an infection is seen. There is pain and erythema in the area of exposed bone. Purulent exudates may or may not be evident. Management consists of oral antibiotics, oral antibacterial rinse, pain control, superficial debridement to relieve soft tissue irritation

Stage 3: exposed and necrotic bone with pain, infection, and one or more of the following: pathological fracture, extraoral fistula, or osteolysis extending to the inferior border of the alveolar bone. Management consists of an antibacterial oral rinse, antibiotic therapy and pain control, and surgical debridement or resection for longer-term control of infection and pain.

Source: Reprinted from American Association of Oral and Maxillofacial Surgeons (2009) with permission from John Wiley & Sons, Inc.

Q. What guidelines should be followed before a patient initiates oral bisphosphonate therapy?

A. Patients should have a complete dental examination and any major dental procedures including extractions and implants should be completed before bisphosphonate therapy is started. It is best to delay dental treatment until there is optimal dental health. While on bisphosphonate therapy, patients should have routine maintenance dental visits. Meticulous oral hygiene should be reinforced with the patient (International Academy of Oral Medicine and Toxicology 2007).

7.12 HIV/AIDS Research and Medications (Cheryl Barber, MPH, MSOD)

Q. What is the origin of HIV?

A. International scientists discovered that simian immunodeficiency virus or SIV, the chimpanzee version of the immunodeficiency virus, was most likely to have mutated into HIV transmittable to humans. Humans hunted these chimpanzees, native to West Equatorial Africa, and the virus may have been transmitted from their infected blood (Lihana et al. 2014). Genetic analysis of a blood sample in 1959 from a man in Kinshasa, in the Democratic Republic of Congo, suggested that HIV-1 possibly stemmed from a single virus in the late 1940s or early 1950s though the mode of transmission is unknown (AIDS Institute 2011). The virus spread across Africa as a result of behaviors that included migration, intra- and international commerce, housing, travel, sexual practices, drug use, and war, and eventually began to spread to other parts of the world.

Q. What is the history and etiology of HIV/AIDS?

A. Medical professionals started seeing young homosexual males presenting with unusual malignancies in 1981 and since then HIV has infected tens of millions of people around the world. Their immune systems were not fending off infections as normally expected and they presented with symptoms such as diarrhea, anorexia, wasting, premature aging, and alopecia. In addition, some presented with Kaposi sarcoma, exhibiting dark purple lesions on their faces and other parts of their bodies. Because those presenting with symptoms were homosexuals, the syndrome was tagged the "gay plague." Their health deteriorated and many died before doctors were able to diagnose the condition. By 1982, scientists had found epidemiological evidence that it was an infectious disease transferred by body fluids and by exposure to contaminated blood or blood products (CDC 2018a). Around the same time, medical professionals observed the disease being spread in patients with hemophilia who were receiving blood transfusions, infants of infected mothers, intravenous drug users, and sexually active women. One consequence was that in 1984, the first needle exchange program started in Amsterdam as heterosexual immigrants from Central Africa started presenting with the disease. In 1983, lymphadenopathy-associated virus was identified at the Pasteur Institute as Gallo of the National Institutes of Health made the link between the virus and disease. The disease was named "human immunodeficiency virus" (HIV) in 1986 along with the isolation of the virus and identification of its genomic sequence. These discoveries finally gave scientists the tools necessary to develop tests for the disease.

The HIV virus binds to a CD4 receptor on CD4+ T cells and infects and kills these cells which are needed by the host to combat it (Figure 7.1). And because of transcription errors, the virus produces progeny possessing different genomic structures, rendering them undetectable to body defense systems thus allowing them to continually infect new cells. Over time, a person develops an immunodeficiency and becomes vulnerable to many parasitic infections, resulting in the disease we call "acquired immunodeficiency syndrome" (AIDS). Untreated AIDS means

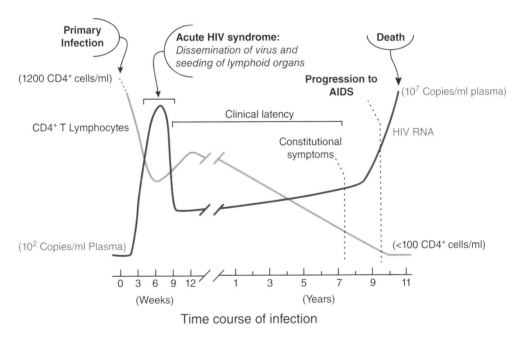

Figure 7.1 Schematic indicating the relationship between the levels of virus and CD4+ T cells, the acute phase, clinical latency, the progression from HIV infection to AIDS and death. Modified from: File: Hiv-timecourse copy.svg|thumb|Hiv-timecourse copy at http://commons.wikimedia.org/wiki/File%3AHiv-timecourse_copy.svg.

the infected individual has no protection from other diseases that healthy people easily fight. Zidovudine (AZT), FDA approved in 1987, possessed some ability to inhibit viral transcription but because of the mutation rate it lacked the capacity to contain the disease. Scientists later identified the CD4 receptor as the HIV binding site and determined that additional cofactors, CXCR4 and CCR5, were required for binding.

Before the advent of highly active antiretroviral therapy (HAART), many people died of secondary infections. HAART resulted in a substantial decline in the HIV-associated mortality rate but a person must strictly adhere to the treatment regimen for the treatment to be successful. A diagnosis of AIDS requires the presence of the HIV virus and opportunistic infections/AIDS-defining illnesses and CD4 count <200 specific conditions or diseases and must be made by a licensed medical provider. It is important to note that a person diagnosed with AIDS must have had contact with the virus, but there are individuals who have had contact with the virus but do not progress to AIDS.

Unchecked, the HIV virus spreads through unprotected anal, vaginal, or oral sex, needle sharing, and infected blood supplies. An infected woman can infect her baby during pregnancy, birth, or breastfeeding and the viruses will reproduce in both the mother and child as the disease progresses.

The virus entering the bloodstream triggers an immune response causing other cells to produce antibodies. These antibodies start to rid of the body of these disease-causing molecules. Antibodies recognize HIV's surface molecules then tags them as "different" and targets them for destruction by the immune system. When the system is working efficiently, the production of antibodies is an essential part of the immune response. However, HIV ultimately infects and destroys the very cells needed to signal this response, which renders the immune system unable to stop the progression to AIDS (Figure 7.2).

Primary HIV infection is the first stage of the disease and typically lasts 1–2 weeks. During this period, the virus rapidly reproduces before the immune response has started. The resulting high viral load and the death of the CD4 cells are indicative of an acute infection. Some people experience flu-like symptoms such as fever, swollen glands, headaches, rashes, and muscle or joint pain during primary infection, but the symptoms can be mild and may be representative of other minor illnesses. Early symptoms start to manifest 1–2 months after transmission but can occur as early as two weeks after exposure. Some people never experience symptoms. It is important to note that the immune response has not yet begun and that at this point antibody detection tests are unable to diagnose the infection. For this reason, and because newly infected people are highly contagious, it is essential to develop tests capable of diagnosing these early infections. Since newly infected people are generally unaware of their HIV status, they pose a substantial risk of infecting their sexual partners. The term "window period" describes the span between viral entry and the point when the host starts to respond and produce antibodies, which can take anywhere from two to 12 weeks. HIV seroconversion is defined as the point when the body produces enough antibodies to result in a positive HIV antibody test.

Following the acute stage of the disease, infected individuals may look and feel completely healthy for many years. However, the virus integrates its genetic information into the host's DNA and continuously replicates. Without medical treatment, the immune system progressively deteriorates. This late stage is called clinical latency and as with the acute stage, a person can look and feel perfectly healthy but can still be infectious. Without antiretroviral therapy, an average of 10 years may elapse from the time of initial infection to the onset of AIDS.

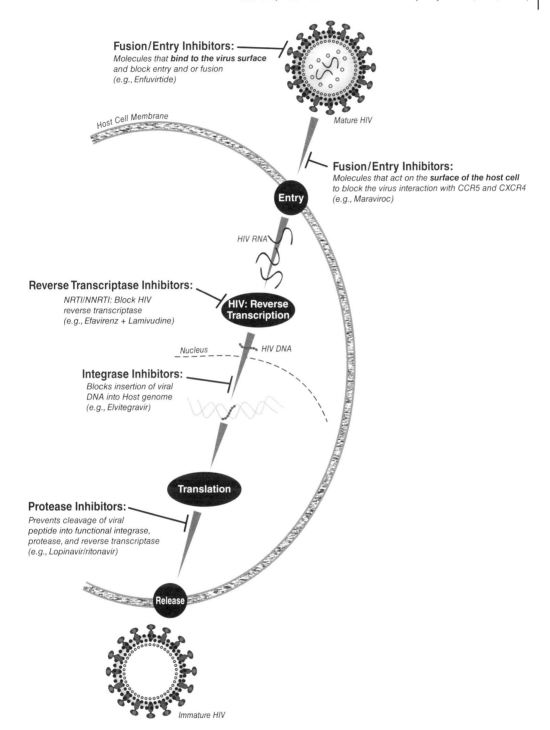

Figure 7.2 Cartoon showing the sites of inhibition for five different ARVs approved for HIV treatment. *Source:* Courtesy of Dr William Abrams.

Q. What is the epidemiology of HIV and AIDS?

A. Since its discovery, the number of AIDS cases has continued to increase both in the United States and around the world even after decades of programs designed to increase disease awareness. The cases span all races, countries, sexual orientations, genders, and income levels. There are still many reasons why infected people remain untested and therefore unaware of their HIV status. The main reasons people put off testing include having to cope with the disease, the stigma associated with being HIV positive, they feel they are protected because they usually use condoms, or they haven't engaged in what they perceive as risky behavior.

An estimated 1.1 million people in the US were living with HIV at the end of 2015, the most recent year for which this information was available. Of those people, about 15%, or one in seven, did not know they were infected (CDC 2018a).

The rate of new infections declined from 25% in 2003 to 20% in 2012. In 2015, there were an estimated 38 500 new HIV infections, down from 41 800 in 2010 (CDC 2014). The annual number of new HIV infections in the US has not increased and has actually declined by 5% from 2011 to 2015. This decrease correlates with the use of effective HIV medications (CDC 2013). Studies have shown that people aware of their status avoid behaviors that would spread the infection; they seek medical care and take combination antiretroviral therapy (cART), reducing the spread of HIV (CDC 2014). Gay, bisexual, and other men who have sex with men continued to bear the greatest burden by risk group, representing an estimated 26 200 of these new HIV infections (CDC 2018b). The US started listing HIV as a cause of death on death certificates in 1987 and by 2015, 507 351 people had died of the disease. In 2015 alone, 6465 people died from the disease and it was the ninth leading cause of death for those aged 25–34 (CDC 2018c).

Worldwide, there were about 2.1 million new cases of HIV in 2013, but new infections have fallen 38% since 2001 and new infections among children have fallen by 58% in the same period (CDC 2018b; UNAIDS 2014b). There were about 35 million people living with HIV around the world and of those, 3.2 million were children, 2.1 million adolescents, and 4.2 million people over age 50 (CDC 2018c; UNAIDS 2014b). Children below the age of 15 years old had an estimated 1.8 million new infections, or about 5000 new infections per day (UNAIDS 2018).

Globally, AIDS-related deaths peaked in 2005 at 2.4 million, have declined steadily since then, and were estimated at 1.5 million in 2013 (UNAIDS 2014a). Even though sub-Saharan Africa carried the biggest burden of HIV/AIDS, countries in South Asia, Southeast Asia, Eastern Europe, Central Asia, and Latin America are still significantly affected by the disease (CDC 2014; UNAIDS 2014b).

Q. What is the description of the HIV life cycle and the drugs that interfere with its progression?

A. The viral life cycle consists of several stages: viral attachment, fusion, viral uncoating, transcription and translation, integration, assembly, and maturation and budding.

Viral Attachment
The virus enters the body through sexual contact, blood exposure, or mother-to-child transmission (MTCT), and binds to CD4+ cells. The binding, called viral attachment, results when proteins on the surface of the virus recognize specific proteins on the surface of the cells (NIH 2013). Entry inhibitor class drugs block this attachment by binding themselves to the proteins on the surface of the cells or on the surface of the virus. Drug inhibition at this stage is different from many of the other anti-HIV drugs in that the other drugs inhibit the virus after it has entered the cell. Monoclonal antibodies can also block infection at this stage by binding to proteins on the surface of the cells or on the surface of the virus. One such antibody, W614A-3S,

recognizes a specific form of a highly conserved motif of the gp41 envelope protein, elicits viral neutralization to protect CD4+ T cells and was inversely correlated with viral load and viral DNA (Lucar et al. 2017). Killick reported that in an animal model, vaccine immunogens based on Env bound to a two domain CD4 variant, 2dCD4^{S60C}, were capable of consistently eliciting potent, broadly neutralizing antibody responses in New Zealand white rabbits against a panel of clinically relevant HIV-1 pseudoviruses (Killick et al. 2015).

Fusion

Once attached, the virus fuses with the cell by merging the cell membrane to the outer envelope of the virus and then injects its genetic material. This process can be blocked by a fusion-inhibiting drug, which has the ability to bind to an envelope protein and prevent the structural changes necessary for the virus to fuse with the cell.

Viral Uncoating

The virus then reproduces by commandeering the genetic machinery of the host cell and creating multiple copies of itself. This process begins by dissolving the protective layer surrounding the viral RNA (Mamede et al. 2017). Eliminating infection at this step precludes the conversion of viral RNA to DNA and stops the infection process, but the localization and mechanism of the uncoating process remain poorly understood. Recent studies suggest that the uncoating process is at or in the nucleus and additional research will be required to clearly understand this process.

Transcription and Translation

Viral reverse transcriptase is the first essential enzyme of HIV replication; reverse transcriptase inhibitors drugs were the first drugs available to treat HIV and are still an effective backbone drug used in treating HIV when combined with other targeted drugs.

HIV's single-stranded viral RNA (ssRNA) is converted to double-stranded DNA (dsDNA) by the enzyme reverse transcriptase. This enzyme uses the host cell's own building blocks to change/transcribe its genetic material to the dsDNA that then begins to replicate. Three types of reverse transcriptase inhibitors drugs can block this process. Nucleotide transcriptase inhibitors (NtRTIs) and nucleoside reverse transcriptase inhibitors (NRTIs) are structurally similar to the building blocks of DNA. Transcription will be reduced when thymidine analogs and cytidine analogs lacking the 3′-OH group on the deoxyribose sugar compete for bases on the DNA molecule. To be active, the NRTIs must be metabolized by host cell kinases to their triphosphate forms (NRTI-TPs). NRTIs require a three-step activation while the NtRTIs require only a two-step phosphorylation. When the viral RT incorporates them into the DNA strand, they are able to block the next nucleotide from attaching, thus terminating viral replication. Drug resistance can occur when amino acid substitutions cause mutations that block the binding of the NRTIs/NtRTIs inhibitors to the viral enzyme. Pyrophosphorolysis is another pathway whereby the virus develops resistance to NRTIs/NtRTIs by removing the incorporated NRTIs from the DNA strand.

Nonnucleoside reverse transcriptase inhibitors (NNRTIs) have a high level of specificity and do not competitively bind to the DNA strand. Instead, they bind directly to the reverse transcriptase molecule and alter its structure so that it is unable to function properly. Their binding site is a specific "pocket" site associated with but distinct both spatially and functionally from the NRTI binding site (Clercq 2004) and unlike NRTIs, the NNRTIs do not require phosphorylation steps for activation. Monotherapy with NNRTI can lead to drug-resistant virus so the NNRTIs should be used in combination with other antiretrovirals. Drug resistance is usually a result of genetic variability due to multiple substitutions to the amino acids forming the hydrophobic pocket binding site. One approach to addressing this problem is the generation of NNRTIs based on pyrimidine derivatives utilizing a combination of various substituents within multiple fragments of the parent NNRTI molecule that results in the development of highly potent inhibitory compounds (Elliston and Kochetkov 2017).

Integration

The virus can only use the host cell's genetic machinery after it incorporates or integrates the newly transcribed viral DNA into the host cell's nucleus. Integrase strand transfer inhibitors (INSTI) block this stage by competing with the active Mg2+ sites needed by integrase. This inhibits 3'end processing and prevents the virus from transferring its viral genetic material. These integrase inhibitors drugs are a vital part of the HAART or cART regimens especially for those people who have developed resistance to drugs that target the other enzymes. Two other mechanisms utilized by integrase inhibitors are lens epithelial-derived growth factor (LEDGF/p75) and integrase binding inhibitors (INBIs).

Assembly

Following integration, the virus uses the host cell's protein manufacturing capability to make the proteins needed to assemble new viruses. A key step is processing the viral protein strands into functional components with a proteolytic enzyme. The viral protein fragments then assemble into fully formed virions. Protease inhibitors (PIs) block the action of the viral enzyme aspartyl protease, which prevents the immature viral proteins from assembling into mature virions that are able to infect other cells. These three enzymes, reverse transcriptase, integrase, and protease, are the basis of most current HAART treatment regimens.

Maturation and Budding

Mature virions break off from the host cell, freely circulate, and infect CD4+ T cells, which initiates a new replication cycle. Currently, there are no drugs capable of preventing the maturation and budding process though several budding inhibitor drugs are currently in development. A historical timeline of HIV therapeutic approaches is provided in Table 7.20.

Q. HIV and pregnancy?

A. Of the 3.5 million adults living with HIV globally in 2016, 15.3 million (44%) were women of reproductive age who could become pregnant and were taking or in need of antiretroviral therapy (ART). Providing ART to these women before pregnancy, during pregnancy, and while breastfeeding would prevent MTCT and improve the survival of both the mother and child (Gilbert et al. 2015; WHO 2016). Without maternal ART, 15–30% of formula-fed babies and up to 45% of those breastfed would become infected (UNAIDS 2018). Earlier studies found that rapid adoption of Zidovudine monotherapy given antenatally, intrapartum, and to neonates resulted in a 68% reduction in MTCT (Townsend et al. 2014). In high-income countries, the implementation of ART has reduced MTCT rates to less than 1–2% since 2000, with extremely low rates being reported among women who conceive while receiving ART (0.2% in France from 2000 to 2010) (Mandelbrot and Tubiana 2015).

    Preexposure prophylaxis (PrEP) is one of several strategies that support safer conception in serodiscordant couples, alongside several behavioral and biomedical interventions, including fully suppressive treatment of either partner's HIV infection. Existing evidence, albeit scarce, supports the safety of PrEP in the preconception period and during pregnancy (Heffron et al. 2016; Mofenson et al. 2017). Adherence to a therapeutic drug regimen is crucial in pregnancy, as missed ART might lead to virological failure or breakthrough, increased risk of MTCT, and potential transmission of drug-resistant virus to fetuses (Yeganeh et al. 2017).

Table 7.20 Historical timeline of HIV treatment

Years	NRTI	PI	NNRTI	INSTI	Entry inhibitors	Pharmacokinetic booster
1980–1990	AZT Zidovudine					
1991–2000	ddI Didanosine ddC Zalcitabine d4T Stavudine 3TC Lamivudine ABC Abacavir ABC/3TC/AZT Trizivir	SQV Saquinavir hard gel RTV Ritonavir IDV Indinavir NFV Nelfinavir SQV Saquinavir soft gel APV Amprenavir ddIEC DidanosineEC 3TC/AZT Combivir LPV/RTV Kaletra	NVP Nevirapine EFV Efavirenz			LPV/RTV Kaletra
2001–2010	FTC Emtricitabine ABC/3TC Epzicom TDF/FTC Truvada	ATV Atazanavir FPV Fosamprenavir TPV Tipranavir DRV Darunavir	ETR Etravirine	RAL Raltegravir	T-20 Enfuviritide MVC Maraviro	
2011-present	TDF/FTC/RPV Complera(STR) TDF/FTC/ EVG/ COBI Stribild(STR) ABC/3TC/DTG Triumeq(STR) TAF/FTC/ EVG/ COBI Genvoya(STR)	ATV/COBI Evotaz DRV/COBI Prezcobix	NPVXR Nevirapine RPV Rilpivirine TDF/FTC/RPV Complera(STR)	TDF/FTC/ EVG/COBI Stribild(STR) DTG Dolutegravir EVG Elvitegravir ABC/3TC/DTG Triumeq(STR) TAF/FTC/ EVG/COBI Genvoya(STR)		TDF/FTC/ EVG/COBI Stribild(STR) COBI** Cobicistat ATV/COBI Evotaz DRV/COBI Prezcobix TAF/FTC/ EVG/COBI Genvoya(STR)

Source: Adapted from Cihlar and Fordyce (2016).
INSTI, integrase strand transfer inhibitor; NNRTI, nonnucleoside reverse transcriptase inhibitor; NRTI, nucleoside reverse transcriptase inhibitor; PI, protease inhibitors.

The Antiretroviral Pregnancy Registry (APR) collects prospective data where ART exposure is assessed before birth outcomes are reported, predominantly through voluntary reports from mainly US-based healthcare providers. The APR has sufficient statistical power to rule out an increased risk of 1.5 times or greater in overall birth defects in infants exposed to zidovudine, lamivudine, tenofovir, disoproxil, fumarate, abacavir, emtricitabine, nevirapine, ritonavir, lopinavir, and didovudine, and an increased risk of two times in those exposed to darunavir, rilpivirine, efavirenz, and raltegravir, compared with the general US population (UNAIDS 2018). Some studies have identified potential safety signals that require continued monitoring. For example, a US study reported a significantly increased risk of congenital abnormalities associated with zidovudine exposure in the first trimester, and an increase in skin and musculoskeletal defects, while the French Perinatal Cohort reported a twofold increased risk of congenital heart defects associated with first-trimester zidovudine exposure (although this increase was not found in the APR study) (Antiretroviral PregRegis 2016; Sibiude et al. 2015; Williams et al. 2015). Specific guidelines are available from the US Department of Human Services (AIDSinfo 2018b).

The relationship between antenatal ART and adverse pregnancy and birth outcomes is complex and not completely understood. Adverse effects in these children include increased mortality and infectious disease morbidity, impaired growth, metabolic changes, neurodevelopmental delays, altered immunity, and mitochondrial abnormalities, so we need to better understand the potential causal pathways to improve health risks (Desmonde et al. 2016; Slogrove et al. 2016; Zash et al. 2016). The Pregnancy and HIV/AIDS: Seeking Equitable Study (PHASES) initiative is an ongoing initiative to develop guidance for ethical HIV research among pregnant women, with the goal of providing accelerated access to treatment (Krubiner et al. 2016). Additional research is needed to understand potential effects of cART through breast milk or intrauterine exposure. Furthermore, this knowledge is of vital importance since the number of HIV-exposed uninfected children will undoubtedly increase as better drugs and treatments are developed (Coelho et al. 2017).

Q. What are the long-term issues associated with HIV?

A. Some patients suffer from HIV medicinal side effects months after starting medication and these effects can continue for years. Examples of long-term side effects include kidney problems, including kidney failure; liver damage (hepatotoxicity); heart disease; diabetes or insulin resistance; and/or an increase in fat levels in the blood (hyperlipidemia) (AIDSinfo 2018c). Additional changes include how the body uses and stores fat (lipodystrophy), weakening of the bones (osteoporosis), nerve damage (peripheral neuropathy), and mental health-related effects, including insomnia, depression, and/or thoughts of suicide. Some of the medications, particularly therapies used in the past, caused changes in body shape and appearance, including increased fat in the belly, neck, shoulders, breasts, or face, or loss of fat in the face, legs, or arms. However, these changes rarely occur with the HIV medicines currently in use (CDC 2018b; NIH 2018).

When patients experience adverse effects that are life-threatening, their HAART must be modified (Table 7.21). These effects can require the patient to immediately discontinue the ARV drugs and begin an alternative regimen to alleviate the toxicity. If the patient experiences symptoms less than life-threatening, one drug is substituted for another. However, when serious life-threatening events do occur the underlying principle is to maintain viral suppression. Providers must be aware when selecting a new regimen that resistance mutations are sequestered in HIV reservoirs throughout the body and though mutations did not show up in previous

Table 7.21 Common or severe adverse effects associated with HAART

Effect	Drug class
Bleeding	PIs
Heart disease	NRTIs and PIs
Cholelithiasis	PIs
Bone density effects	NRTIs
Bone marrow suppression	NRTIs
Diabetes mellitus and insulin resistance	NRTIs and PIs
Dyslipidemia	NRTI, NNRTIs, PIs, INSTIs
Gastrointestinal effects	NRTIs, PIs, INSTIs, EIs
Hepatic effects	NRTIs, NNRTIs, PIs, EIs
Hypersensitivity reaction	NRTIs, NNRTIs, INSTIs, EIs
Lactic acidosis	NRTIs
Lipodystrophy	NRTIs
Myopathy	INSTIs
Elevated creatine phosphokinase	INSTIs
Rash	All types
Renal effects/urolithiasis	All types
Stevens–Johnson syndrome	
	NRTIs, NNRTIs, PIs, INSTIs
Toxic epidermal necrosis	NRTIs, NNRTIs, PIs, INSTIs

Source: Adapted from the Guidelines for the Use of Antiretroviral Agents in Adults and Adolescents Living with HIV. Limitations to Treatment Safety and Efficacy. Adverse Effects of Antiretroviral Agents. https://aidsinfo.nih. gov/guidelines/html/1/adult-and-adolescent-arv/31/adverse-effects-of-arv
EI, entry inhibitor; INSTI, integrase strand transfer inhibitor; NNRTI, nonnucleoside reverse transcriptase inhibitor; NRTI, nucleoside reverse transcriptase inhibitor; PI, protease inhibitors.

resistance test results they can appear in subsequent testing. Before switching from one regimen to another, providers must check:

- medical history and complete ARV history, including prior virological responses to ART
- all previous resistance test results
- viral tropism (if Maroviroc® is being considered)
- HLA-B*5701 status (if Abstinence, Be faithful, and use Condoms [ABC] is being considered)
- comorbidities
- pregnancy status, use of contraceptives, and desire for pregnancy (if dolutegravir is being considered for patients of child-bearing potential)
- HBV status, since patients with evidence of chronic HBV infection should not discontinue tenofovir disoproxil fumarate or tenofovir alafenamide unless a regimen contains another agent that is active against HBV
- adherence history
- prior intolerances to any ARVs
- concomitant medications and supplements to consider drug interactions with ARVs.

Q. What is latency and how does it affect the cure for HIV?

A. Latency refers to integrated provirus in the host's cellular DNA that is not actively replicating. However, antiviral medications as well as the immune system only react to actively replicating and infecting virus and fail to inactivate HIV in the latent state. Latency begins when the virus sequesters itself in memory CD4+ T cells within days of infection. The dormant cells, termed reservoirs, allow the virus to hide in the body for years without causing any symptoms or expressing viral antigens that would elicit an immune response causing detection. While CD4+ memory T cells are clearly the major viral reservoir, other sites including peripheral blood and bone marrow (Hill et al. 2014), lymphoid tissue and the GI tract (Chun et al. 2008) have been shown to harbor HIV viral genetic code. For reasons that are not clearly understood, the virus retains the ability to reactivate when therapy is interrupted and even in the presence of medication to start new and productive infections.

It is essential that any cure for HIV rids the body of these latent reservoirs. There is evidence that reactivation is under the direction of the virus rather than the host cell. There is also evidence that very early initiation of cART has been associated with a reduced number of latently infected cells, which limits the extent or size of the reservoir.

Additional efforts to cure HIV focus on gene therapy, boosting HIV-specific immunity, reducing inflammation, preventing latency, gene editing, and stem cell transplantation/generation of cells resistant to HIV-1 infection. Researchers are also developing several long-acting ART therapies capable of suppressing HIV over extended periods of time, thereby reducing the burden of current regimens. These agents may be delivered by several methods: inserted as intravaginal rings, implanted as time-release medications, or as injectable antibodies with potencies spanning anywhere from one month to one year. Several of these agents have reached the stage of human studies.

Another method gaining increased focus is "shock and kill" that involves reactivation and purging of HIV latently infected cells (Melkova et al. 2017). HIV latency is probably a heterogeneous process involving many immunological and environmental factors (e.g., T cell subsets, size of the reservoir, anatomical sanctuaries, cytokine environment, and immunological synapses) (Dahabieh et al. 2015; Melkova et al. 2017) so it is important to understand the properties of the reservoir and how virus reactivation will affect those cells as well as healthy cells. This strategy involves using latency-reversing agents (LRAs) such as disulfiram, vorinostat, or romidepsin to eliminate latently infected cells by stimulating HIV transcription and targeting these cells to be killed by the immune system. The proof of concept would demonstrate that the drugs could increase virus transcription in patients while on ART who at baseline had undetectable levels. Once reactive, the virus could then be killed by the ART medication. Reactivation was measured by the increase in cell-associated HIV RNA and/or plasma HIV RNA in total and resting CD4+ T cells after the drug was administered and compare to predrug levels (Petravic et al. 2017). However, the results were disappointing since all the investigated LRAs showed increased viral RNA (Elliott 2014, 2015) without decrease in the size of the latent reservoir or the proportion of inducible latently infected cells "kicked out of" latency," the number of HIV-specific T cells or any inhibition of T cell cytokine production (Sogaard et al. 2015).

In July 2014, results from the first-phase drug trial containing a combination of "shock & kill" –Reduction of the Latent HIV-1 Reservoir (REDUC) with Vacc-4x and Romidepsin – were announced at the International AIDS Conference in Melbourne. Individuals infected with HIV received the vaccine to establish a base-level immune response. They then received the drug to coax the virus out of their hidden reservoirs. Results from the Phase 1 trial were positive because the drug was able to kick some amount of HIV out of the reservoirs. The next phase of the trial, to demonstrate whether or not the vaccine was effective at disabling HIV-infected cells, was completed in 2015. Between May 19, 2014, and October 8, 2014, researchers enrolled 20 individuals; 17 subjects completed the drug infusions. Results showed that 16 subjects exhibited total HIV-1 DNA, 15 subjects had integrated HIV-1 DNA, and six had infectious units per million cells (IUPM) at baseline and at one or more points in time after the study treatment, total HIV-1 DNA declined from screening to six weeks after romidepsin treatment (mean reduction 39.7%, 95% CI −59.7 to −11.5; p = 0.012). The decrease in integrated HIV-1 DNA from baseline to eight weeks after romidepsin treatment was not significant (19.2%, −38.6 to 6.3; p = 0.123) (Solomon 2015). Among the six assessable participants, the mean reduction in IUPM from screening to six weeks after romidepsin treatment was 38.0% (95% CI −67.0 to −8.0; p = 0.019). There were 141 adverse events: 134 (95%) were grade 1 and 7 (5%) were grade 2–3 (Solomon 2015). This *in vivo* combinatorial approach provided the first evidence for the feasibility of a combined "shock and kill" strategy, but also emphasized that further optimization of this strategy was needed to achieve a sizeable effect on the latent reservoir, that could translate into a clinically measurable benefit for people living with HIV-1 (Kelly-Sell et al. 2012; Leth et al. 2016; Solomon 2015).

Q. What is a PrEP?

A. PrEP is daily medications taken by people who are at high risk of coming in contact with the HIV virus. When taken as directed, the medication is highly effective in reducing the risk of infection by sexual contact, by more than 90% (Petry 1999), and is 70% effective in reducing the risk of HIV for IV drug users. PrEP is sold as Truvada® and is a combination of tenofovir and emtricitabine, both NRTIs. Users must adhere to the regimen because the effectiveness of the medication is directly correlated with the precise dosage and the circulating drug concentration. Prospective users must first confirm a negative status before starting Truvada and be reconfirmed every three months thereafter. Federal guidelines recommend PrEP for HIV-negative people who are in a sexual relationship with an HIV-positive person; people who have injected drugs in the past six months or have shared needles; and someone who works at or has been in a drug treatment center in the past six months (AIDSinfo 2018a). Recent tests estimated the protective effects of PrEP at 91% (95% CI 47–98%; p = 0.008) when the TDF levels were consistent with daily dosage (Portman 2018). It was felt that lack of efficacy in earlier trials might have been the result of insufficient drug levels due to diversion from the rigid regimen.

CDC researchers have estimated that the risk of infection through a single sex act with a person who has HIV ranges from 1 in 72 for receptive anal intercourse to 1 in 2500 for oral sex, though this figure assumes the HIV-positive partner is not on antiretroviral treatment and the couple is not using condoms, PrEP, or any other prevention method (CDC 2018c). CDC, in collaboration with the Health Services Administration (HRSA) and the University of California, has recently launched its first PrEP support hotline for providers, offering clinical guidelines and expert assistance to physicians, nurse practitioners, and physician assistants to help familiarize them with treatments and procedures. The PREPLINE number is 855-448-7737 and is available from 11 a.m.–6 p.m., weekdays only. In partnerships with community-based organizations, the Division of HIV/AIDS Prevention has announced a new five-year, $215 million funding opportunity to support HIV prevention efforts of organizations like this one.

Q. What is postexposure prophylaxis (PEP)?

A. PEP refers to taking HIV medications after a person has been exposed to the virus, in an effort to prevent infection. Anyone who has been exposed to the virus through sexual contact, experienced occupational exposure through the sharing of needles used in a drug treatment center or who has been sexually assaulted should strongly consider requesting this medication. It should only be used in emergency situations and must be taken within three days of exposure. The sooner one starts the medication, the better the results. The person will need to take the medication once or twice daily for 28 days. PEP usually consists of three anti-HIV drugs: Truvada (a fixed-dose combination tablet combining emtricitabine and tenofovir) and raltegravir, an integrase inhibitor. This is the preferred regimen but others are available, including those for children, persons with reduced renal functions, and pregnant women.

Q. What is HAND? What are the connections between HIV and dementia or neurocognitive impairment?

A. Neuropsychological impairment has accompanied HIV/AIDS throughout the years (Buhler and Mann 2011). However, the advent of HARRT has produced better medical outcomes and reduced the severity of the neurological effects. Symptoms include decline in brain function, movement skills, and shifts in behavior and moods. Screening tools for these conditions are not yet well established. It is known that after conversion, the virus crosses the blood–brain barrier through infected macrophages, microglia, and multinucleated giant cells (Gonzalez and Martin-Garcia 2005; Harbison et al. 2014; Langford et al. 2014; McArthur et al. 2005) and if untreated could develop into HIV encephalitis and HIV leukoencephalopathy. Studies have found that subjects with prolonged untreated HIV infection experienced loss in volume in various parts of the brain including the thalamus, caudate, and cerebellum, and untreated HIV for even longer periods of time was linked with cortical thinning in the frontal lobe, temporal lobes, and cingulate cortex (Sanford et al. 2018). The virus also causes generalized inflammation, which can be the precursor for numerous other conditions or exacerbate the neurological condition. Unfortunately, the blood–brain barrier resists crossover of some antiretroviral medications, which possibly allows untreated virus to replicate (Koob 2018; McAuthur et al. 2010). However, several medications do cross the blood–brain barrier; abacavir, darunavir, emtricitabine, efavirenz, fosamprenavir, indinavir, lopinavir, lopinavir, maraviroc, nevirapine, raltegravir, and zidovudine.

AIDS dementia complex (ADC) is usually associated with late HIV-1 infection and with severe immunosuppression or CD4 counts below 200 cells/μL. The condition HIV-associated neurocognitive disorder (HAND) presents as a mild form of dementia yet is very similar to ADC. HAND is classified into three distinct categories depending on the severity of symptoms. The mildest form is asymptomatic neurocognitive impairment (ANI) characterized by the lowest level of impairment that barely compromises daily functions. People with ANI show impairment on neuropsychological tests but do not usually recognize or acknowledge having symptoms. However, ANI is clinically relevant because people with ANI can progress to one of the more severe forms of HAND. Participants in the CNS HIV Antiretroviral Therapy Effects Research (CHARTER) study who had ANI at baseline were 2–6 times more likely to develop symptomatic HAND during several years of follow-up than those who were neurocognitively normal at baseline (Saylor et al. 2016). When daily functions were impaired to a greater extent such as behavior changes, decision-making difficulties, tremors or loss of coordination, problems with learning, attention, and concentration, and memory difficulties, the disease was classified as a mid-level impairment or mild neurocognitive disorder (MND).

The most severe case, HIV-associated dementia (HAD), was characterized by major cognitive impairment where the symptoms were severe enough to interfere with everyday activity (Esmaeili et al. 2015). Very rare symptoms included psychosis, mania, and seizures. Sometimes a person deteriorated to the point where they entered a vegetative state incapable of human interaction. A study conducted in South Africa researching HAD found a positive correlation between current alcohol dependence disorders and low CD4 counts (200 and below) with positive HAD results (Robbins et al. 2011). This study used the cutoff defined on the International HIV Dementia Scale (IHDS). Currently neuropsychological tests are the gold standard for diagnosing HAND. Tools such as CogState and the revised HIV dementia scale are adequate for diagnosing HAND but have less sensitivity in detecting the milder forms (Joska et al. 2016; Kimani 2018).

HAART has reduced HAD to about 5%, but milder impairments are still prevalent in the HIV community. Even for those on cART medication, there is no cure for the impairment and no clear understanding of the risk factors and disease progression; 30–50% of people living with HIV still demonstrate the effects of HAND in their lives. Increased age and comorbidities appear to increase the risk of developing HAND and managing it is difficult because of the contributions from other infections, nutritional imbalances, depression, anxiety, and the gradual development of the symptoms.

Diagnosing the disease is difficult since the ailment has no typical progression or documented course of action. Since no single test can diagnose HAND, an accurate diagnosis requires an extensive examination evaluating a combination of mental status tests, radiology studies, electrophysiological tests, brain scans, and the biochemical analysis of the cerebrospinal fluid.

HAART has significantly increased the lifespan of the HIV-infected population and many patients who contracted the virus decades ago have lived to enjoy their senior years with few or no symptoms. But even when a person is on medication, HIV-associated cognitive impairment can worsen with the duration of the infection, with age and age-related conditions such as cardiovascular disease. Since it is generally believed that virus replication in the brain is a necessary prerequisite for the development of HAND (Langford et al. 2017) and that the virus entered the brain at an early stage of infection, it is quite possible that the brain functions as a reservoir capable of sustaining latent viral infections (Fois and Brew 2015). To this end, it is important to define new predictive disease markers, develop clear screening and diagnostic protocols, and include CNS-penetrating medications in future treatment plans (Eggers et al. 2017; Ellis et al. 2014). It has not yet been established if CNS-penetrating drugs can prevent the development of HAND so for now, the best course of action is for the person to strictly adhere to their antiviral therapy.

A number of studies have successfully used intranasal insulin to improve cognitive function in healthy individuals, and in individuals with impaired cognitive performance as a result of aging or Alzheimer disease (Craft et al. 2012). The mechanism for this protective effect is not well understood, but insulin has a variety of metabolic and trophic effects and might directly protect neurons and dampen inflammatory cytokine expression (Craft et al. 2013). These multitarget effects of insulin, coupled with intranasal delivery to selectively target the CNS, make intranasal insulin an attractive candidate for a neuroprotective therapy against HAND (Saylor et al. 2016).

Q. What do we know about alcohol abuse and HIV?

A. HIV medications are extremely hard on the body, so it is important that the liver, which is responsible for removing waste products, works efficiently while a person is being therapeutically treated. Once infected and on medication, the body may react differently to alcohol and drugs. It may even take longer to recover from marijuana, alcohol, or other recreational drug usage. Certain HIV medications can alter recreational drug levels in unexpected and potentially dangerous ways. For example, crystal methamphetamine can be present at many times its normal level in the bloodstream when mixed with an HIV drug called ritonavir (Norvir®) because ritonavir lowers the body's ability to break down the recreational drug. Also, an interaction between alcohol and efavirenz was observed resulting in no change in intoxication or drowsiness before and after efavirenz despite lower blood-alcohol concentration (McCance-Katz et al. 2013). Yet there is no direct scientific evidence of an interaction between HIV medication and alcohol and unlike other recreational drugs, alcohol does not directly increase or decrease the levels of HIV drugs. Therefore, while on cART men should not have more than 2–3 drinks of alcohol a day and women not drink more than 1–2 drinks a day (AIDSinfo 2018a).

There has always been a high incidence of alcohol abuse in people with HIV, with a prevalence rate from 29% to 60% (Petry 1999; Samet et al. 2004). Alcohol misuse exerts broad damage to multiple neurotransmitter systems and alcohol may also weaken the resistance of the blood–brain barrier to leukocytes, providing a means of ingress for HIV into the brain (Persidsky et al. 2011). To some extent, the effects of alcohol abuse parallel pathology associated with HIV (Norman and Basso 2015), including effects on the frontal temporal and parietal lobes (Wilkinson et al. 1987); significant white matter degeneration (Monnig et al. 2013); and reduced subcortical volumes and thickness (Momenan et al. 2012). These types of abnormalities usually correlate with diminished cognitive function (Park et al. 2010). Chronic alcohol abusers can be disinclined to follow their medical regimens, which exacerbates their condition, and since chronic alcohol misuse has been shown to cause immunosuppression (Cook 1998; Kronfol et al. 1993; Spies et al. 2004; Szabo et al. and Saha 2015), it can accelerate their disease (Spies et al. 2004; Miguez et al. 2003). It is possible that HIV and alcohol interaction may have a synergistic effect on the disease, causing a disease progression rate higher than would have been expected from the disease alone. Alcohol abuse is also linked with anemia, cancer, cardiovascular disease, cirrhosis, and several other conditions (Garbutt 2018).

Research protocols have not yet uncovered a comprehensive technique capable of deciphering the direct connection between HIV and alcohol misuse. Earlier studies reported that compared to seronegative subjects, HIV-seropositive subjects demonstrated poorer performance on measures of verbal intelligence, concept formation, and visual reaction time. Furthermore, HIV-positive subjects with a history of alcohol abuse demonstrated an even higher level of impairment (Fama 2009). The study also showed that subjects with comorbid alcoholism and HIV infection performed in the impaired range on measures of new learning, while HIV-negative, control subjects misusing alcohol alone performed within the normal range of function (Fama 2009). Additional studies resulted in similar data, where HIV-positive individuals who misused alcohol showed increased impairment compared to HIV-negative or nonalcohol-abusing individuals (Fama 2011).

Q. Are there different strains or subtypes of HIV?

A. There are two primary human strains, HIV-1 and HIV-2, along with SIVs (simian immunodeficiency viruses). HIV-1 is the predominant strain and accounts for 95% of all worldwide infections. HIV-2 is a milder version of the disease. It progresses slower than HIV-1, results in fewer deaths, and is relatively uncommon. HIV-2 is mostly concentrated in West Africa in countries such as Cape Verde, Ivory Coast, Gambia, Guinea-Bissau, Mali, Mauritania, Nigeria, and Sierra Leone (Hemelaar 2012) but cases have been reported in France, Portugal, and Spain.

The virus is classified into types, groups, and subtypes. The high transcription error rate of HIV causes it to mutate very readily and accounts for the diversity in the groups. Therefore, the blood of an infected person can contain several different strains and subtypes. The HIV-1 and HIV-2 viruses have several different subtypes and it is entirely probable that more subtypes will emerge in the future. According to the Joint United Nations Programme on HIV/AIDS (UNAIDS), diagnostic tests detect all known subtypes of the virus. The HIV-1 virus consists of the following four groups: Group M has nine subgroups A1, A2, A3, A4, A6, B, C, D, F1, F2, G, H, J, and K; Group N; Group O; and Group P (HIV Sequence 2017; Taylor et al. 2008).

Of the four groups of HIV, M is responsible for most of the global epidemic. The other three groups, N, O, and P, are relatively uncommon. Group O accounts for about 5% of infections in several West and Central African countries. Group N is a very distinctive form of the virus and not clearly defined because few isolates have been identified and sequenced (HIV Sequence 2017; Lihana et al. 2014). Group P is a human isolate resembling SIV and both Groups N and P localize to individuals in Cameroon.

There are over 60 diverse strains within HIV-1 found throughout the world yet it is rare to find more than one or two strains occupying the same geographic region. Different subtypes in the same person can combine genetic material to form hybrids known as circulating recombinant forms (CRFs) (database 2018). Intersubtype recombinant genomes can happen; they are usually found within a person who is dually or multiply infected. These recombinants are classified as unique recombinant forms (URF) and when highly transmitted along with the other circulating strains, their classification is changed to CRF. To date, we know of approximately 89 CRFs (database 2018).

Subtype B is the dominant HIV subtype in the United States and Western Europe. It represents only 12% of global HIV infections yet is the focus of the majority of HIV research. There is less research available for subtype C, although 50% of people living with HIV have this subtype since it has a high prevalence in southern Africa, eastern areas of Africa, and India (Taylor et al. 2008).

Since scientists believe the HIV-1 epidemic originated in Cameroon and the Democratic Republic of Congo, it is no surprise that the greatest diversity of subtypes predominate in these regions (Hemelaar 2012). Migration and population mixing dictated the geographical patterns in the distribution of subtypes and since these patterns are continually changing, predicting transmission patterns in these areas has become a daunting task.

Q. What does protective immunity look like?

A. In the past, scientists have been able to correlate protective immunity from one response in the design of another response. Here, scientists cannot avail themselves of paradigms used in other vaccine developments because they lack a model to follow since there are no closely related diseases. This leaves several questions about how the immune response would proceed, such as which cells would be more important in the response: specific T-cells or specific antibodies? Answering this question would be instrumental in designing and validating a vaccine. Also, researchers have not yet identified an animal model that reliably predicts efficacy in humans, though they are testing vaccines against SIV and genetically engineered hybrids of SIV and HIV.

There are several other factors that can cause difficulty in designing effective vaccines. In most diseases, the person survives by developing naturally derived immunity after infection, and this immune response is generally sufficient to prevent future infection. This type of response would provide a model illustrating the amount of protection a successful vaccine should provide. Since the body cannot achieve natural immunity against HIV disease, researchers have limited knowledge in identifying the level of immune response necessary to effectively fight the virus. Another impediment to vaccine design is the variability and number of HIV types. There are numerous HIV subtypes and each is genetically distinct from the other. A vaccine could protect against one subtype but not against the others, thus limiting its ability to contain the disease, and since new subtypes are continuously emerging this problem can only worsen.

In 2009, the results of the largest HIV vaccine trial in history were announced. Referred to as "RV144," the trial had more than 16 000 participants and took six years to complete (Kim 2015). The trial used a "prime-boost" strategy with two experimental HIV vaccines: (i) a recombinant vaccine using a canarypox virus with inserted genes that code for antigenic proteins from HIV intended to stimulate T cell-mediated immunity, and (ii) the "boost," which was composed of a genetically engineered antigenic surface protein from HIV intended to stimulate B cell production (Buchbinder et al. 2009; Haynes et al. 2012; HIV trial 2018).

This was the first prime vaccine (Lu 2009), defined as a vaccine given in multiple immunizations, to be tested for efficacy against HIV in humans. The individual boost vaccines showed no efficacy in previous tests but when they were combined in the RV144 trial, they showed a modest effect, 31%, in preventing HIV infection. This level of efficacy was not sufficient for medical use, yet it was the first HIV vaccine trial to actually show promise in protection against the virus (Kim 2010). A study published in 2012 indicated that T cell responses likely did not play a role in the vaccine's protection against infection but that the vaccine's efficacy was related to antibody responses to certain regions of viral envelope proteins (Haynes et al. 2012).

An additional obstacle to overcome in vaccine design is in the V3 or variable loop regions. These regions can mutate and change in structure, enabling the virus to escape immune responses. There have been modest successes in producing stronger antibodies by removing and altering the peptide areas within this region. A vaccine containing the V3 sequences from several strains of HIV was used in animals and produced antibodies able to neutralize several laboratory-adapted virus strains (Hatziioannou and Evans 2012).

Other vaccine candidates consist of proteins administered with an adjuvant, which is an agent included to further stimulate the immune system. Positive results of an SIV vaccine trial in rhesus macaques proposed using cytomegalovirus (CMV) as a vector to stimulate the ability of killer T cells to attack the infected cells (Hansen et al. 2011).

A different avenue of research includes therapeutic vaccines that would be administered after an infection has occurred. This treatment would probably not be a cure but would be sufficient to lower the viral load, boost the body's immune response, delay progression to disease, and hopefully eliminate the need for antiretroviral drugs. Several such therapeutic vaccines are undergoing clinical trials where people living with HIV are testing investigational vaccines made from their own white blood cells. Proof-of-principle would determine whether or not the procedure is safe and well tolerated, and whether it could stimulate the body's immune response via the vaccine. Then the vaccines would have to be tested in several different formulations to determine the formulation that resulted in the best immune system response.

Additional research strategies have included the use of live attenuated vaccines that would hopefully weaken the virus, be harmless to the body, and elicit an immune response. Though attenuated, these vaccines should still be considered risky because they could retain the ability to integrate viral DNA into the host genome. The measles vaccine is a good model for this type of vaccine because it generates a long-lasting immune response.

Recombinant subunit vaccines designed to stimulate antibodies to HIV by mimicking proteins on the surface of the virus are also considered risky because if the inactivation process fails, surviving virus could infect the recipient. Previous attempts have produced little or no success other than Remune, a preparation based on the killed whole virus approach. These preparations were investigated as possible therapeutic vaccines for people already infected with HIV (Lai and Jones 2002) and even though they showed dramatic increases in CD4+ lymphocyte counts, they showed no enhancement of the immunization response (Valdez et al. 2003).

Several other strategies have been used in the design of vaccines. One example is a modified-envelope vaccine that mimics the way HIV protein interacts with host cells. Since HIV surface proteins are often hidden from the immune system by a coating of sugar molecules (NIH 2013; Nicholson 2016), removing or altering some of these surface molecules could lead to more potent neutralizing antibodies.

Peptide vaccines, made by linking peptides to lipids, were tested as an HIV vaccine designed so that the lipid would carry the peptide directly into cell membranes where it could be presented to the immune system with maximum efficiency. A Phase 1/2 randomized trial of safety and immunogenicity of ALVAC-HIV (vCP1452) alone, and ALVAC-HIV (vCP1452) Prime/ LIPO-5 boost was launched but the study was halted due to a case of myelitis possibly related to the LIPO-5 vaccine; the researchers detected no appreciable cell-mediated immunity and antibody responses were limited (Peiperl et al. 2014).

DNA vaccines are engineered by cloning small pieces of genetically modified viral DNA into bacteria to give hosts the ability to express HIV genes capable of mounting an immune response. The technique has worked well in mice but not in larger primates or humans and safety considerations remain since the viral DNA might retain the ability to infect (Jacobson et al. 2017) and possible future genetic mutations could result in reduction of the vaccine efficacy.

Replicons are pieces of DNA or RNA that replicate from a single origin and are being studied as carriers of modified HIV genetic material because they have properties similar to viruses in their ability to enter cells. Replicons do not reproduce in host cells and generate little or no immune response. This strategy should allow a single type of replicon system to be used to deliver different therapeutic agents repeatedly in the same person without itself initiating an immune response.

Recombinant vectored vaccines, used to stimulate cellular immunity, were constructed by incorporating fragments of HIV into empty canarypox viruses or adenoviruses that could infect cells while causing few or no symptoms. The modified vectors were designed to initiate the expansion of HIV vector-specific CD4+ T cells (Auclair et al. 2018). This type of vaccine closely resembles an actual infection more than vaccines containing proteins or DNA. The premise is that the vaccine would produce a harmless infection of the host cells, which would display immunogenic epitopes on their surface and produce a long-lasting immune response. They have been shown to produce stronger HIV-specific cytotoxic T cell (CD8) responses in animals (Arrode-Bruses et al. 2010), but unexpected outcomes suggested that the vaccination caused potentially detrimental immune responses to the very cells required to mount the response.

Rabies, measles, poliovirus, herpes simplex, human rhinovirus, influenza, and pertussis viruses are also being evaluated as vectors for HIV vaccines. Current efficacy trials are listed in Table 7.22.

Q. Who is the Berlin patient?

A. In 2008, an HIV patient was cured of the disease for the first time. The "Berlin patient," Timothy Ray Brown, received a bone marrow transplant from a donor who was an "elite controller" who was naturally resistant to HIV because he was homozygous for the CCR5 delta 32 mutation that renders immune cells resistant to infection by most HIV viruses. Brown has remained off ART since the day of his transplant (Lederman and Pike 2017). When the case was announced, the medical world was amazed and encouraged, but it has not yet led to a cure.

Table 7.22 HIV vaccine efficacy trials

Study	Site	Vaccine	Volunteers	Vaccine/Placebo randomization	Results
Vax004	USA and Netherlands	AIDSVAX B/B gp120 with alum	5100 MSM & 300 women	2 : 1	No vaccine efficacy
Vax003	Thailand	AIDSVAX B/E gp120 with alum	2500 men & women IDUs	1:1	No vaccine efficacy
HVTN 502 Step trial	North America, Caribbean, South America, Australia	MRKAd5 HIV-1 gag/pol/nef trivalent Vaccine based on adenovirus type 5	3.00 MSM & heterosexual women and men	1:1	No vaccine efficacy
HVTN 503 Phambili trial	South Africa	MRKAd5 HIV-1 gag/pol/nef trivalent vaccine based on adenovirus type 5	801 heterosexual men & women	1:1	No vaccine efficacy
HVTN 505	USA	6-plasmid DNA vaccine and rAd5 vector boost	2504 men or transgender women who have sex with men	1:1	No vaccine efficacy
HIV-V-A004	USA, Rwanda, South Africa, Thailand, Uganda	Homologous Ad26 mosaic vector regimens or AD26 mosaic and MVA mosaic heterologous vector regimens, with high-dose, low-dose or no clade C gp140 protein plus adjuvant	400 men & women	–	Results pending
HVTN 100	South Africa	ALVAC-HIV and bivalent subtype C gp120/MF59	252 men & women	5:1	Results pending
HVTN 702	South Africa	ALVAC-HIV and bivalent subtype C gp120/MF59	5400 men & women	1:1	Results pending
HVTN 703 / HPTN 081	South America, sub-Saharan Africa	VRC01 broadly neutralizing monoclonal antibody	2400 MSM, transgender & 1500 women	2:1	Results pending
RV144	Thailand	Recombinant canarypox vector vaccine (ALVAC-HIV [vCP1521]) and recombinant glycoprotein 120 subunit vaccine (AIDSVAX B/E)	16402 community-risk men & women	1:1	31.2% vaccine efficacy at 42 months

Source: Adapted from Rubins M, Venkatarghavan R, Saxena A, et al. HIV vaccine: recent advances, current roadblocks, and future directions. http://dx.doi.org/10.1155/2015/560347.

HIV-infected persons known as "elite controllers" possess a gene mutation capable of naturally controlling the virus, thus preventing it from progressing to AIDS, and researchers thought this mechanism could offer a route to vaccine development. The RV144 trials were studies involving these individuals, whose HIV infections never progress to AIDS despite repeated exposure. The premise was to determine a way to emulate their innate ability to control the virus. A trial of this vaccine approach (HVTN 505) was halted in July 2013 because the vaccine failed to lower risk of infection in the recipients (Portman 2018).

Q. Are any vaccines available now?

A. Scientists are actively searching for a HIV-1 vaccine capable of effectively preventing infection. Over the years, a number of scientific approaches have gained popularity in vaccine development, including the induction of neutralizing antibodies in the late 1980s, induction of CD8 T cells in the early 1990s, and currently, combination approaches. To date, there are no therapeutic HIV vaccines approved by the FDA. The ideal therapeutic would (i) slow down the progression of HIV infection; (ii) eliminate the need for ART while still keeping undetectable levels of HIV; and (iii) eliminate all HIV from the body (NIAID 2016). In 2016 an NIH-supported clinical trial was launched to test a modified HIV vaccine called HVTN 702, testing whether an experimental vaccine regimen could safely prevent HIV infection among South African adults. The data are still pending.

Q. What is CRISPR and how does it fit into HIV research?

A. CRISPR/Cas9, described in 2012, is designed to generate cells carrying precise gene mutations, including rearrangement and deletion within chromosomes. It also has the ability to remove entire chromosomes. This opens new avenues for modeling and generating therapies for HIV research. One approach focuses on using CRISPR to cut HIV virus out of the DNA of immune cells while another approach makes human cells resistant to HIV infections similar to the delta 32 mutation. In 2016, Kaminski et al., using lentivirus delivered by CRISPR/Cas9, showed that gene editing significantly diminished HIV-1 replication in infected primary CD4+ T cell cultures and drastically reduced viral load in cultures of CD4+ T cells obtained from HIV-1-infected patients (Kaminski et al. 2016). This protocol could provide a new therapeutic platform for curing AIDS. Ophinni's group designed RNA-guided CRISPR/Cas9 targeting the HIV-1 regulatory genes *tat* and *rev* with guide RNAs (gRNA) cloned into lentiCRISPRv2 and transduced into 293 T and HeLa cells. The expressed Tat and Rev proteins successfully abolished the expression of each protein relative to the control cells. CRISPR/Cas9 was further tested in persistently and latently HIV-1-infected T cell lines in culture, in which p24 levels were significantly suppressed even after cytokine reactivation (Ophinni et al. 2018).

Q. Where do we go from here?

A. Dr Fauci, NIAID Director, noted at a plenary lecture titled "Ending the HIV/AIDS Pandemic: The Critical Role of HIV Prevention Science" that despite the availability of HIV prevention modalities such as treatment as prevention and PrEP, the rate of new HIV infections worldwide has declined minimally in recent years (Fauci 2018). He went on to say that a durable end to the HIV/AIDS pandemic would require the development and widespread implementation of new and improved HIV prevention tools.

Current treatments have dramatically reduced HIV-associated morbidity and mortality, prolonged survival, and prevented HIV transmission. However, eradication of the disease cannot be achieved with current HIV treatments due to latently infected CD4+ T cells. US and

European guidelines have begun to emphasize INSTIs because of their high levels of efficacy, safety, and tolerability. These treatment regimens are based on many factors including drug efficacy, pill and dosing requirements, drug–drug interaction, adverse effects, individual resistance test results, comorbid conditions, and/or economic status. Yet, due to viral latency, the ability to sustain viral suppression still depends on the patient adhering to treatment regimens for decades because of the sequestered virus. An effective cure must possess the ability to locate these dormant viruses and eradicate them.

To that end, medical research is focused on latency-reversing agents to activate the viral reservoirs involving techniques such as immunotherapies, innate immunity activators, effector antibodies, gene therapies, and therapeutic vaccines to eliminate the persistent viral reservoirs and/or induce effective immune control of HIV infection (Archin et al. 2014; Chun et al. 2015). There are currently ~52 medicines, drugs and/or vaccines in development, including novel combination treatments, improved therapies, and preventive vaccines; 32 are antiretrovirals and antivirals, 16 are vaccines and four are cell therapies and all are in some stage of clinical trials or awaiting review by the FDA (PhRMA 2017). One has to believe that there are strategies yet to be developed that will unlock the cure that has to date evaded our best efforts.

You may have read about the new drug Gammora. Preliminary trials indicated that it could substantially reduce viral load by 99% within four weeks by killing infected cells without harming the healthy ones (All Africa 2018). The treatment consisted of a synthetic peptide compound derived from the HIV-derived integrase that stimulated the integration of multiple HIV DNA fragments into the host cell's genomic DNA and triggered the infected cell's apoptosis or self-destruction (Papadopoulos 2018). The researchers did not suggest that the drug was effective in eliminating viral reservoirs and it was not clear if the drug was more effective than the cART that the subjects were also taking. The study was conducted by researchers at Zion Medical and the Hebrew University of Jerusalem. However, it only included nine subjects, Phase 2 trials have not yet been initiated, and the data have not been peer reviewed. Substantiating the data will involve many steps and could take several years, but there is hope.

Individuals can help those infected with HIV by working to reduce the stigma associated with the disease, by reaching out to local HIV service organizations, and/or engaging with others through www.hiv.gov/digital-tools. People can also engage through social media like Facebook, Twitter, Instagram or Snapchat, to connect with others who are interested and involved in HIV issues. Or they can get involved in HIV awareness days to stay abreast of developments in HIV research. These steps will ensure an educated and engaged electorate.

Acknowledgments

I wish to thank Dr Daniel Malamud and Dr William Abrams for generously sharing their knowledge and expertise.

References

AIDS Institute (2011). Where did HIV come from? www.theaidsinstitute.org/education/aids-101/where-did-hiv-come-0.

AIDSinfo (2018a). HIV and Drug and Alcohol Users. HIV and Specific Populations. https://aidsinfo.nih.gov/understanding-hiv-aids/fact-sheets/22/63/hiv-medicines-and-side-effects.

AIDSinfo (2018b). Recommendations for Use of Antiretroviral Drugs During Pregnancy. https://aidsinfo.nih.gov/guidelines/html/3/perinatal/488/overview.

AIDSinfo (2018c). Side Effects of HIV Medicines. HIV Medicines and Side Effects. https://aidsinfo.nih.gov/understanding-hiv-aids/fact-sheets/22/63/hiv-medicines-and-side-effects.

Alford, D.P., Compton, P., and Samet, J.H. (2006). Acute pain management for patients receiving maintenance methadone or buprenorphine therapy [published correction appears in Ann Intern Med 2006 Mar 21;144(6):460]. *Annals of Internal Medicine* 144 (2): 127–134.

All Africa (2018). Kenya: Study – New HIV Drug Gammora is 99% Effective. https://allafrica.com/stories/201811050278.html.

Almiñana-Pastor, P.J., Segarra-Vidal, M., López-Roldán, A., and Alpiste-Illueca, F.M. (2017). A controlled clinical study of periodontal health in anticoagulated patients: assessment of bleeding on probing. *Journal of Clinical and Experimental Dentistry* 9 (12): e1431–e1438.

Alvarez, P.A. and Pahissa, J. (2010). QT alterations in psychopharmacology: proven candidates and suspects. *Current Drug Safety* 5 (1): 97–104.

American Academy of Periodontology (1996). Periodontal management of patients with cardiovascular diseases. *Journal of Periodontology* 67: 627–635.

American Academy of Periodontology (2004a). Position paper. Systemic antibiotics in periodontics. *Journal of Periodontology* 75: 1553–1565.

American Academy of Periodontology (2004b). Task force on periodontal treatment of pregnant women. *Journal of Periodontology* 75: 495.

American Association of Oral and Maxillofacial Surgeons (2009). Position Paper on Bisphosphonate-Related Osteonecrosis of the Jaw – 2009 Update. Advisory Task Force on Bisphosphonate-Related Osteonecrosis of the Jaws. *Journal of Oral and Maxillofacial Surgery* 67: 2–12.

American Dental Association (2002). Gingival retraction cord. *Journal of the American Dental Association* 133: 653.

American Dental Association (2011). ADA professional product review. *Journal of the American Dental Association* 6: 1–16.

American Dental Association: American Academy of Orthopaedic Surgeons. Advisory Statement (2003). Antibiotic prophylaxis for dental patients with total joint replacements. *Journal of the American Dental Association* 134: 895–898.

American Dental Hygiene Association (2011). www.adha.org/ce_course15/oral_antiplatelet_agents.htm.

Antiretroviral PregRegis (2016). Prenatal exposure to zidovudine and risk for ventricular septal defects and congenital heart defects: data from the antiretroviral pregnancy registry. *European Journal of Obstetrics & Gynecology and Reproductive Biology* 197: 6–10.

Archin, N.M., Sung, J., Garrido, C. et al. (2014). Eradicating HIV-1 infection: seeking to clear a persistent pathogen. *Nature Reviews Microbiology* 11: 750–764.

Ardekian, L., Gaspar, R., Peled, M. et al. (2000). Does low-dose aspirin therapy complicate oral surgical procedures? *Journal of the American Dental Association* 131: 331–335.

Arrode-Brusés, G., Sheffer, D. et al. (2010). Characterization of T-cell responses in macaques immunized with a single dose of HIV DNA vaccine. *Journal of Virology* 84 (3): 1243–1253.

Auclair, S., Liu, F., Niu, Q. et al. (2018). Distinct susceptibility of HIV vaccine vector-induced CD4 T cells to HIV infection. *PLOS Pathogens* 14 (2): e100688.

Awtry, E.H. and Loscalzo, J. (2000). Aspirin. *Circulation* 101: 1206–1218.

Baddour, L.M., Epstein, A.E., Erickson, C.C. et al. (2011). A summary of the update on cardiovascular implantable electronic device infections and their management. *Journal of the American Dental Association* 142: 159–165.

Barasch, A., Cunha-Cruz, J., Curro, F.A. et al. (2011). Risk factors for osteonecrosis of the jaws: a case-control study from the CONDOR dental PBRN. *Journal of Dental Research* 90: 439–444.

Beach, S.R., Celano, C.M., Noseworthy, P.A. et al. (2013). QTc prolongation, torsades de pointes, and psychotropic medications. *Psychosomatics* 54 (1): 1–13.

Bell, W.R. (1998). Acetaminophen and warfarin. Undesirable synergy. *Journal of the American Medical Association* 279: 702–703.

Bradley, J.G. and Davis, K.A. (2003). Orthostatic hypotension. *American Family Physician* 68: 2393–2399.

Brennan, M.T., Valerin, M.A., Noll, J.L. et al. (2008). Aspirin use and post-operative bleeding from dental extractions. *Journal of Dental Research* 87: 740–744.

Buchbinder, S.P., Mehrotra, D.V., Duerr, A. et al. (2009). Efficacy assessment of a cell-mediated immunity HIV-1 vaccine (the step study): a double-blind, randomized, placebo-controlled, test-of-concept trial. *Lancet* 374 (9696): 1119.

Budenz, A.W. (2008). Local anesthetics and medically complex patients. *Journal of the California Dental Association* 28: 611–619.

Buhler, M. and Mann, K. (2011). Alcohol and the human brain: a systematic review of different neuroimaging methods. *Alcoholism: Clinical and Experimental Research* 35 (10): 1771–1793.

Cardona-Tortajada, F., Sainz-Gómez, E., Figuerido-Garmendia, J. et al. (2009). Dental extractions in patients on antiplatelet therapy. A study conducted by the Oral Health Department of the Navarre Health Service (Spain). *Medicina Oral Patologia Oral y Cirugia Bucal* 14: e588–e592.

CDC (2013). *HIV Surveillance Report*, Diagnoses of HIV Infection in the United States and Dependent Areas, vol. 25. www.cdc.gov/hiv/pdf/library/reports/surveillance/cdc-hiv-surveillance-report-2013-vol-25.pdf.

CDC (2014). Closing the Gaps in HIV Prevention & Care. Annual Report, Prevention D.O.H.A. www.cdc.gov/hiv/pdf/policies/cdc-hiv-2014-dhap-annual-report.pdf.

CDC (2018a). Division of HIV/AIDS Prevention, National Center for HIV/AIDS, Viral Hepatitis, STD, and TB Prevention. www.cdc.gov/hiv/basics/transmission.html.

CDC (2018b). Persons with HIV: Prevention and Care. www.cdc.gov/hiv/guidelines/index.html.

CDC (2018c). Preexposure prophylaxis for the prevention of HIV infection in the United States, A clinical practice guideline. https://jamanetwork.com/journals/jama/fullarticle/2735509.

Cho, C.M., Hirsch, R., and Johnstone, S. (2005). General and oral health implications of cannabis use. *Australian Dental Journal* 50: 70–74.

Chun, T.W., Nickle, D.C., Justement, J.S. et al. (2008). Persistence of HIV in gut-associated lymphoid tissue despite long-term antiretroviral therapy. *Journal of Infectious Diseases* 197: 714–720.

Chun, T., Moir, S., and Fauci, A.S. (2015). HIV reservoirs as obstacles and opportunities for an HIV cure. *Nature Immunology* 16: 584–589.

Ciancio, S.G. (2004). Medications' impact on oral health. *Journal of the American Dental Association* 135: 1440–1448.

Cihlar, T. and Fordyce, M. (2016). Current status and prospects of HIV treatment. *Current Opinion in Virology* 18: 50–56.

Cipriani, A., Hawton, K., Stockton, S., and Geddes, J.R. (2013). Lithium in the prevention of suicide in mood disorders: updated systematic review and metanalysis. *British Journal of Medicine* 346: f3646.

Clercq, E.D. (2004). Non-nucleoside reverse transcriptase inhibitors (NNRTI): past, present, and future. *Chemistry & Biodiversity* 1 (1): 44–64.

Coelho, A.V.C., Celsi, F., Tricarico, O.M., and Crovella, S. (2017). Antiretroviral treatment in HIV-1-positive mothers: neurological implications in virus-free children. *International Journal of Molecular Sciences* 18 (2): 423.

Cook, R.T. (1998). Alcohol abuse, alcoholism, and damage to the immune system. *Alcoholism: Clinical and Experimental Research* 22 (9): 1927–1942.

Craft, S., Baker, L., Montine, T. et al. (2012). Intranasal insulin therapy for Alzheimer disease and amnestic mild cognitive impairment: a pilot clinical trial. *Archives of Neurology* 69: 29–38.

Craft, S., Cholerton, B., and Baker, L.D. (2013). Insulin and Alzheimer's disease: untangling the web. *Journal of Alzheimers Disease* 33: S263–S275.

Dahabieh, M., Battivelli, E., and Verdin, E. (2015). Understanding HIV latency: the road to an HIV cure. *Annual Review of Medicine* 66: 407–421.

Dajani, A.S., Taubert, K.A., Wilson, W. et al. (1997). Prevention of bacterial endocarditis. Recommendations by the American Heart Association. *Circulation* 96: 358–366.

Daly, C. (2016). Treating patients on new anticoagulant drugs. *Australian Prescriber* 39: 205–207.

database (2018). HIV Circulating Recombinant Forms (CRFs). www.hiv.lanl.gov/content/sequence/HIV/CRFs/CRFs.html.

Deacon, J.M., Pagliaro, A.J., Zelicof, S.B. et al. (1996). Prophylactic use of antibiotics for procedures after total joint replacement. *Journal of Bone and Joint Surgery* 78: 1755–1770.

Desmonde, S., Goetghebuer, T., Thorne, C., and Leroy, V. (2016). Health and survival of HIV perinatally exposed but uninfected children born to HIV-infected mothers. *Current Opinion in HIV and AIDS* 11: 465–476.

Donaldson, M. and Goodchild, J.H. (2006). Oral health of the methamphetamine abuser. *American Journal of Health-System Pharmacy* 63: 2078–2082.

Eastell, R. and Walsh, J.S. (2017). Anabolic treatment for osteoporosis: teriparatide. *Clinical Cases in Mineral and Bone Metabolism* 14 (2): 173–178.

Eggers, C., Arendt, G., Hahn, K. et al. (2017). HIV-1-associated neurocognitive disorder: epidemiology, pathogenesis, diagnosis, and treatment. *Journal of Neurology* 264: 1715–1727.

Elliott, J.H., Wightman, F., Solomon, A. et al. (2014). Activation of HIV transcription with short-course vorinostat in HIV-infected patients on suppressive antiretroviral therapy. *PLoS Pathogens* 10 (10): e1004473.

Elliott, J.H., McMahon, J.H., Chang, C.C. et al. (2015). Short-term administration of disulfiram for reversal of latent HIV infection: a phase 2 dose-escalation study. *Lancet HIV* 2 (12): e520–e529.

Ellis, R.J., Letendre, S., Vaida, F. et al. (2014). Randomized trial of central nervous system-targeted antiretrovirals for HIV-associated neurocognitive disorder. *Clinical Infectious Diseases* 58: 1015–1022.

Elliston, V.T.V. and Kochetkov, S.N. (2017). Novel HIV 1 non-nucleoside reverse transcriptase inhibitors: a combinatorial approach. *Biochemistry* 82 (13): 1716–1743.

Esmaeili, P., Boissier, N., and Valcour, V. (2015). HIV-associated Neurocognitive Disorder (HAND). www.caregiver.org/hiv-associated-neurocognitive-disorder-hand.

Fama, R. (2009). Working and episodic memory in HIV infection, alcoholism, and their comorbidity: baseline and 1-year follow-up examinations. *Alcoholism: Clinical and Experimental Research* 33: 1815–1824.

Fama, R. (2011). Remote semantic memory for public figures in HIV infection, alcoholism, and their comorbidity. *Alcoholism: Clinical and Experimental Research* 35 (2): 265–276.

Fauci, S. (2018). HIV remission free of antiretroviral therapy is a feasible goal. 22nd International AIDS Conference. www.eurekalert.org/pub_releases/2018-07/nioa-fhr072418.php.

Fois, A.F. and Brew, B.J. (2015). The potential of the CNS as a reservoir for HIV-1 infection: implications for HIV eradication. *Current HIV/AIDS Reports* 12: 299–303.

Fugazzotto, P.A., Lightfoot, W.S., Jaffin, R. et al. (2007). Implant placement with or without simultaneous tooth extraction in patients taking oral bisphosphonates: postoperative healing, early follow-up, and the incidence of complications in two private practices. *Journal of Periodontology* 78: 1664–1669.

Ganda, K. (2008). Anticoagulants warfarin (Coumadin), standard heparin, and low molecular weight heparin (LMWH): assessment, analysis, and associated dental management guidelines. In: *Dentist's Guide to Medical Conditions and Complications*, 169–174. Ames, IA: Wiley Blackwell.

Garbutt, J.C. (2018). 12 Health Risks of Chronic Heavy Drinking. www.onhealth.com/content/1/heavy_drinking_alcohol_abuse.

Georgakopoulou, E.A., Achtari, M.D., and Afentoulide, N. (2011). Dental management of patients before and after renal transplantation. *Stomatologija, Baltic Dental and Maxillofacial Journal* 13: 107–112.

Gibson, N. and Ferguson, J.W. (2004). Steroid cover for dental patients on long-term steroid medication: proposed clinical guidelines based upon a critical review of the literature. *British Dental Journal* 197: 681–685.

Giglio, J.A. and Laskin, D.M. (2010). Prevalence of psychiatric disorders in a group of adult patients seeking general dental care. *Quintessence International* 41 (5): 433–437.

Gilbert, E.M., Darin, K.M., Scarsi, K.K., and McLaughlin, M.M. (2015). Antiretroviral pharmacokinetics in pregnant women. *Pharmacotherapy* 35: 838–855.

Gonzalez, S.F. and Martin-Garcia, J. (2005). The neuropathogenesis of aids. *Nature Reviews Immunology* 5: 69–81.

Goodchild, J.H. and Donaldson, M. (2007). Methamphetamine abuse and dentistry: a review of the literature and presentation of a clinical case. *Quintessence International* 38: 583–590.

Goss, A., Bartold, M., Smabrook, P., and Hawker, P. (2010). The nature and frequency of bisphosphonate-associated ostenecrosis of the jaws in dental implant patients: a south Australian case series. *Journal of Oral and Maxillofacial Surgery* 68: 337–343.

Grewal, V.S. and Fayans, E.P. (2008). Bisphosphonate-associated osteonecrosis. A clinician's reference to patient management. *New York State Dental Journal* 74 (1): 38–44.

Hansen, S.G., Ford, J.C., Lewis, M.S. et al. (2011). Profound early control of highly pathogenic SIV by an effector memory T-cell vaccine. *Nature* 473: 523–527.

Harbison, C., Zhuang, K., and Westmoreland, S. (2014). Giant cell encephalitis and microglial infection with mucosally transmitted simian-human immunodeficiency virus SHIVSF162P3N in rhesus macaques. *Journal of Neurovirology* 20 (1): 62–72.

Hatziioannou, T. and Evans, D.T. (2012). Animal models for HIV/AIDS research. *Nature Reviews Microbiology* 10 (12): 852–867.

Haynes, B.F., Gilbert, P.B., McElrath, M.J. et al. (2012). Immune-correlates analysis of an HIV-1 vaccine efficacy. *New England Journal of Medicine* 366: 1275–1286.

Hayward, K.L., Powell, E.E., Irvine, K.M., and Martin, J.H. (2016). Can paracetamol (acetaminophen) be administered to patients with liver impairment? *British Journal of Clinical Pharmacology* 81 (2): 210–222.

Heffron, R., Pintye, J., Matthews, L.T. et al. (2016). PrEP as peri-conception HIV prevention for women and men. *Current HIV/AIDS Reports* 13: 131–139.

Hemelaar, J. (2012). The origin and diversity of the HIV-1 pandemic. *Trends in Molecular Medicine* 18 (3): 182–192.

Higuchi, H., Yabuki, A., Ishii-Maruhama, M. et al. (2014). Hemodynamic changes by drug interaction of adrenaline with chlorpromazine. *Anesthesia Progress* 61 (4): 150–154.

Hill, A.L., Rosenbloom, D.I., Fu, F. et al. (2014). Predicting the outcomes of treatment to eradicate the latent reservoir for HIV-1. *Proceedings of the National Academy of Sciences of the United States of America* 111: 13475–13480.

HIV Sequence (2017). HIV and SIV Nomenclature. www.hiv.lanl.gov/content/sequence/HelpDocs/subtypes-more.html.

Horn, J.R. and Hansten, P.D. (2009) The dangers of beta-blockers and epinephrine. www. pharmacytimes.com/publications/issue/2009/2009-05/druginteractionsbetablockers-0509.

Horowitz, L.G. and Nersasian, R.R. (1978). A review of marijuana in relations to stress-response mechanisms in the dental patient. *Journal of the American Dental Association* 96 (6): 983–986.

Hughes, G.J., Patel, P.N., and Saxena, N. (2011). Effect of acetaminophen on international normalized raio in patients receiving warfarin therapy. *Pharmacotherapy* 31 (6): 591–597.

Hylek, E.M., Heiman, H., Skates, S.J. et al. (1998). Acetaminophen and other risk factors for excessive warfarin anticoagulation. *Journal of the American Medical Association* 279: 657–662.

International Academy of Oral Medicine and Toxicology (2007). IAOMT Position Paper on Human Jawbone Osteonecrosis. https://iaomt.org/wp-content/uploads/JON-Position-Paper.pdf.

Jacobson, J.M., Routy, J., Welles, S. et al. (2017). Dendritic cell immunotherapy for HIV-1 infection using autologous HIV-1 RNA: a randomized, double-blind, placebo-controlled clinical trial. *Journal of Acquired Immune Deficiency Syndromes* 72 (1): 31–38.

Jeffcoat, M., Sedghizadeh, P.P., and Subramanian G. (2011). International Association of Dental Research (IADR) 89th General Session and Exhibition: Abstract 890. San Diego, CA.

Jeske, A.H. and Suchko, G.D. (2003). Lack of a scientific basis for routine discontinuation of oral anticoagulation therapy before dental treatment. *Journal of the American Dental Association* 134: 1492–1497.

Jones, A., Seghizadeh, P., and Khuat, C. (2011). New light shed on bisphosphonates and BRONJ. *Academy News. Academy of Osseointegration* 22 (8): 10.

Joska, J.A., Witten, J., Thomas, K.G. et al. (2016). A comparison of five brief screening tools for HIV-associated neurocognitive disorders in the USA and South Africa. *AIDS and Behavior* 20 (8): 1621–1631.

Kalmar, J. (2009). Oral manifestations of drug reactions. http://emedicine.medscape.com/article/1080772-overview.

Kaminski, R., Chen, Y., Fischer, T. et al. (2016). Elimination of HIV-1 genomes from human T-lymphoid cells by CRISPR/ Cas9 gene editing. *Scientific Reports* 6: 22555.

Kassab, M.M., Radmer, T.W., Glore, J.W. et al. (2011). A retrospective review of clinical international normalized ratio results and their implications. *Journal of the American Dental Association* 142: 1252–1257.

Kelly-Sell, M.J., Kim, Y.H., Strauss, S. et al. (2012). The histone deacetylase inhibitor, romidepsin, suppresses cellular immune functions of cutaneous T cell lymphoma patients. *American Journal of Hematology* 87 (4): 354–360.

Killick, M., Grant, M.L., Cerutti, N.M. et al. (2015). Env–2dCD4S60C complexes act as super immunogens and elicit potent, broadly neutralizing antibodies against clinically relevant human immunodeficiency virus type 1 (HIV-1). *Vaccine* 33 (46): 6298–6306.

Kim, J.H., Rerks-Ngarm, S., Excler, J., and Michael, N. (2010). HIV vaccines: lessons learned and the way forward. *Current Opinion in HIV and AIDS* 5 (5): 428–434.

Kim, J.H., Excler, J., and Michael, N. (2015). Lessons from the RV144 Thai phase III HIV-1 vaccine trial and the search for correlates of protection. *Annual Review of Medicine* 66: 423–437.

Kimani, R.W. (2018). Assessment and diagnosis of HIV-associated dementia. *Journal for Nurse Practitioners* 14 (3): 190–195.

Kisely, S. (2016). No mental health without oral health. *Canadian Journal of Psychiatry* 61 (5): 277–282.

Klasser, G.D. and Epstein, J.B. (2006). The methamphetamine epidemic and dentistry. *General Dentisty* 54: 431–439.

Koka, S., Babu, N.M.S., and Norell, A. (2010). Survival of dental implants in post-menopausal bisphosphonate users. *Journal of Prosthodontic Research* 54: 108–111.

Koob, G.F. (2018). Alcohol and the aging brain. https://niaaa.scienceblog.com/103/alcohol-and-the-aging-brain.

Kronfol, A., Nair, M., and Goel, K. (1993). Lymphocyte subset and natural killer cytoxicity in alcoholism. *Advances in Biosciences* 86: 115–119.

Krubiner, C.B., Faden, R.R., Cadigan, R.J. et al. (2016). Advancing HIV research with pregnant women: navigating challenges and opportunities. *AIDS Patient Care and STDs* 30: 2261–2265.

Kuruvilla, M. and Gurk-Turner, C. (2001). A review of warfarin dosing and monitoring. *Proceedings (Baylor University Medical Center)* 14: 305–306.

Lai, D. and Jones, T. (2002). Remune. Immune Response. *Current Opinion in Investigational Drugs* 3 (3): 391–398.

Lambrecht, J.T., Greuter, C., and Surber, C. (2013). Antidepressants relevant to oral and maxillofacial surgical practice. *Annals of Maxillofacial Surgery* 3 (2): 160–166.

Lamster, I.B., Lalla, E., Borgnakke, W.S. et al. (2008). The relationship between oral health and diabetes mellitus. *Journal of the American Dental Association* 139 (Suppl 5): 19 s–24 s.

Landesberg, R., Cozin, M., Cremers, S. et al. (2008). Inhibition of oral mucosal cell wound healing by bisphosphonates. *Journal of Oral and Maxillofacial Surgery* 61: 1115–1117.

Langford, D., Marquie-Beck, J., de Almeida, S. et al. (2014). Giant cell encephalitis and microglial infection with mucosally transmitted simian-human immunodeficiency virus SHIVSF162P3N in rhesus macaques. *Journal of NeuroVirology* 20 (1): 62–72.

Langford, D., Marquie-Beck, J., de Almeida, S. et al. (2017). Relationship of antiretroviral treatment to postmortem brain tissue viral load in HIV-infected patients. *Journal of Neurology* 264: 1715–1727.

Lederman, M.M. and Pike, E. (2017). Ten years HIV free: an interview with "the Berlin patient," Timothy Ray Brown. *Pathogens and Immunity* 2 (3): 422–430.

Lee, J.M. and Shin, T.J. (2017). Use of local anesthetics for dental treatment during pregnancy; safety for parturient. *Journal of Dental Anesthesia and Pain Medicine* 17 (2): 81–90.

Lee, C.Y. and Suzuki, J.B. (2010). CTX biochemical marker of bone metabolism. Is it a reliable predictor of bisphosphonate-associated osteonecrosis of the jaws after surgery? Part II: a prospective clinical study. *Implant Dentistry* 19 (1): 29–38.

Leth, S., Schleimann, M.H., Nissen, S.K. et al. (2016). Combined effect of Vacc-4x, recombinant human granulocyte macrophage colony-stimulating factor vaccination, and romidepsin on the HIV-1 reservoir (REDUC): a single arm, phase 1B/2A trial. *Lancet* 3 (10): e463–e472.

Lifshey, F.M. (2004). Evaluation of and treatment considerations for the dental patient with cardiac disease. *New York State Dental Journal* 70: 16–19.

Lihana, R.W., Ssemwanga, D., Abimiku, A., and Ndembi, N. (2014). Update on HIV-1 diversity in Africa: a decade in review. *AIDS Patient Care and STDs* 14 (2): 83–100.

Little, J.W., Miller, C., Robert, H. et al. (2002). Antithrombotic agents: implications in dentistry. *Oral Surgery Oral Medicine Oral Pathology Oral Radiology Endotontology* 93: 544–551.

Little, J.W., Fallace, D.A., Miller, C.S., and Rhodus, N.L. (2008). *Dental Management of the Medically Compromised Patient*, 7e, 236–247. St Louis: Mosby.

Little, J.W., Jacobson, J.J., and Lockhart, P.B. (2010). The dental treatment of patients with joint replacements. *Journal of the American Dental Association* 141: 667–671.

Lockhart, P.B., Loven, B., Brennan, M.T. et al. (2007). The evidence base for the efficacy of antibiotic prophylaxis in dental practice. *Journal of the American Dental Association* 138 (4): 458–474.

Lu, S. (2009). Heterologous prime-boost vaccination. *Current Opinions in Immunology* 21 (3): 346–351.

Lucar, O., Su, B., Potard, V. et al. (2017). Neutralizing antibodies against a specific human immunodeficiency virus gp41 epitope are associated with long-term non-progressor status. *EBioMedicine* 22: 122–132.

Madan, G.A., Madan, S.G., Madan, G. et al. (2005). Minor oral surgery without stopping daily low-dose aspirin therapy: a study of 51 patients. *Journal of Oral and Maxillofacial Surgery* 63: 1262–1265.

Malamed, S.F. (1993). Physical evaluation and the prevention of medical emergencies: vital signs. *Anesthesia & Pain Control in Dentistry* 2: 107–113.

Malik, M. and Camm, A.J. (2001). Evaluation of drug-induced QT interval prolongation: implications for drug approval and labelling. *Drug Safety* 24 (5): 323–351.

Mamede, J.I., Cianci, G.C., Anderson, M.R., and Hope, T.J. (2017). Early cytoplasmic uncoating is associated with infectivity of HIV-1. *Proceedings of the National Academy of Sciences of the United States of America* 114 (34): 7169–7178.

Mandelbrot, L. and Tubiana, R. (2015). No perinatal HIV-1 transmission from women with effective antiretroviral therapy starting before conception. *Clinical Infectious Diseases* 61: 1715–1725.

Marx, R.E., Cillo, J.E. Jr., and Ulloa, J.J. (2007). Oral bisphosphonate-induced osteonecrosis: risk factors, prediction of risk using serum CTx testing, prevention, and treatment. *Journal of Oral and Maxillofacial Surgery* 65: 2397–2410.

McArthur, J.C., Brew, B.J., and Nath, A. (2005). Neurological complications of HIV infection. *Lancet* 4: 543–555.

McAuthur, J.C., Steiner, J., Sacktor, N., and Nath, A. (2010). Human immunodeficiency virus-associated neurocognitive disorder: mind the gap. *Annals of Neurology* 67: 699–714.

McCance-Katz, E.F., Gruber, V.A., Beatty, G. et al. (2013). Interactions between alcohol and the antiretroviral medications ritonavir or efavirenz. *Journal of Addiction Medicine* 4: 264–270.

Mealey, B.L. and Oates, T.W. (2006). Diabetes mellitus and periodontal diseases. *Journal of Periodontology* 77: 1289–1303.

Melkova, Z., Shankaran, P., Madlenakova, M., and Bodor, J. (2017). Current views on HIV-1 latency, persistence, and cure. *Folia Microbiologica* 62 (1): 73–87.

Michalowicz, B.S., DiAngelis, A.J., Novak, M.J. et al. (2008). Examining the safety of dental treatment in pregnant women. *Journal of the American Dental Association* 139: 686–695.

Miguez, M.J., Posner, G., Morales, G. et al. (2003). HIV treatment in drug abusers: impact of alcohol use. *Addiction Biology* 8: 33–37.

Mofenson, L.M., Baggaley, R.C., and Mameletzis, I. (2017). Tenofovir disoproxil fumarate safety for women and their infants during pregnancy and breastfeeding. *AIDS Patient Care and STDs* 31: 213–232.

Momenan, R., Steckler, L.E., Saad, Z.S. et al. (2012). Effects of alcohol dependence on cortical thickness as determined by magnetic resonance imaging. *Psychiatry Research* 204: 101–111.

Monnig, M.A., Tonigan, J.S., Yeo, R.A. et al. (2013). White matter volume in alcohol use disorders: a meta-analysis. *Addiction Biology* 18: 581–592.

Muzzin, K.B. and O'Brien, C. (2010). Dealing with the devastation. How to provide oral heath care to patients with a history of methamphetamine abuse. *Dimensions of Dental Hygiene* 8: 42–45.

Nahas, G. and Latour, C. (1992). The human toxicity of marijuana. *Medical Journal of Australia* 3: 163–184.

Napeñas, J.J., Hong, C.H.L., Brennan, M.T. et al. (2009). The frequency of bleeding complications after invasive dental treatment in patients receiving single and dual antiplatelet therapy. *Journal of the American Dental Association* 140: 690–695.

Napenas, J.J., Hong, C.H., Kempter, E. et al. (2011). Selective serotonin reuptake inhibitors and oral bleeding complications after invasive dental treatment. *Oral Surgery, Oral Medicine, Oral Pathology, Oral Radiology, and Endodontics* 112 (4): 463–467.

New York State Department of Health (2006). Oral Health Care During Pregnancy and Early Childhood. Practice Guidelines. www.health.ny.gov/publications/0824.pdf.

Newton, T.F., de La Garza, R. 2nd, Kalechstein, A.D. et al. (2005). Cocaine and methamphetamine produce different patterns of subjective and cardiovascular effects. *Pharmacology, Biochemistry, and Behavior* 82: 90–97.

NIAID (2016). First New HIV Vaccine Efficacy Study in Seven Years Has Begun. South Africa Hosts Historic NIH-Supported Clinical Trial. www.niaid.nih.gov/news-events/first-new-hiv-vaccine-efficacy-study-seven-years-has-begun.

Nicholson, J.B. (2016). The immune system. *Essays in Biochemistry* 60 (3): 275–301.

Nicolatou-Galitis, O., Papadopoulou, E., Sarri, T. et al. (2011). Osteoneocrosis of the jaw in oncology patients treated with bisphosphonates: prospective experience of a dental oncology referral center. *Oral Surgery Oral Medicine Oral Pathology Oral Radiology and Endodontology* 112: 195–202.

NIH (2013). Key HIV Protein Structure Revealed. www.nih.gov/news-events/nih-research-matters/key-hiv-protein-structure-revealed.

NIH (2018). HIV and Lipodystrophy. https://aidsinfo.nih.gov/understanding-hiv-aids/fact-sheets/22/61/hiv-and-lipodystrophy.

Nishimura, R.A., Otto, C.M., Bonow, R.O. et al. (2017). 2017 AHA/ACC focused update of the 2014 AHA/ACC guideline for the Management of Patients with Valvular Heart Disease: a report of the American College of Cardiology/American Heart Association Task Force on Clinical Practice Guidelines. *Circulation* 135 (25): e1159–e1195.

Norman, L.R. and Basso, M. (2015). An update of the review of neuropsychological consequence of HIV and substance abuse: a Litature review and implications for treatment and future research. *Current Drug Abuse Reviews* 8: 50–71.

Ophinni, Y., Inoue, M., Kotaki, T., and Kameoka, M. (2018). CRISPR/Cas9 system targeting regulatory genes of HIV-1 inhibits viral replication in infected T-cell cultures. *Scientific Reports* 8: 7784.

Paauw, D.S. (2017). Antibiotic prophylaxis for artificial joints. www.mdedge.com/internalmedicine/article/132023/infectious-diseases/antibiotic-prophylaxis-artificial-joints.

Page II, R.L. (2005). Weighing the cardiovascular benefits of low-dose aspirin. ACPE Program ID Number: 290–000–05-H01. www.pharmacytimes.com.

Pallasch, T.J. (1998). Vasoconstrictors and the heart. *Journal of the California Dental Association* 26: 668–673, 676.

Papadopoulos. L. (2018). First Human Clinical Trial of HIV Drug Gammora Offers Potential Cure. https://interestingengineering.com/first-human-clinical-trial-of-hiv-drug-gammora-offers-potential-cure.

Park, S.Q., Kahnt, T., Beck, A. et al. (2010). Prefrontal cortex fails to learn from reward prediction errors in alcohol dependence. *Journal of Neuroscience* 30 (22): 7749–7753.

Patel, R. and Paya, C.V. (1997). Infections in solid organ transplant recipients. *Clinical Microbiology Reviews* 10: 86–124.

Patrono, C., Collar, B., Dalen, J. et al. (1998). Platelet-active drugs: the relationships among dose, effectiveness, and side effects. *Chest* 114: 470S–488S.

Patrono, C., Coller, B., FitzGerald, G.A. et al. (2004). Platelet-active drugs: the relationships among dose, effectiveness, and side effects. The seventh ACCP conference on antithrombotic and thrombolytic therapy. *Chest* 126 (3 Suppl): 234 S–264 S.

Peiperl, L., McElrath, M.J., Kalams, S. et al. (2014). Phase I/II randomized trial of safety and immunogenicity of LIPO-5 alone, ALVAC-HIV (vCP1452) alone, and ALVAC-HIV (vCP1452) prime/LIPO-5 boost in healthy, HIV-1-uninfected adult participants. *Clinical and Vaccine Immunology* 21 (11): 1589–1599.

Persidsky, Y., Ho, Y., Ramirez, S.H. et al. (2011). HIV-1 infection and alcohol abuse: neurocognitive impairment, mechanisms of neurodegeneration and therapeutic intervention. *Brain, Behavior, and Immunity* 25 (Suppl): 561–570.

Pérusse, R., Goulet, J.P., and Turcotte, J.Y. (1992). Contraindications to vasoconstrictors in dentistry: part II. *Oral Surgery Oral Medicine Oral Pathology* 74: 687–691.

Petravic, J., Rasmussen, T.A., Lewis, S.R. et al. (2017). Relationship between measures of HIV reactivation and decline of the latent reservoir under latency-reversing agents. *Jounal of Virology* 91 (9): ii.

Petry, N. (1999). Alcohol use in HIV patients: what we don't know may hurt us. *International Journal of STD & AIDS* 10: 561–570.

PhRMA (2017). More Than 50 Medicines and Vaccines in Development for HIV/AIDS Infection Treatment and Prevention. www.phrma.org/press-release/more-than-50-medicines-and-vaccines-in-development-for-hiv-infection-treatment-and-prevention.

Pinto, A., Farrar, J.T., and Hersh, E.V. (2009). Prescribing NSAIDs to patients on SSRIs: possible adverse drug interaction of importance to dental practitioners. *Compendium of Continuing Education in Dentistry* 30 (3): 142–151; quiz 52, 54.

Portman, M. (2018). HIV prevention strategies. *Medicine* 46 (5): 293–299.

Randall, C. (2007). Surgical management of the primary care dental patient on antiplatelet medication. www.ukmi.nhs.uk/activities/specialistServices.

Rees, S.R. and Gibson, J. (1997). Angioedema and swellings of the orofacial region. *Oral Diseases* 3: 39–42.

Rieder, M.J. and Spino, M. (1988). The theophylline-erythromycin interaction. *Journal of Asthma* 25 (4): 195–204.

Rinchuse, D.J., Rinchuse, D.J., Sosovicka, M.F. et al. (2007). Orthodontic treatment of patients using bisphosphhonates: a report of 2 cases. *American Journal of Orthodontics and Dentofacial Orthopedics* 131: 321–326.

Robbins, R.N., Remien, R.H., Mellins, C.A. et al. (2011). Screening for HIV-associated dementia in South Africa: potentials and pitfalls of task-shifting. *AIDS Patient Care and STDs* 25: 587–593.

Roden, D.M. (2008). Clinical practice. Long-QT syndrome. *New England Journal of Medicine* 358 (2): 169–176.

Rubin, R., Salvati, E.A., and Lewis, R. (1976). Infected total hip replacement after dental procedures. *Oral Surgery Oral Medicine Oral Pathology* 41: 13–23.

Rubin, R.H., Young, L.S., and Rubin, R.H. (1994). Infection in the organ transplant recipient. In: *Clinical Approach to Infection in the Compromised Host*, 3e (eds. R.H. Rubin and L.S. Young), 629–705. New York: Plenum.

Ruggiero, S.L., Mehrotra, B., Rosenberg, T.J. et al. (2004). Osteonecrosis of the jaws associated with the use of bisphosphonates: a review of 63 cases. *Journal of Oral and Maxillofacial Surgery* 62: 527–534.

Sadock, B.J., Sadock, V.A., and Ruiz, P. (2017). *Kaplan & Sadock's Comprehensive Textbook of Psychiatry*, 10e. The Hague: Wolters Kluwer.

Samet, J.H., Phillips, S.J., Horton, N.J. et al. (2004). Detecting alcohol problems in HIV-infected patients: use of the CAGE questionnaire. *AIDS Research and Human Retroviruses* 20: 151–155.

Sanford, R., Ances, B.M., Meyerhoff, D.J. et al. (2018). Longitudinal trajectories of brain volume and cortical thickness in treated and untreated primary human immunodeficiency virus infection. *Clinical Infectious Diseases* 67 (11): 1697–1704.

Saraghi, M., Golden, L., and Hersh, E.V. (2018). Anesthetic considerations for patients on anti-depressant therapy – part I. *Anesthesia Progress* 64: 253–261.

Saylor, D., Dickens, A.M., Sacktor, N. et al. (2016). HIV-associated neurocognitive disorder – pathogenesis and prospects for treatment. *Nature Reviews Neurology* 12 (5, 309): 234–248.

Scully, C. and Bagan-Sebastian, J.V. (2004). Adverse drug reactions in the orofacial region. *Critical Reviews of Oral Biology & Medicine* 15: 221–240.

Scully, C. and Porter, S. (2003). Lumps and swelling of the mouth. In: *Orofacial Disease. Update for the Dental Clinical Team* (ed. C. Scully), 69–74. Philadelphia: Churchill Livingstone.

Segelnick, S.L. and Weinberg, M.A. (2006). Reevaluation of initial therapy: when is the appropriate time? *Journal of Periodontology* 77: 1598–1601.

Segelnick, S.L. and Weinberg, M.A. (2009). The periodontist's role in obtaining clearance prior to patients undergoing a kidney transplant. *Journal of Periodontology* 80: 874–877.

Ship, J.A. (2003). Diabetes and oral health: an overview. *Journal of the American Dental Association* 134 (Suppl 1): 4s–10s.

Sibiude, J., Le Chenadec, J., Bonnet, D. et al. (2015). In utero exposure to zidovudine and heart anomalies in the ANRS French perinatal cohort and the nested PRIMEVA randomized trial. *Clinical Infectious Diseases* 61: 270–280.

Singh, B., Sinha, N., Giri, T. et al. (2015). Management of edentulous orofacial dyskinesia. *Journal of Contemporary Dental Practice* 16 (7): 607–611.

Skaar, D.D., O'Connor, H., Hodges, J.S. et al. (2011). Dental procedures and subsequent prosthetic joint infections. *Journal of the American Dental Association* 142: 1343–1351.

Slogrove, A.L., Goetghebuer, T., Cotton, M.F. et al. (2016). Pattern of infectious morbidity in HIV-exposed uninfected infants and children. *Frontiers in Immunology* 7: 164.

Smith, H.S. (2009). Opioid metabolism. *Mayo Clinic Proceedings* 84 (7): 613–624.

Soave, R. (2001). Prophylaxis strategies for solid-organ transplantation. *Clinical Infectious Diseases* 33 (Supplement 1): S26–S31.

Sogaard, O.S., Graversen, M.E., Leth, S. et al. (2015). The depsipeptide romidepsin reverses HIV-1 latency in vivo. *PLoS Pathogens* 11 (9) https://doi.org/10.1371/journal.ppat.1005142.

Sollecito, T.P., Abt, E., Lockhart, P.B. et al. (2015). The use of prophylactic antibiotics prior to dental procedures in patients with prosthetic joints. *Journal of the American Dental Association* 146 (1): 11–16.e8.

Solomon, D.H. (2015). Bionor announces that the HIV 'Shock & Kill' trial REDUC with Vacc-4x and romidepsin meets its primary endpoint by significantly reducing latent HIV reservoir and demonstrates control of viral load. https://globenewswire.com/news-release/2015/12/21/797102/10158683/en/Bionor-announces-that-the-HIV-Shock-Kill-trial-REDUC-with-Vacc-4x-and-romidepsin-meets-its-primary-endpoint-by-significantly-reducing-latent-HIV-reservoir-and-demonstrates-control-.html.

Spies, C.D., von Dossow, V., Eggers, V. et al. (2004). Altered cell-mediated immunity and increased postoperative infection rate in long-term alcohol patients. *Anesthesiology* 100 (5): 1088–1100.

Stahl, S.M. (2008). *Stahl's Essential Psychopharmacology: Neuroscientific Basis and Practical Applications.* Cambridge: Cambridge University Press.

Steinbacher, D.M. and Glick, M. (2001). The dental patient with asthma. *Journal of the American Dental Association* 132: 1229–1239.

Strassler, H.E. and Boksman, L. (2011). Tissue management, gingival retraction and hemostasis. www.oralhealthgroup.com/features/tissue-management-gingival-retraction-and-hemostasis.

Szabo, G. and Saha, B. (2015). Alcohol's effect on host defense. *Alcohol Research: Current Reviews* 37 (2): 159–170.

Taylor, B.S., Sobieszczyk, M.E., McCutchan, F.E., and Hammer, S.M. (2008). The challenge of HIV-1 subtype diversity. *New England Journal of Medicine* 358 (15): 1590–1602.

Teicher, M.H., Altesman, R.I., Cole, J.O. et al. (1987). Possible nephrotoxic Interaction of lithium and metronidazole. *Journal of the American Medical Association* 257 (24): 3365–3366.

Townsend, C.L., Byrne, L., Cortina-Borja, M. et al. (2014). Earlier initiation of ART and further decline in mother-to-child HIV transmission rates, 2000–2011. *AIDS Patient Care and STDs* 28: 1049–1057.

Townsend, R.R. (2017). NSAIDs and acetaminophen: effects on blood pressure and hypertension. www.uptodate.com/contents/nsaids-and-acetaminophen-effects-on-blood-pressure-and-hypertension.

trial, HIV vaccine (2018). The prime-boost phase III HIV vaccine trial. https://clinicaltrials.gov/ct2/show/NCT00223080.

UNAIDS (2018). On the fast-track to an AIDS-free generation. www.unaids.org/en/resources/documents/2016/GlobalPlan2016.

Valdez, H., Mitsuyasu, R., Landay, A. et al. (2003). Interleukin-2 increases CD4+ lymphocyte numbers but does not enhance responses to immunization: results of A5046s. *Journal of Infectious Diseases* 187 (2): 320–325.

Weinberg, M.A. (2002). Fundamentals of drug action. In: *Oral Pharmacology* (eds. M.A. Weinberg, C. Westphal and J.B. Fine), 224, 337–368. New Jersey: Pearson Education Inc.

Whelton, P.K., Carey, R.M., Aronow, W.S. et al. (2018). 2017 ACC/AHA/AAPA/ABC/ACPM/AGS/APhA/ASH/ASPC/NMA/PCNA Guideline for the Prevention, Detection, Evaluation, and Management of High Blood Pressure in Adults: A Report of the American College of Cardiology/American Heart Association Task Force on Clinical Practice Guidelines. *Journal of American College of Cardiology* 71: e127–e248.

WHO (2016). *Consolidated Guidelines on the Use of Antiretroviral Drugs for Treating and Preventing HIV Infection: Recommendations for a Public Health Approach*, 2e. Geneva: World Health Organization.

Wilkinson, A.N., Nathan, P.E., and Butters, N. (1987). *CT Scan and Neuropsychological Assessments of Alcoholics*. New York: Guilford.

Williams, P.L., Crain, M.J., Yildirim, C. et al. (2015). Congenital anomalies and in utero antiretroviral exposure in human immunodeficiency virus-exposed uninfected infants. *JAMA Pediatrics* 169: 48–55.

Wilson, W., Taubert, K.A., Gewitz, M. et al. (2007). Prevention of infective endocarditis: Guidelines from the American Heart Association Rheumatic Fever, Endocarditis, and Kawasaki Disease Committee, Council on Cardiovascular Disease in the Young, and the Council on Clinical Cardiology, Council on Cardiovascular Surgery and Anesthesia, and the Quality of Care and Outcomes Research Interdisciplinary Working Group. *Circulation* 116: 1736–1754.

Yagiela, J.A. (1999). Adverse drug interactions in dental practice: interactions associated with vasoconstrictors. *Journal of the American Dental Association* 130: 701–709.

Yagiela, J.A. and Haymore, T.L. (2007). Management of the hypertensive dental patient. *Journal of the California Dental Association* 35: 51–59.

Yajnik, S., Thapar, P., Lichtor, J.L. et al. (1994). Effects of marijuana history on the subjective, psychomotor, and reinforcing effects of nitrous oxide in humans. *Drug and Alcohol Dependence* 36: 227–236.

Yap, Y.G. and Camm, A.J. (2003). Drug induced QT prolongation and torsades de pointes. *Heart* 89 (11): 1363–1372.

Yeganeh, N., Kerin, T., Ank, B. et al. (2017). HIV antiretroviral resistance and transmission in mother-infant pairs enrolled in a large perinatal study. *Clinical Infectious Diseases* 66: 1770–1777.

Yip, J.K., Borrell, L.N., Cho, S.-C. et al. (2012). Association between oral bisphosphonate use and dental implant failure among middle-aged women. *Journal of Clinical Periodontology* 39: 408–411.

Zash, R., Souda, S., Chen, J. et al. (2016). Reassuring birth outcomes with tenofovir/emtricitabine/efavirenz used for prevention of mother to child transmission of HIV in Botswana. *Journal of Acquired Immune Deficiency Syndromes* 71 (4): 428–436.

Zemrak, W.R. and Kenna, G.A. (2008). Association of antipsychotic and antidepressant drugs with Q-T interval prolongation. *American Journal of Health-System Pharmacy* 65 (11): 1029–1038.

8

Herbal, Dietary, and Natural Remedies

8.1 Herbal–Drug Interactions

Q. Do herbal products have any harmful effects?

A. One of the major skepticisms is whether these products are safe and effective. One of the most worrisome adverse effects of herbal products is anticoagulation. Most herbal medicines are unapproved drugs being sold as dietary supplements. In 1990, the Food and Drug Administration (FDA) classified herbal medicines as food supplements. The Dietary Supplement and Health Education Act (DSHEA) of 1994 classifies vitamins, minerals, amino acids, and herbs as dietary supplements, which allows the marketing of these "food supplements" without the approval of any government agency or testing for safety, efficacy, or standards of manufacturing. The FDA is only required to prove that these products are unsafe. Thus, the burden of proof is on the FDA to prove a product is unsafe before it can be removed from the market. Dietary supplements do not have to be tested prior to marketing, and the effectiveness of the product does not have to be demonstrated by the manufacturer. The product label must include a disclaimer that the product is not FDA evaluated or approved and it is not intended to diagnose, treat, or prevent any disease (Cupp 1999). The DSHEA does not regulate the accuracy of the label; the product may or may not contain the product listed in the amounts claimed. Herbal products therefore cannot be marketed for the diagnosis, treatment, cure, or prevention of disease. However, these products can be labeled explaining their proposed effect on the human body (e.g. alleviation of fatigue) or their role in promoting general well-being (e.g. enhancement of mood). Dietary supplement labeling requires the wording "dietary supplement" as part of the product name, and it must include a "supplement facts" panel on the ingredients. Also, products derived from plants must designate the plant part and the Latin binomial.

Q. What are herbal medications made from?

A. Herbal medications are made from natural ingredients extracted from a plant and are either in the original form or refined, where the essential extract is removed from the plant, concentrated, and then added back into the original form to make it more concentrated. The active ingredients in an herbal product may be present in only one specific part of the plant or in all parts. For example, the active ingredient in ginger is composed of roots found below ground, whereas in St John's wort it comes from leaves and stems that are above the ground. Every herb contains many active chemicals. Most of these chemicals have not been isolated and identified so that the strength of the product varies considerably, which makes standardization difficult. Additionally, the chemical composition of herbal supplements is unpredictable. Some standardizations are printed on the product label and may differ from one manufacturer to another.

Q. What are some adverse effects of herbal medications that are of concern especially for dental surgery?

A. Most reactions are due to filler substances added to the herbal product but not listed on the label. Commonly encountered adverse effects include sedation and bleeding, which manifests either via direct effects on capillaries, by interfering with platelet adhesion, or by increasing fibrinolytic activity. Caution should be used when nonsteroidal antiinflammatory drugs (NSAIDs) are recommended to patients taking herbs that could increase bleeding, including ginger, garlic, and ginkgo. Another adverse effect is an allergic reaction to the herb, which can manifest in the oral cavity (e.g., gingiva, tongue).

Q. What herbal products can be taken by patients for dental problems?

A. See Table 8.1.

Table 8.1 Common herbal products taken by patients for dental problems

Oral condition	Herbal supplement
Aphthous ulcer	*Aloe vera*, red raspberry
Caries	Licorice root
Oral inflammation in cancer patients	Chamomile, vitamin E
Oral fungal infections	Tea tree oil, garlic, cinnamon
Periodontal diseases	Coenzyme Q10, sanguinaria

Q. Are there any dental drug interactions with St John's wort?

A. St John's wort is indicated for depression. It has many drug interactions, but none pertain to dentistry. Most of the interactions are primarily due to induction of CYP3A4, CPY1A2, and CYP2C9. These drugs include warfarin, cyclosporine, HIV protease inhibitors, theophylline, digoxin, and oral contraceptives, resulting in a decrease in concentration or effect of the medicines.

Q. What steps should be taken if a drug–herbal interaction is suspected?

A. Adjust the dosage of the herb, temporarily discontinue the herb, closely monitor the patient, or change the drug therapy.

Q. What are some important drug–herbal product interactions in dentistry?

A. See Table 8.2.

Table 8.2 Common herbal–drug interactions in dentistry

Herbal supplement	Interacting dental drug	How to manage
St John's wort	Alprazolam (Xanax®), diazepam, midazolam (Versed®), ibuprofen, codeine, ketoconazole, clarithromycin, erythromycin	Don't take the two medications together. The active ingredient in St John's wort has a half-life of 24–48 hours
Khat	Penicillins (amoxicillin, ampicillin)	Avoid chewing khat or take the penicillin 2 hours after chewing khat
Kava	Alprazolam, acetaminophen, NSAIDs	Avoid concurrent use because of additive effect

Source: Cupp (1999); Fugh-Berman (2000); Izzo and Ernst (2001).

8.2 Implications in Dentistry

Q. Why is it important to ask patients if they are taking any herbal medications?

A. Patients should be questioned about taking any herbal supplement. Prolonged bleeding may occur during dental procedures (e.g., surgery) in patients taking ginger, ginkgo, ginseng, St John's wort, garlic, green tea, glucosamine/chondroitin, omega-3 fatty acids, and saw palmetto. Bleeding will most likely be controlled in healthy patients. If the patient is also taking aspirin or other blood thinner, consult with the patient's physician. These medications should be stopped at least seven days before periodontal/implant/extraction surgery.

Q. Can herbal medications interfere with dental anesthesia?

A. Yes. There are many herbs that can act as sedatives or stimulants that could modify anesthesia, including valerian, kava, St John's wort and ginseng (Tweddell and Boyle 2009).

Q. Are there any dental-related adverse effects of herbal products?

A. Yes, there are dental-related adverse effects (Cupp 1999) – see Table 8.3.

Table 8.3 Dental-related adverse effects of herbal products

Herbal product	Adverse effect
St John's wort	Xerostomia
Echinacea	Tongue numbness
Garlic	Gingival bleeding
Feverfew	Gingival bleeding and mouth ulcerations
Ginger	Gingival bleeding
Ginkgo	Gingival bleeding
Ginseng	Gingival bleeding
Kava	Tongue numbness

Q. Which herbal products interact with warfarin and increase bleeding?

A. Many dietary/herbal supplements act similarly to antiplatelet/anticoagulant drugs. Ginkgo (*Ginkgo biloba*), ginseng (*Panax ginseng*), licorice (*Glycyrrhiza*), garlic (*Allium sativum*), Dong quai (*Angelica sinensis*), and Danshen (*Salvia miltiorrhiza*) should be discontinued before performing invasive dental procedures that could cause postoperative bleeding. It has been recommended to stop all herbals that can cause increased bleeding about 7–14 days prior to the dental procedure. No interactions were found for echinacea (*Echinacea angustifolia*, *Echinacea purpurea*, *Echinacea pallida*) or saw palmetto (*Serenoa repens*) (Izzo and Ernst 2001). Vitamin A or E in high doses interacts with warfarin and increases the anticoagulation effects. It is important to take only the recommended daily requirements (Terrie 2013).

Q. Are there any herbal drugs that could interfere with dental anesthesia?

A. Yes. Some herbals can be sedating or stimulating which can interfere with moderate sedation and general anesthesia with a potential for prolongation or interference with anesthetic agents. Most likely there are no interactions with local dental anesthesia.

References

Cupp, M.J. (1999). Herbal remedies: adverse effects and drug interactions. *American Family Physician* 59: 1239–1244.

Fugh-Berman, A. (2000). Herb–drug interactions. *Lancet* 355: 134–138.

Izzo, A.A. and Ernst, E. (2001). Interactions between herbal medicines and prescribed drugs: a systematic review. *Drugs* 61: 2163–2165.

Terrie, Y.C. (2013). Drug–supplement interactions: patient awareness is key. www.pharmacytimes. com/publications/issue/2013/october2013/drug-supplement-interactions-patient-awareness-is-key.

Tweddell, P. and Boyle, C. (2009). Potential interactions with herbal medications and midazolam. *Dental Update* 36 (3): 175–178.

Appendix 1

Smoking Cessation Therapy

Q. Can a dentist prescribe medications for smoking cessation?

A. Yes. Dentists are encouraged to help patients with smoking cessation by counseling and prescribing smoking cessation medications.

Q. Should only one product be recommended or prescribed?

A. Combination therapy with or without behavioral therapy is recommended for smoking cessation. Combination drug therapy is usually more effective than monotherapy, particularly for more heavily tobacco-dependent patients. Preferred combinations are nicotine replacement therapy (NRT) plus bupropion (Zyban®) or high-dose NRT using a nicotine patch plus nicotine gum or lozenges.

Q. Is Nicorette® gum sugar free?

A. Yes. Nicorette gum does not contain sugar.

Q. What is Chantix®?

A. Chantix (varenicline) is a nicotine receptor partial agonist and the first designer drug for tobacco dependence. One serious adverse effect is increased risk for suicidal thoughts and actions. The dentist should know the following about Chantix: (i) patient history of depression or other mental health problems, because these symptoms may worsen while taking Chantix; (ii) experienced nicotine withdrawal symptoms with prior quit attempts, with or without Chantix quitting smoking, with or without Chantix, can result in nicotine withdrawal symptoms such as depressed mood, agitation or a worsening of existing mental health problems, such as depression; (iii) patient has kidney problems or has kidney dialysis (a lower dose may be necessary; obtain a medical consult); (iv) patient has a history of heart or blood vessel problems because these problems and new or worse symptoms can occur while taking Chantix – obtain a medical consult; (v) if patient is pregnant or plans to become pregnant; and (vi) if patient is breast feeding (www.chantix.com/getting-started-with-chantix/what-to-expect).

Q. What medications can the dentist recommend or prescribe for smoking cessation?

A. See Table A1.1.

The Dentist's Drug and Prescription Guide, Second Edition. Mea A. Weinberg, Stuart J. Froum and Stuart L. Segelnick.
© 2020 John Wiley & Sons, Inc. Published 2020 by John Wiley & Sons, Inc.

Table A1.1 Pharmacological agents used for smoking cessation

Product	Directions for use	Supplied	Adverse effects	Rx or OTC
Nicotine gum Generics Nicorette	Do not smoke during treatment because of risk of nicotine overdose. Chew one piece of gum every 1–2 hours for weeks 1–6; every 2–4 hours for weeks 7–9; and every 4–8 hours for weeks 10–12. Do not eat or drink for 15 minutes before chewing gum, and do not eat or drink while chewing gum	2 mg, 4 mg gum; starter kit has 108 pieces and refill kits have 48 pieces	Mouth soreness, sore jaw, dyspepsia (stomach pain or discomfort), bronchospasm, nausea, vomiting	OTC
Nicotine transdermal system Generics Nicotine patch (generic) Nicoderm CQ® Nicotrol® Habitrol® Prostep®	Do not smoke during treatment because of risk of nicotine overdose. Nicoderm CQ: use one patch daily; start at 21 mg/day for 6 weeks, then 14 mg/day for 2 weeks, then 7 mg/day for 2 weeks. Maximum therapy is 3 months. Habitrol: if you smoke >10 cigarettes a day: use 21 mg patch for 4 weeks, then the 14 mg patch for 2 weeks, and the 7 mg patch for 2 weeks. If you smoke ≤10 cigarettes a day: start with 14 mg patch for 6 weeks, then 7 mg patch for 2 weeksTreatment ends at 8 weeks.	Nicoderm CQ (28-day supply): 21 mg, 14 mg, 7 mg patches Nicotrol: 15 mg (worn only while awake), 10 mg and 5 mg patches Habitrol: 21 mg, 14 mg, 7 mg Prostep: 22 mg or 11 mg patches	Local skin irritation, insomnia (difficulty in sleeping)	OTC
Nicotine lozenge Commit®	If patient smokes the first cigarette more than 30 minutes after waking, then use 2 mg lozenge; use 4 mg if smokes first cigarette within 30 minutes of waking. Maximum: not more than 20 lozenges a day. Allow lozenge to dissolve slowly over 20–30 minutes, swallow as little as possible	2 mg (72 pieces), 4 mg (72 pieces)	Xerostomia, indigestion and irritated throat	OTC
Nicorette	If the first cigarette is smoked more than 30 minutes after waking, use the 2 mg strength; if the first cigarette is smoked within 30 minutes after waking up, use the 4 mg strength. Weeks 1–6: 1 lozenge every 1–2 hours. Weeks 7–9 : 1 lozenge every 2–4 hours. Weeks 10–12 : 1 lozenge every 4–8 hours	2 mg lozenge 4 mg lozenge	Cardiovascular changes, increased heart rate, dizziness, nausea, vomiting, bronchospasm	OTC
Nicotine nasal spray Nicotrol NS®	Start with two sprays in each nostril every hour, which may be increased to 80 sprays per day for heavy smokers; maximum dose 40 doses/day. Maximum therapy is 6 months. Taper after 4–6 weeks. Patient should tilt head back when using the spray	Prescription product Easy spray delivers 0.5 mg nicotine; available in 10 mL bottles	Irritation of nasal mucosa, cough, sneezing, bronchospasm in patients with preexisting asthma. Tolerance to adverse effects develops after the first week of using the inhaler. Contraindicated in patients with reactive airway disease (e.g., wheezing or allergic reactions) or chronic nasal disease such as nasal polyps or sinusitis	Rx (prescription only)

Product	Instructions	Description	Adverse effects	Availability
Nicotine inhalation system Nicotrol Inhaler®	Less nicotine per puff is released with the inhaler than with a cigarette. Best effect is achieved by frequent continuous puffing for about 20 minutes (that is 6–16 cartridges per day; use 1 cartridge per hour). The recommended treatment is up to 3 months and, if needed, a gradual reduction over the next 6–12 weeks. Total treatment should not exceed 6 months. Avoid food and acidic drinks before and during use of inhaler	Prescription product Inhaler uses nicotine cartridges (10 mg/cartridge) that provide about 20 minutes of active puffing, or approximately 80 deep draws	Irritation of mouth and throat, cough Contraindicated in patients with reactive airway disease	Rx (prescription only)
Oral medications (nonnicotine drugs Zyban (bupropion HCl) (does not contain nicotine)	Patient should stop smoking within 2 weeks of start of therapy. Option 1: initial dose is 150 mg/day for 3 days, then 150 mg twice a day (at least 8 hours apart). Option 2: 150 mg every morning (this option has fewer adverse effects and is better tolerated). Maximum daily dose is 300 mg. Continue drug therapy for 7–12 weeks after the patient stops smoking and can be maintained up to 6 months. Can be used with nicotine patches	Prescription 150 mg sustained-release tablets	Insomnia, xerostomia, anxiety. Contraindicated in seizures, those currently using Wellbutrin®, eating disorder, alcohol dependence or head trauma. Additionally, blood pressure should be monitored	Rx (prescription only)
Chantix (varenicline) (does not contain nicotine)	FDA approved in 2006. Not used for patients younger than 18 years old. Caution in patients with renal impairment. Packs: first month: 1 card – 0.5 mg × 11 tabs and 3 cards – 1 mg × 14 tabs Bottles: 0.5 mg, 1.0 mg	Starting one week before the patient quits smoking. 0.5 mg/day for 3 days then 0.5 mg twice a day (am and pm) for the next 4 days. Then after the first 7 days, 1 mg twice a day. No tapering needed. Approved for maintenance up to 6 months. Take after eating and with a full glass of water. Do not double the dose if the dose is missed	Nausea, trouble sleeping, headache, *changes in behavior, hostility, agitation, depressed mood, suicidal thoughts or actions*	Prescription

Source: Fiore et al. (2008).

Q. Can the patient smoke while using a patch or other products?

A. No. Smoking while using a nicotine patch or other nicotine products increases the risk of nicotine overdose.

Q. How often is Nicorette gum used?

A. The 2 mg gum is for smokers <25 cigarettes/day and the 4 mg gum for smokers ≥25 cigarettes/day. It is recommended to chew a piece every 1–2 hours during the first six weeks of quitting (a minimum of nine per day). An additional piece can be used if there is a craving. Not more than 24 pieces can be used in one day.

Q. How is the nicotine patch used?

A. If the patient smokes more than 10 cigarettes a day.

1) For the first six weeks, 21 mg per day.
2) For weeks 7 and 8, switch to a moderate-dosage patch, about 14 mg per day.
3) For weeks 9 and 10, change to a low-dosage patch that delivers 7 mg of nicotine per day (www.nicodermcq.com/about-nicoderm-cq.html).

If the patient smokes less than 10 cigarettes a day.

1) Begin with 14 mg for six weeks
2) Then switch to 7 mg for two weeks

Q. Are there any adverse effects of NRT products?

A. Yes (www.drugs.com/sfx/nicotine-side-effects.html)

Patch: if increased heartbeat and dizziness occur, it is best to switch to a lower-dose patch. Other adverse effects include skin irritation (medical attention is needed if there is swelling or persistent redness lasting more than four days at the application site), abnormal dreams, headache, muscle aches, nausea and vomiting. If the patient has a history of heart disease, refer the patient to their physician.

- *Gum*: abnormal dreams, diarrhea, difficulty sleeping, dry mouth, joint pain, muscle pain, nervousness, sweating, weakness, mouth, teeth, or jaw problems, allergic reaction, irregular or fast heartbeat, diarrhea, nausea, vomiting.
- *Lozenge*: warm or tingling sensation in the mouth, allergic reaction, persistent indigestion, irregular or fast heartbeat, pain, swelling or sores in the mouth.
- *Inhaler*: coughing, diarrhea, flu-like symptoms, headache, hiccups, indigestion, mouth or throat irritation, muscle aches, nausea, pain in the jaw and neck, runny nose, taste changes, allergic reaction, irregular or fast heartbeat.
- *Spray*: back pain, burning or irritation of the mouth, nose, or eyes, changes in taste and smell, constipation, cough, earache, facial flushing, gas, headache, hoarseness, indigestion, irritability, joint pain, sores in the mouth, ulcers or blisters in the nose, nose bleed, nausea, runny nose, sneezing, sore throat, stuffy nose, watery eyes, irregular or fast heartbeat, memory loss.

Q. Are there any drug interactions with smoking cessation products?

A. The following medications may need dosage adjustment when taking nicotine patch, gum, lozenge, or spray.

- Acetaminophen (Tylenol®)
- Beta-blockers (atenolol, pindolol, metoprolol, timolol, nadolol, and propranolol)

- Caffeine (coffee, tea, colas)
- Furosemide
- Phenylephrine (Neo-Synephrine®)
- Prazosin (Minipress®)
- Theophylline
- Tricyclic antidepressants (amitriptyline, nortriptyline, imipramine)

Reference

Fiore, M.C., Jaen, C.R., Baker, T.B. et al. (2008). *Treating Tobacco Use and Dependence: 2008 Update. Clinical Practice Guideline*. Rockville, MD: US Department of Health and Human Services, Public Health Service.

Appendix 2

Oral Manifestation of Drugs

See Table A2.1.

Q. Are there any drugs that cause a "drug-induced vesiculobullous reaction"?

A. Yes. There are some drugs that induce the development of oral lesions that clinically and histologically resemble idiopathic vesiculobullous conditions such as lichen planus, lupus erythematosus (LE), pemphigoid, and erythema multiforme. A differential diagnosis of a vesiculobullous disorder is drug eruptions. If a patient is diagnosed with a bullous disorder, be sure to check for the possibility that a drug the patient is taking is causing a reaction.

Q. What is the treatment for drug-induced vesiculobullous disorders?

A. Treatment is primarily based on symptoms and highly dependent on the individual case. Some patients require topical steroids and in severe cases systemic steroids or cyclosporine. Contact the patient's physician.

Q. Do cardiovascular drugs have a high incidence of oral manifestations?

A. Yes. Cardiovascular drugs have a high incidence of oral manifestations, up to 14.1% (Habbab et al. 2010). The incidence increases with the number of drugs taken and if the patient is diabetic.

Q. What is the definition of fixed drug eruptions?

A. Fixed drug eruptions, sometimes called contact stomatitis, occur when there is repeated ulceration at the same site in response to the same drug. It can be caused by many drugs including tetracycline or ingredients of products including toothpastes, oral rinses, chewing gum, and dental materials (Scully and Bagan 2004). Once the offending drug is determined, the medication should be stopped.

Q. What prescription medications can be prescribed for severe decreased salivary flow because of radiation to the head and neck region or patients with Sjögren syndrome?

A. Pilocarpine (Salagen®) is only indicated for (i) the treatment of symptoms of dry mouth from salivary gland hypofunction caused by radiotherapy for cancer of the head and neck; and (ii) the treatment of symptoms of dry mouth in patients with Sjögren syndrome.

Table A2.1 Oral manifestation of drugs

Oral condition	Linked to the following medications	Notes
Candidiasis (fungal/yeast infection) Shows up intraorally as a white plaque-like lesion that can be wiped off with gauze Fungal infections are found on the maxillary palatal gingival when patients do not remove and clean their maxillary denture as directed	Inhalation steroids (in asthma)	Patient should rinse mouth after use of inhaled asthma drugs
Tardive dyskinesia (abnormal mouth and tongue movements including lip puckering and tongue protrusion)	Antipsychotics	There is no definitive treatment; patient management is important
Esophageal burning/ulcers	Tetracycline/doxycycline	Take with a full glass of water while sitting or standing in an upright position
Gingival enlargement	Phenytoin (Dilantin®) Nifedipine (Procardia®, Adalat®) and other calcium channel blockers Cyclosporine	Maintain meticulous oral hygiene; sometimes surgical removal of gingival is necessary but the enlargement will eventually return
Gingival hemorrhages	Warfarin (Coumadin®) Clopidogrel (Plavix®)	Note petechiae on chart; consult with patient's physician
Hairy tongue	Mouth rinses Antibiotics (especially broad spectrum) Steroids	Brush tongue
Taste changes	Lithium Metronidazole (Flagyl®)	Taste changes are transient for metronidazole (metallic taste) but chronic for lithium because the patient will be on lithium for a long time
Exaggerated gag reflex	Digitalis/cardiac glycosides	Patient management with impression and radiographs
Xerostomia	Many. See next column	Many OTC products: Orajel® gel, spray, toothpaste, Biotène® products, Oasis® moisturizing mouth rinses and saliva substitutes (e.g., Xero-Lube®, Salivart®) Prescription sialagogue may be beneficial; pilocarpine HCl (Salagen) and cevimeline (Evoxac®)

Table A2.1 (Continued)

Oral condition	Linked to the following medications	Notes
Drug-induced vesiculobullous conditions	Lichenoid (lichen planus-like) reactions: beta-blockers, ACE inhibitors (captopril) and NSAIDs Pemphigoid-like reactions: amoxicillin, clonidine, furosemide, nadolol, penicillin VK Pemphigus-like reaction: captopril, propranolol Erythema multiforme-like reactions: carbamazepine, clindamycin, codeine, diltiazem, nifedipine, tetracycline, verapamil	It must be determined that the oral lesions are actually due to a drug the patient is taking. Treatment depends on the individual case. The patient's physician may need to be contacted

Source: Adapted from Ciancio (2004).

Q. What are common adverse effects of pilocarpine for the treatment of xerostomia?

A. Headache, visual disturbance, lacrimation, sweating, respiratory distress, gastrointestinal spasm, nausea, vomiting, diarrhea, atrioventricular block, tachycardia, bradycardia, hypotension, hypertension, shock, mental confusion, cardiac arrhythmia, and tremors (www.drugs.com/pro/pilocarpine.html). Pilocarpine should be administered with caution to patients with known or suspected cholelithiasis or biliary tract disease.

Q. What is the dose of pilocarpine HCl?

A. Supplied: 5 mg tab; 5 mg tid or qid, may increase up to 10 mg tid. It can take up to six weeks for the drug to have the maximum effect.

Q. What is the dose in patients with hepatic impairment?

A. In patients with moderate hepatic impairment, the starting dose should be 5 mg twice daily, followed by adjustment based on therapeutic response and tolerability. Patients with mild hepatic insufficiency (Child–Pugh score of 5–6) do not require dosage reductions. Consult with the patient's physician.

Q. Are there any drug interactions with pilocarpine?

A. Yes. Pilocarpine should be administered with caution to patients taking beta-adrenergic antagonists because of the possibility of conduction disturbances. Pilocarpine is a cholinergic agonist drug so it might antagonize the anticholinergic effects of drugs used concomitantly.

Q. What is cevimeline HCL (Evoxac)?

A. Cevimeline is indicated for alleviation of symptoms in patients with Sjögren syndrome.

Q. What is the dose for cevimeline?

A. Supplied: 30 mg caps: 30 mg tid. It can take up to six weeks for the drug to have its maximum effect.

Q. When is the best time of day to take a sialagogue such as pilocarpine or cevimeline?

A. It is advantageous to take a sialagogue before meals to aid in salivary production which will also assist with mastication.

Q. What are common adverse effects of cevimeline?

A. Shortness of breath, wheezing, chest pain, uneven heart rate, stomach pain on the right side extending up to the shoulder, nausea, vomiting, bloating, and fever.

Q. Is cevimeline contraindicated in certain patients?

A. Yes, patients with uncontrolled asthma, allergies to cevimeline, narrow-angle glaucoma, and inflammation of the iris.

Q. Are there any drug interactions with cevimeline?

A. Yes. Cevimeline should be administered with caution to patients taking beta-adrenergic antagonists, because of the possibility of cardiac conduction disturbances. There are synergistic effects with other cholinergic drugs. Cevimeline might interfere with desirable anticholinergic effects of drugs used concomitantly.

Q. Which drugs can cause xerostomia?

A. Classification of drugs causing xerostomia is listed in Table A2.2. If medication cannot be changed or dose altered, it is recommended to increase water intake, or the patient can suck on sugarless candy or chew sugarless gum. Oral OTC products such as Oasis and Biotène (e.g., oral rinses, toothpaste, and gel) may be helpful.

Table A2.2 Common drugs that cause xerostomia

Drug classification	Drugs
Antiacne	Accutane® (isotretinoin)
Antianxiety	Xanax® (alprazolam), Tranxene® (clorazepate), Valium® (diazepam), Atarax®, Vistaril® (hydroxyzine), Ativan® (lorazepam), Serax® (oxazepam)
Anticonvulsants	Tegretol® (carbamazepine), Neurontin® (gabapentin), Lamictal® (lamotrigine)
Antidepressants	Elavil® (amitriptyline), Wellbutrin® (bupropion), Anafranil® (clomipramine), Norpramin® (desipramine), Sinequan® (doxepin), Prozac® (fluoxetine), Luvox® (fluvoxamine), Tofranil® (imipramine)
Antipsychotics	Clozaril® (clozapine), Zyprexa® (olanzapine), lithium, Haldol® (haloperidol)
Antihistamines	Benadryl® (diphendydramine), Actifed® (triprolidine/pseudoephedrine), Claritin® (loratadine), Dimetane® (brompheniramine), Dimetapp® (brompheniramine/phenylpropanolamine), Phenergan® (promethazine)
Anticholinergic (antispasmodic/ antimotion sickness)	Bellergal® (belladonna alkaloids), Bentyl® (dicyclomine, hyoscyamine with atropine), Donnatal® (belladonna alkaloids and phenobarbital), Transderm-Scop® (scopolamine)
Antidiarrheal	Imodium AD® (loperamide), Lomotil® (diphenoxylate with atropine)
Bronchodilator	Atrovent® (ipratropium), Isuprel® (isoproterenol), Proventil® (salbutamol), Ventolin® (albuterol)
Diuretics	Diuril® (chlorthiazide), Lasix® (furosemide), Hydrodiuril® (hydrochlorothiazide), Dyazide® (triamterene), Maxzide® (triamterene/hydrochlorothiazide)
Sedative/hypnotics	Restoril® (temazepam), Halcion® (triazolam)

References

Ciancio, S.G. (2004). Medications impact on oral health. *Journal of the American Dental Association* 135: 1440–1448.

Habbab, K.M., Moles, D.R., and Porter, S.R. (2010). Potential oral manifestations of cardiovascular drugs. *Oral Diseases* 16 (8): 769–773.

Scully, C. and Bagan, J.V. (2004). Adverse drug reactions in the orofacial region. *Critical Reviews in Oral Biology and Medicine* 15 (4): 221–239.

Appendix 3

American Heart Association Antibiotic Prophylaxis Guidelines

Table A3.1   Prophylactic antibiotic regimens for oral and dental procedures

Situation	Drug	Regimen (to be taken 30–60 min before dental procedure)
Oral	Amoxicillin	Adults: 2 g Children: 50 mg/kg
Unable to take oral medications	Ampicillin or cefazolin, or ceftriaxone[a]	Adults: 2 g IM or IV Children: 50 mg/kg IM or IV Adults: 1 g IM or IV Children: 50 mg/kg IM or IV
Allergic to penicillins or ampicillin – oral	Cephalexin[a] or clindamycin or azithromycin or clarithromycin	Adults: 2 g Children: 50 mg/kg Adults: 600 mg Children: 20 mg/kg Adults: 500 mg Children: 15 mg/kg
Allergic to penicillins or ampicillin and unable to take oral medications	Cefazolin or ceftriaxone[a] or clindamycin	Adults: 1 g IM or IV Children: 50 mg/kg IM or IV Adults: 600 mg IM or IV Children: 20 mg/kg IM or IV

Source: Reprinted from Wilson et al. (2007) with permission from Lippincott, Williams & Wilkins.
[a] Cephalosporins should not be given to an individual with a history of anaphylaxis, angioedema, or urticaria with penicillins or ampicillin.

The Dentist's Drug and Prescription Guide, Second Edition. Mea A. Weinberg, Stuart J. Froum and Stuart L. Segelnick.
© 2020 John Wiley & Sons, Inc. Published 2020 by John Wiley & Sons, Inc.

References

Sollecito, T.P., Abt, E., Lockhart, P.B. et al. (2015). The use of prophylactic antibiotics prior to dental procedures in patients with prosthetic joints. *Journal of the American Dental Association* 146 (1): 11–16.e8.

Wilson, W., Taubert, K.A., Gewitz, M. et al. (2007). Prevention of infective endocarditis: guidelines from the American Heart Association Rheumatic Fever, Endocarditis, and Kawasaki Disease Committee, Council on Cardiovascular Disease in the Young, and the Council on Clinical Cardiology, Council on Cardiovascular Surgery and Anesthesia, and the Quality of Care and Outcomes Research Interdisciplinary Working Group. *Circulation* 116: 1736–1754.

Index

The Dentist's Drug and Prescription Guide, Second Edition. Mea A. Weinberg, Stuart J. Froum and Stuart L. Segelnick.
© 2020 John Wiley & Sons, Inc. Published 2020 by John Wiley & Sons, Inc.